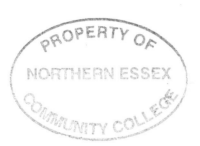

Osteoporosis

Reiner Bartl • Bertha Frisch

Osteoporosis

Diagnosis, Prevention, Therapy

Second Revised Edition

In Collaboration with Christoph Bartl

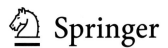 Springer

Prof. Dr. Reiner Bartl
Bavarian Center of Osteoporosis
University of Munich
Marchioninistraße 15
81377 Munich
Germany
reiner.bartl@med.uni-muenchen.de

Christoph Bartl, MD
Department of Orthopaedic and Trauma Surgery
University of Ulm
Steinhövelstraße 9
89075 Ulm
Germany

Prof. Dr. Bertha Frisch
Professor of Hematology
Departments of Pathology and Hematology
Sourasky Medical Center
University of Tel-Aviv
6 Weizmann Street
64233 Tel-Aviv
Israel
bertha-f@013.net.il

ISBN: 978-3-540-79526-1   e-ISBN: 978-3-540-79527-8

DOI: 10.1007/978-3-540-79527-8

Library of Congress Control Number: 2009922223

Cover design: Frido Steinen-Broo, eStudio Calamar, Spain

Printed on acid-free paper

9 8 7 6 5 4 3 2 1

springer.com

Preface

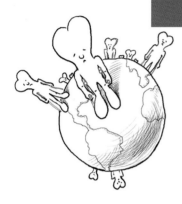

With the dawn of the 21th century has come the realization that bone and joint diseases are the major cause of pain and physical disability worldwide. Moreover, according to the WHO Scientific Group, there are more than 150 musculoskeletal diseases and syndromes, all of which are usually associated with pain and loss of function. It is undoubtedly these insights that prompted the WHO to declare the first 10 years of the new century as "The Bone and Joint Decade 2000–2010". This declaration obviously made a highly significant impact on international, national and medical authorities, as well as on physicians, scientists and citizens worldwide as evidenced by an overwhelming flood (a regular tsunami) of articles, studies and books on the subject in the last few years alone! That is not to mention the coverage in newspapers and journals, on the radio and television and of course all the up-to-date information freely available on the Internet. The number of people suffering from these diseases – already many millions in the developed and underdeveloped countries of the world is expected to double within the next 20 years. In many countries this increase will be even greater due to the longer survival and consequently larger numbers of older people in the population. It is therefore inevitable that the already astronomical costs of health care will rise proportionally. According to the National Osteoporosis Foundation (NOF), the worldwide incidence of hip fracture is projected to increase by 240% in women and 310% in men by 2050, unless appropriate preventive measures are taken on sufficiently large national and international scales, for which, hopefully, this book will provide a stimulus!

On the positive side, the enormous amount of work, research and study of bone disorders over the past 10–20 years or so has contributed greatly to our understanding of the causes, treatment and prevention of osteoporosis and other disorders. Most importantly perhaps, the skeleton is now regarded in a new light, as a dynamic organ undergoing constant renewal throughout life from start to finish, from the cradle to the grave. And what is more: it is now abundantly clear that the skeleton participates, usually not to its advantage, in almost every condition that may affect the organs and tissues in the body! This applies especially to osteoporosis, which is now under control! How did this come about?

- Because of the elucidation of many of the factors involved in osseous remodelling.
- Because of the development of simple, fast, reliable and non-invasive methods for measuring bone density and for testing other factors such as mineralization, trabecular architecture, cortical thickness and the bone cells themselves.
- Because of the identification of general and individual risk factors, such that appropriate measures can be taken to prevent development of osteoporosis and/or its progression, if and when fractures have already occurred.
- And finally, because effective medication for prevention and therapy is now readily available worldwide.

The efficacy of the classes of compounds known as 'bisphosphonates' as well as of selective oestrogen receptor modulators (SERMs) and, more recently, of the anabolic parathyroid hormones has now been unequivocally established by numerous large multicentre trials involving literally millions of patients. In addition, simple methods such as a healthy lifestyle, adequate nutrition, sufficient physical activity and vitamin D and calcium supplements, as required, can be recommended and adopted on a large scale, beginning with the responsible authorities and reaching to the individual citizens. Introduction and acceptance of these methods requires public awareness and support and the realization that every individual is the guardian and caretaker of his/her own bones and responsible for their structural and functional integrity. Fortunately, some progress has been made, as shown by the numerous articles recently published from the "four corners of the globe" which unequivocally establish the epidemic proportions of the problem. Well-founded diagnostic techniques and effective therapies – both antiresorptive and osteo-anabolic – are now available for the prevention, diagnosis and treatment of osteoporosis. It should be emphasized that the treatments recommended in this text are all founded on "evidence-based medicine" (unless otherwise stated) for which the appropriate references are given at the end of the text.

The aim of this book is to demonstrate that "bone is everybody's business" and especially every patient's and doctor's, and to provide guidelines for the diagnosis, therapy and prevention of osteoporosis – from paediatrics to geriatrics. It is hoped and anticipated that this book will raise awareness and provide information to anyone seeking it, and especially to doctors across all disciplines concerned with this preventable and treatable disease.

The main subjects of the first edition of this book were primary and involutional osteoporoses, while the secondary osteoporoses only received 'secondary' attention. However, statistics published some years ago estimated that 40% of osteoporoses in women and 50% in men are secondary. Most probably with the increase in survival and therefore the number of older people in many populations, these proportions have also increased. In addition, the increase in survival of patients with co-morbidities due to improved therapeutic and management strategies must also be taken into account. Therefore, in this edition, more attention has been paid to the recognition of metabolic interactions, risk factors, diagnosis, therapy and management of secondary osteoporoses.

Novel directions in classifications and inter-relationships of major diseases and their subtypes, including osteoporosis, as well as in the application of the particular up-to-date criteria required by systems biology and by the relatively novel fields of genomics, metabolomics and pharmacogenomics, among others, are briefly mentioned but not actually utilized in this text. All of the above have been developed, confirmed and published and many have gained recognition and approval, although widespread acceptance and utilization is only just beginning. Consequently, we have adhered stringently to simplicity, comprehensiveness, and practicality of approach to examinations, methods and implementation of up-to-date testing, prevention strategies, diagnosis criteria, and presentation of therapeutic possibilities, as well as to our own particular goal which is to keep this text as "user-friendly" as possible, so that any doctor seeking information on a particular topic in osteoporosis and associated and secondary osteopathies has uncomplicated and time-saving access to such information. We wish all our readers success in their endeavours to help patients and to reduce suffering in this strife-ridden, beautiful planet of ours. God bless you all!

Munich, Tel-Aviv and Ulm   Reiner Bartl
                                            Bertha Frisch
                                            Christoph Bartl

Contents

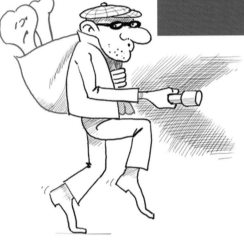

1.1
Osteoporosis: A Silent Thief!

A young healthy adult can hardly imagine that he/she will ever suffer from osteoporosis.

Moreover, when an older individual sustains a fracture or notices a gradual decrease in height, the first reaction is: "This cannot be true, this can't be happening to me. Why should I have osteoporosis? I never had a single problem with my bones in all my life!" And that is just the problem!

Osteoporosis slowly but surely nibbles away at the bones, possibly unnoticed for years, until finally it is exposed by the occurrence of a fracture almost without cause! And so the vicious circle begins and the patient is suddenly confronted by many psychological, social and possibly financial problems, which at times may appear overwhelming: starting from the fracture itself, leading to pain, possibly deformities, anger, anxiety, frustration, depression, loss of self-esteem, decreased mobility and finally even social isolation. One of the most appropriate and effective sources of help is the local osteoporosis support group, where patients can learn from other patients who have had similar experiences, how best to cope with their new challenges. Unfortunately, many people who are at risk are unaware of it and have not yet adopted preventive measures or received treatment. Some estimates suggest that less than 30% of women with osteopenia/osteoporosis are correctly diagnosed, and less than 15% of those diagnosed receive treatment for prevention in cases of osteopenia or therapy in established osteoporosis.

The situation is even worse for men, because it has only recently been recognized that osteoporosis shows no gender discrimination – it only attacks men later than women; that is to say, at the time of the andropause when the levels of male hormones start to decrease and androgen deficiency occurs – from about 50–60 years of age onwards. It has now been calculated that men >50 years have a 13% lifetime risk for fractures!

Regrettably, some doctors still regard osteoporosis as a "normal" aspect of ageing; a process whereby organisms gradually "lose the capacity to deal with life's stresses effectively". The "ageing process" includes pathophysiological changes such as decreases in muscle and bone mass; and these in turn are brought about by quantitative, structural and functional alterations in mechanisms participating in the control of all the systems in the body. These changes may affect the structure of individual cells and their constituents such as mitochondria, as well as changes in cytokines and other factors produced by cells. However, many of these mechanisms can be favourably influenced by outside interventions! We can no longer accept osteoporosis as a "normal component" of ageing, which impinges on, or even ruins, the active life of more than half of all women over 50 years of age, and nearly as many men over 70 years! The purpose of this book is to unmask the bone robbers and to provide guidelines for the early prevention, correct diagnosis and successful treatment of osteoporosis.

R. Bartl, B. Frisch, *Osteoporosis,* DOI 10.1007/978-3-540-79527-8_1,
© Springer-Verlag Berlin Heidelberg 2009

1.2
Osteoporosis: The Global Scope of the Problem

Today many in the medical profession and in health care authorities have come to the realization that osteoporosis can affect everybody from newborn babies to the oldest of the old; and significantly, that both sexes are equally prone and vulnerable, and under similar conditions the difference is mainly a temporal one! Osteoporosis is now identified as one of the 10 most important conditions affecting the entire human race, along with others such as cardio-vascular disorders, hypertension, stroke and diabetes mellitus, and it is essential to take into consideration that each of these disorders is itself a risk factor for osteoporosis! In some cases there is an independent association between two diseases, not related to age or any other known factor: for example, atherosclerosis and osteoporosis, both degenerative chronic diseases, prevalent in developed countries. An estimated 44 million people suffer from osteoporosis in the US alone, as do equally high percentages of the populations in many other countries in the Americas, Europe and Asia. Moreover, it has been estimated that the numbers of people with osteopenia/osteoporosis in the US will increase to 52 million by the year 2010 and to 61 million by the year 2020. Other calculations claim that there are already over 200 million osteoporotic people in the world today: one in three women and one in eight men! With global awareness and participation in preventive measures, these numbers could be reduced, not permitted to increase! It has been pointed out that understanding the epidemiology of osteoporosis is essential for the development of strategies suitable for application to large segments of whole populations if this epidemic is to be contained and finally eradicated!

Fracture of a bone is the most significant consequence of osteoporosis. For comparison, while every eighth woman suffers from breast cancer, every third woman sustains a fracture due to osteoporosis. Although osteoporosis can attack any bone in the body, the typical sites of osteoporotic fractures are the hip, the spine and the wrist. Of the 1.3 million fractures that occur annually in the US in patients aged over 45 years, 70% are attributable to osteoporosis. From the age of 50 years onwards, a woman has the following risk for a fracture:

- Vertebral 32%
- Lower arm 16%
- Hip 15%

Furthermore, a hip fracture poses an increased risk of mortality (Fig. 1.1a,b) related to possible co-morbidities such as rheumatism, chronic cardiovascular disease, stroke, chronic lung disorders, as well as the complications secondary to surgical treatment of the fracture itself. Nearly 50% of patients with hip fractures never fully recover the mobility and independence they previously had, and an additional 25% require a long-term nursing facility or home care. Mortality after a hip fracture is estimated to range from 12 to 35% which is higher than that expected in the general population. The risk of a woman dying from a hip fracture (2.8%) is equal to that of dying from breast cancer and four times greater than that of dying from endometrial cancer (0.7%). The highest mortal-

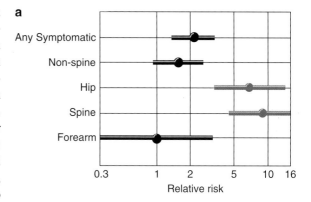

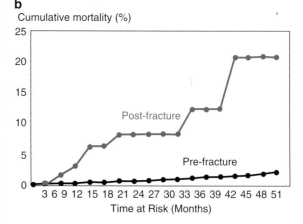

Fig. 1.1a, b. (**a**) Risk of mortality following clinical fractures (modified from Cauley et al. [2000]). (**b**) Risk of mortality in the pre- and post-fracture setting

ity typically occurs within the first 6 months after a fracture, but some studies have shown a sustained effect over a longer period. It has been estimated that the respective figures for men are worse than those given above for women.

A general approach to quantify the burden of any disease is to assess the disability it incurs, including deaths due to the disease itself, as well as the disability that remains in survivors. The approach based on disability-adjusted life years (DALYs) lost allows a comparison with other diseases (Fig. 1.2). Osteoporosis accounts for more DALYs than rheumatoid arthritis, asthma or hypertensive heart disease. With regard to neoplastic disorders, the burden of osteoporosis is greater than that for cancer at all sites, with the exception of pulmonary cancer (Fig. 1.3).

Monetary costs associated with osteoporotic fractures are tremendous: approximately 40 million US dollars daily in the US. The total cost for medical and hospital expenses, possibly nursing-home care and lost productivity reached 17 billion US dollars in 2005 (Fig. 1.4a,b)! Hip fractures alone account for about 60% of these costs, and fractures at other sites for about 40%. In the year 2000, there were estimated to be 620,000 new fractures at the hip and 620,000 clinical spine fractures in men and women aged 50 years

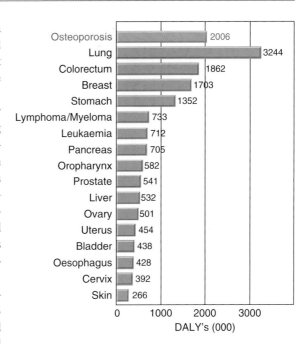

Fig. 1.3. Burden of disease estimated as disability-adjusted life years (DALYs) lost due to selection of neoplastic diseases in Europe (modified from Johnell and Kanis [2006])

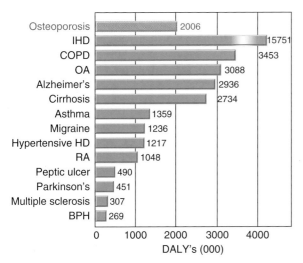

Fig. 1.2. Burden of diseases estimated as disability-adjusted life years (DALYs) lost due to selection of non-communicable diseases in Europe (modified from Johnell and Kanis [2006]). *IHD*, ischaemic heart disease; *COPD*, chronic obstructive pulmonary disease; *OA*, osteoarthritis; *RA*, rheumatoid arthritis; *BPH*, benign prostatic hyperplasia

or over in Europe. In many countries the population as a whole is living longer and the proportion of elderly people is increasing, especially those aged 85 years or more. Global demographic changes are expected to increase the incidence of hip fractures nearly fourfold by the year 2050. Each year, osteoporotic fractures affect more women than heart attacks, strokes and breast cancer combined. Indeed, the economic costs of osteoporosis are as significant as those of chronic obstructive pulmonary disease, myocardial infarction, strokes and breast cancer. The recently updated economic estimate indicates that nationwide measures for osteoporosis prevention and treatment are cost-effective when the 10-year probability of a hip fracture reached 3% of the whole population, as shown in a recent US position paper (2008). Using a value of approximately 63,000 Euros per quality-adjusted life-year (QALY) gained as a threshold for cost effectiveness, treatment of osteoporosis with alendronate, risedronate, ibandronate, zoledronate, strontium or raloxifene was cost-effective in all populations, except for 50-year-old women without a previous vertebral fracture, since the average fracture risks are relatively low in this age group (Fig. 1.5). However, in

1

a

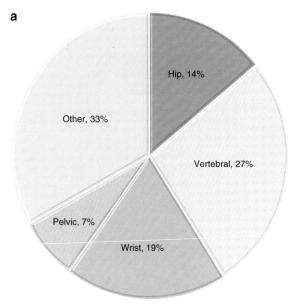

Total fractures = 2.05 M

b

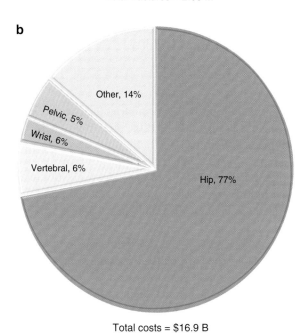

Total costs = $16.9 B

Fig. 1.4a, b. (a) Fracture distribution by type in the US, 2005. (b) Cost distribution by type in the US, 2005 (modified from Burge et al. [2007])

all other cases of postmenopausal women the cost per QALY gained was below 63,000 Euros. The absolute 10-year hip fracture probability at which intervention became cost-effective was similar across race/ethnicity groups, but tended to be slightly higher for men than for women.

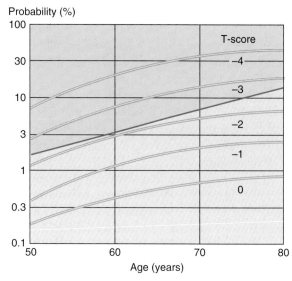

Fig. 1.5. Ten-year probability of hip fracture in Swedish men and women, according to T-scores assessed at the femoral neck by DXA. Probability scale is logarithmic. The *blue line* represents the probability at which interventions are cost-effective (modified from Kanis et al. [2005])

Another highly significant aspect of osteoporosis, as mentioned previously, is the fact that numerous disorders in most medical disciplines have deleterious effects on the bones – primarily involving osteoporosis. Examples of some such conditions include: infections and inflammatory disorders, e.g. AIDS and inflammatory bowel disease, cardiovascular disorders, diabetes mellitus and the metabolic syndrome, neurologic conditions such as Parkinson's disease and epilepsy; in oncology, cancers of the breast, prostate, lung and colon, congenital disorders such as osteogenesis imperfecta and interdisciplinary causes such as effects of drugs – a notable example are the glucocorticoids – and, last but not least, transplantations of cells and of organs. One report listed 60 different processes and conditions in which the New Bone Biology was studied. All may be associated, directly or indirectly, with a decrease in bone mass and bone density. In this context, it should also be stressed that metabolic conditions that cause intrinsic biochemical alterations, and thereby also damage the bones, have initiated the concept and the classification of metabolic bone diseases. Included under this heading are rickets (osteomalacia), renal osteodystrophy, hyperparathyroidism and osteoporosis. Osteoporosis also remains a major public health problem through its association with fragility fractures in the older age groups, which are steadily increasing in many countries. It is now abundantly clear that osteoporosis poses a major public health threat and arresting this disorder should be a primary goal of our preventive efforts in the coming decade.

All physicians (including the family doctor) have a duty to provide the patients with the knowledge they need to make their own informed decisions. Patients, for their part, have the responsibility to learn as much as possible about the preservation of their own health and to cooperate with their doctors to find suitable individual strategies and approaches to build up the structure and protect the strength of their bones; this includes attention to nutrition, exercise and other lifestyle factors such as smoking and alcohol. Different approaches have been tried and, encouragingly, group-based, multidisciplinary education programmes have significantly increased the patients' knowledge of osteoporosis and its consequences.

It is also encouraging to note that, according to one recent poll, public awareness of osteoporosis has increased from 15 to 85% within the last few years, but the consequences, including the personal implications of this knowledge, are not yet fully realized. However, occasional reports do indicate that some progress is being made, such as for example the stabilizing incidence of ankle fractures and the declining incidence of knee fractures since 1970 up to 2008 in elderly people in Finland.

Clinical osteology, (including osteoporosis, the most frequent and widespread disorder) has now become an important and independent specialty which encompasses all aspects of the skeleton and its disorders, including effects of nutrition, lifestyle and exercise. These aspects form an integral part of any program designed to prevent osteoporosis and of any protocols for its treatment. However, a greater degree of active participation in health education and its implementation is still required, as emphasized in many articles published only recently in 2008 from countries around the globe, including the US, Canada, the European Union, Mexico and Japan, among others (Fig. 1.6). Heightened awareness and closer cooperation between family doctors and specialists should result in better functional outcome for the patients as well as in lower national costs.

A change in approach will also facilitate the attainment of these goals, for example by direct-to-

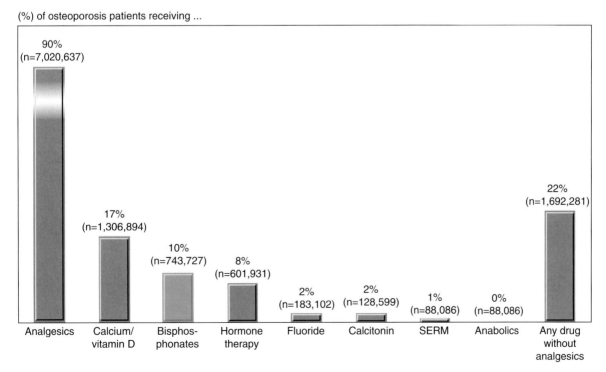

Fig. 1.6. Percentages of osteoporosis patients receiving osteoporosis-specific drugs in Germany (modified from Häussler et al. [2006], Bone EVA study)

consumer availability of densitometry and drugs for the prevention of osteoporosis. This has already been initiated by the establishment of consultation "counters" in pharmacies and drug stores in some cities in the US and Europe. This intervention by clinical pharmacists has already resulted in clinically significant rates of patient identification and treatment. Put simply in other words: people can and should take matters into their own hands! Each and every one of us is obligated to preserve his/her own skeletal structure and function throughout life! Consequently, as individuals, we must be informed and, as parents, we must educate. We are all responsible for ourselves:

"Bone Is Everybody's Business".

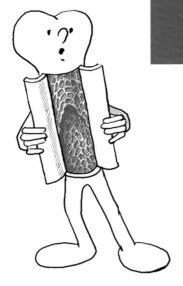

2.1
Bone: An Architectural Masterpiece

The structure, function, physiology, normal processes of preservation and maintenance of the skeleton, as well as the pathologic processes underlying osteodystrophies are briefly outlined in this chapter.

The skeleton consists of about 220 bones and constitutes approximately 15% of the total body weight.

Bone has *five main tasks* to fulfill:

- Support and locomotion: of the body as a whole and of its individual components, e.g. from the smallest (the toes) to the largest (the legs and spine).
- Protection: the skeleton protects internal organs from possibly harmful external effects. For example, the ribs shelter the heart and lungs, while the cranial bones protect the brain.
- Storehouse for minerals: The skeleton is the largest depot for minerals in the body. In total, 99% of calcium, 85% of phosphate and 50% of magnesium are stored in the bones. Approximately 1–1.5 kg calcium is built into the skeleton in the form of hydroxyapatite.
- Storehouse for bone matrix proteins: The mineralized bone substance consists of about 50% organic material: 25% matrix (ground substance) and 25% water. The matrix contains 90% collagen type I and 10% other proteins such as glycoprotein, osteocalcin, osteonectin, bone sialoprotein, osteopontin, fibronectin, as well as various proteoglycans. All these proteins are synthesized and secreted by osteoblasts and have a variety of functions, such as seeding crystal formation, binding calcium crystals and serving as sites for the attachment of bone cells. Collagen also has direct effects on important bone cell functions, including apoptosis, cell proliferation and differentiation, which are under complex control from the cell surface to the nucleus. Although collagen may have less effect on bone strength and stiffness than mineral does, it may still have a profound effect on bone fragility. Collagen changes that occur with age and reduce bone toughness or stiffness may be an important factor in the risk of fracture. Bone matrix also contains proteins such as bone morphogenic proteins (BMPs), thrombospondin-2 and metalloproteinases that stimulate or inhibit the actions of bone cells. Some studies have shown that bone also contains growth factors and cytokines, such as transforming growth factor beta 1 (TGF-β1).
- The skeleton participates in the endocrine regulation of energy by means of mechanisms involving leptin and osteocalcin, by which glucose levels in the serum as well as adiposity are both effected. In this context it is clear that the processes involved in energy balance influence many organs and tissues, while imbalance induces adverse effects in the liver, pancreas and skeletal muscle, which in turn affect the bones.

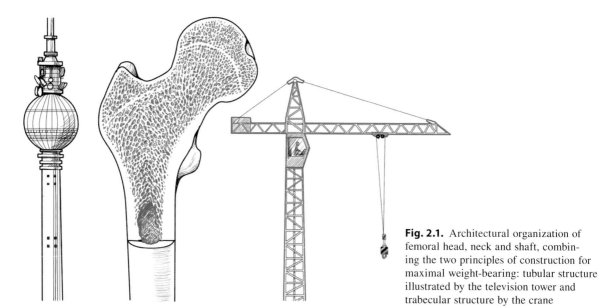

Fig. 2.1. Architectural organization of femoral head, neck and shaft, combining the two principles of construction for maximal weight-bearing: tubular structure illustrated by the television tower and trabecular structure by the crane

Bone has two mechanical functions to fulfill: weight-bearing and flexibility (Fig. 2.1). Specific *structural organizations*, from the macroscopic through the microscopic to the molecular, enable bone to perform these functions:

- Configuration and size of bones
- Proportion of compact (cortical) to cancellous (trabecular) bone; adapted to weight-bearing (Fig. 2.2)
- Trabecular bone structure with "nodes" to support weight (a "node" comprises the nodular junction of three or more trabeculae) (Fig. 2.3)
- Lamellar organization of osseous tissue
- Degree of mineralization of osseous tissue
- Arrangement of collagen fibres and filaments, together with non-collagenous matrix proteins (NCPs)
- Cable-like organization of collagen molecules and their "cross-linking"

The elasticity of bone is achieved mainly by a special mixture of its component parts, known as "two-phase

components" in the building industry. Bone consists of the matrix (the material laid down by the osteoblasts) made up of layers of collagen molecules between which crystalline calcium and phosphate are deposited (Fig. 2.4). This "passive gradual mineralization" increases density as the bone gets older. The new matrix begins to mineralize after about 5–10 days from the time of deposition (*primary mineralization*) (Fig. 2.5). On completion of the bone remodelling cycle, a phase of *secondary mineralization* begins. This process consists of a gradual maturation of the mineral component, including an increase in the amount of crystals and/or an augmentation of crystal size toward its maximum dimension. This secondary mineralization progressively increases the mineral content in

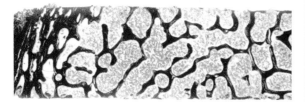

Fig. 2.2. Overview of a section of normal bone biopsy from a middle-aged man showing wide cortex and uniform, connected trabeculae. Gomori staining

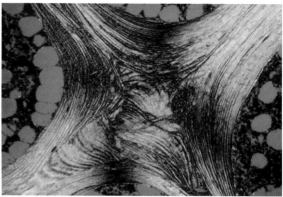

Fig. 2.3. "Node" at the intersection of four trabeculae showing an osteon with concentric lamellae. Gomori staining, polarization

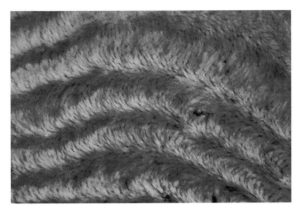

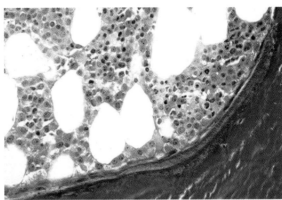

Fig. 2.4. Alternating light and dark "undulating" lamellae due to arrangement of collagen fibres. Giemsa staining, polarization

Fig. 2.5. Flat osteoblasts and layers of newly formed osteoid (*various shades of red*) on mineralized bone (*blue*). Ladewig

bone matrix. At the end of the primary mineralization, mineral content represents only about 50 % of the maximum degree of mineralization obtained at the end of the secondary mineralization phase. Various trace elements, water and mucopolysaccharides serve as binding material (glue) which binds the proteins and minerals firmly together. Collagen is responsible for the elasticity (flexibility) of bone while the minerals provide strength and rigidity. The bundles of collagen fibres are arranged parallel to the layers of matrix and are connected by cement lines. In adult bone, the degree of mineralization depends on the rate of remodelling. That means that the biologic determinant of mineralization is the rate of bone turnover. These

correlations also demonstrate that "bone mass" and "bone mineral density" (BMD), although often used synonymously, are two different entities. Indeed, the term "bone mineral density" has been introduced in the interpretation of the positive effects of the bisphosphonates on fracture risk.

The external aspect of bone conceals its inner architecture (Fig. 2.6). The two main supporting structures of bone are only recognized in X-ray films or bone biopsy sections:

- *Compact, cortical bone*: This forms the outer layer of the long bones, is very densely packed and hard, and has a slow metabolic rate. Therefore, cortical bone is resorbed and replaced at a much slower rate

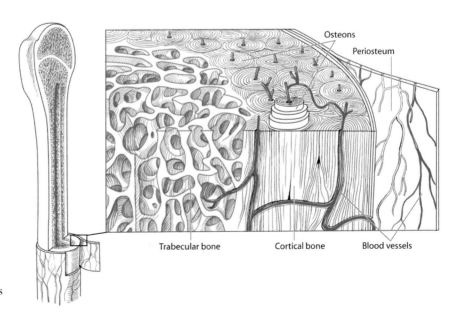

Fig. 2.6. Structure of bone: Cortical bone together with its vascular system surrounds the trabecular network

Osteons

Periosteum

Trabecular bone   Cortical bone   Blood vessels

2

than trabecular bone. The layer of cortical bone of the long tubular bones (femur, humerus) consists of osteons also called Haversian systems, which are longitudinally oriented cylinders about 5 mm long and made up of 5–20 "rings".

- *Spongy, cancellous, trabecular bone, sometimes also known as ossicles*: The axial skeleton (cranium, vertebral column, thorax and pelvis) has a specialized construction. At first glance the trabeculae appear to be randomly distributed, but closer inspection reveals that they are oriented precisely along the lines of stress and weight-bearing ("trajection lines"), producing sponge- and lattice-like structures (Fig. 2.7). The more closely the trabecular "nodes" are spaced, the greater the stability and strength of the bone, while the trabecular plates dominate the elastic properties of the trabecular bone.

Cortical bone has three surfaces and each has different anatomic features:

- The endosteal envelope faces the marrow cavity and comprises a high surface area and therefore supports a high bone turnover.
- The periosteal envelope, the outer surface of the bone to which the tendons, ligaments and muscles are attached, is capable of remodelling, as is the intracortical surface.
- The intracortical envelope, with bone surfaces inside the Haversian system, i.e. the osteons.

The *skeleton* can be divided into two main compartments:

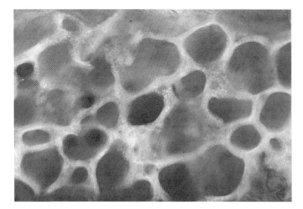

Fig. 2.7. Surface of a trimmed plastic block showing a fairly uniform trabecular network

- *Axial skeleton*: This refers to the spine and proximal femur. The bone in this area is primarily trabecular with a high turnover.
- *Appendicular skeleton*: This refers to the long bones of the legs and arms. The bone in these areas is primarily cortical with a low turnover.

Approximately 80 % of bone is cortical and only 20 % is trabecular and they undergo *different rates of remodelling*:

- Cortical bone is dense, is 90 % calcified, has a low surface:volume ratio and therefore has a slow remodelling rate.
- In contrast, cancellous bone has a porous structure and a large surface area. Approximately 25 % of cancellous bone is remodelled annually compared to only 2.5 % of cortical bone. It therefore follows that any decrease in bone is first manifest in bones with a large proportion of trabeculae and therefore with a higher surface area.

The *proportion of trabecular bone* varies in different skeletal regions:

- Lumbar vertebrae 75 %
- Heels 70 %
- Proximal femur 50–75 %
- Distal radius 25 %
- Middle of the radius <5 %

2.2
Bone: A Permanent Building and Rebuilding Site

Bone is a dynamic organ, highly vascularized and very active metabolically (Fig. 2.8). As bones are not completely developed at birth, they continue to be formed slowly out of cartilage or connective tissue, which are converted into the hard, lamellar components of the skeleton. Growth of bones ("*modelling*") comes to an end at puberty with ossification of the "growth plates". Modelling is of particular interest as bone is much more capable of reacting to external loads during growth than at any other time. About 90 % of adult bone is formed by the end of adolescence and subsequent gains during adulthood are very small.

During adulthood, i.e. throughout life, there is a continuous process of remodelling which maintains

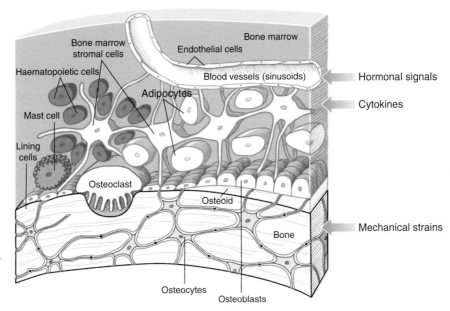

Fig. 2.8. Interdependence of bone and marrow: together they form a single structural and functional entity

the skeleton and adapts the bones to the changing external circumstances (Fig. 2.9). Nevertheless as the body ages, bone loses some of its strength and elasticity and therefore breaks more easily. This is due to loss of mineral and changes in the bone matrix. Bones undergo a constant process of removal and replace-

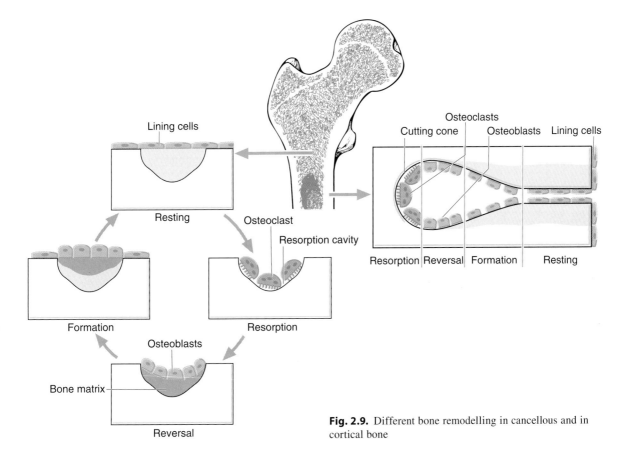

Fig. 2.9. Different bone remodelling in cancellous and in cortical bone

2

Table 2.1. Quantitative parameter of bone remodelling in normal adults

Trabecular bone surface covered with	
Osteoblasts	2–7%
Osteoclasts	1%
Lifespan	
BMU	6–9 Months
Osteoclast	3 Weeks
Osteoblasts	3 Months
Number of active BMUs at any time	1 Million
BMUs initiated per year	3–4 Million/year
BMU size	1–2 mm long and 0.2–0.4 mm wide
Mean time for renewal of the skeleton	10 Years
Renewal per day	0.027% (1 BMU/7 s)

BMU, bone multicellular unit.

ment so that the components of bone are exchanged at regular intervals. This process is called remodelling and serves the following purposes (Table 2.1):
- Mobilization of calcium in the framework of calcium homeostasis
- Replacement of old osseous tissue
- Overall skeletal and individual local adaptation to different loads, weight-bearing and stress

- Repair of damaged bone, both microscopic and macroscopic

The last refers not only to repair or healing of fractures of whole bones, but also to the countless perforations, breaks or cracks of the trabeculae, the "microfractures", "microdamage" or "fatigue damage" which occur constantly and which together with the thickness of the bones determine the fracture risk. As these tiny breaks, cracks or fractures accumulate they weaken older bones and contribute to fracture risk if not quickly and adequately repaired. This, in addition to a slightly negative bone balance over time, eventually leads to reduction in structural continuity of the trabecular network and thereby loss of strength. In cortical bone microcrack density is greater in older individuals and on average the microcracks are shorter in areas of the cortex with more resorption spaces, indicating a relationship with the rate of bone remodelling.

The *bone cells* constitute a specialized osseous cell system responsible for the repair, maintenance and adaptation of bone:
- *Osteoclasts* ("bone resorbers", "bone breakers", "bone carvers") can resorb old, weak bone in a short period of time (Fig. 2.10). These multinucleated giant cells are derived from monocytes of the bone marrow, which is from a haematopoietic cell line. The cell membrane consists of numerous "folds" – the "ruffled border" which faces the surface of the bone (Fig. 2.11). The osteoclasts release quantities of proteolytic and other enzymes into the space between the ruffled membrane and the bone. These substances

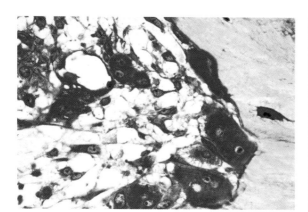

Fig. 2.10. Active osteoclasts in deep resorption bay. Giemsa staining

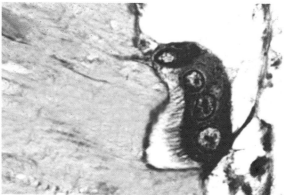

Fig. 2.11. Active osteoclast with ruffled border in lacuna with paratrabecular sinusoid. Giemsa staining

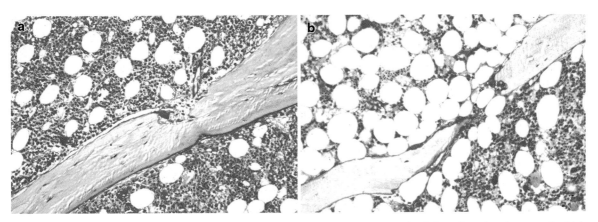

Fig. 2.12a,b. Osteoclasts perforate a trabecula (**a**) and transect it (**b**), thereby disconnecting it from the trabecular network which irreversibly and mechanically weakens that area of bone. Giemsa staining

dissolve the minerals and some of the bone matrix, the rest is phagocytosed and metabolized in the cytoplasm of the osteoclasts. If the trabecula is thin enough, active osteoclasts may perforate and transect it, thereby disconnecting it from the trabecular network which irreversibly weakens that area of bone (Fig. 2.12a,b). Recruitment, differentiation and activation of osteoclasts are accomplished by numerous systemic hormones (such as parathyroid hormones, oestrogens, androgens, leptin and thyroid hormones) as well as cytokines. Various growth factors are also involved. Recent investigations of the RANK/RANKL signalling pathway in the osteoclast have clarified mechanisms of stimulation and activation of resorption. Osteoclasts possess oestrogen receptors, by means of which oestrogen inhibits their recruit-

ment. Androgens also act on osteoclasts. The actions of sex steroids on bone cells are discussed below.

- *Osteoblasts* ("bone builders") are derived from the mesenchyme in the bone marrow. They produce new bone slowly, over several weeks to replace that resorbed by the osteoclasts (Fig. 2.13). Their main function is the synthesis of bone matrix, in particular collagen type I, but also osteocalcin, osteonectin and BMPs. Osteoblasts also possess receptors for oestrogen.

- *Osteocytes* ("bone maintainers", "bone controllers"): The osteocytes are the most numerous of all the bone cells (Fig. 2.14). They develop from osteoblasts. Approximately every tenth osteoblast situated on the surface of the bone is entrapped by the newly formed bone matrix and thus becomes

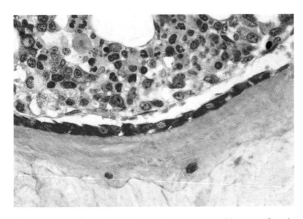

Fig. 2.13. Active cuboidal osteoblasts on osteoid seam of variable width. Giemsa staining

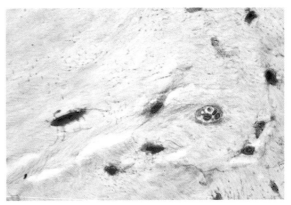

Fig. 2.14. Osteocytes cut at different angles in trabecular bone. Note a narrow trabecular canal containing a blood vessel. Giemsa staining

2

an osteocyte. It possesses receptors for various hormones including PTH and sex hormones. The osteocytes occupy spaces in the bone called "lacunae" and are connected to each other and to the endosteal cells on the surface of the bone by thin channels called "canaliculi" within which long cytoplasmic processes join osteocytes to each other and thus form a circulatory system. Osteocytes posses functional gap junctions enabling them to communicate with one another (like neurons) as well as with the surface lining cells – the endosteal cells. Therefore, osteocytes are in a position to transmit the load-induced signals to pre-osteoblasts which then differentiate and secrete osteoid. The total surface of combined lacunae and canaliculi has been estimated at 1200 m^2. The function of osteocytes has not yet been fully elucidated, but they are known to play an important part in the transport of organic and inorganic materials within the bones. Furthermore, their strategic location enables them to function as mechanosensory cells and thus to detect the need for bone increase or decrease during functional adaptation of the skeleton, as well as the need for repair of microfractures. Osteocytes detect changes in flow of the fluid in the canaliculi and in the levels of circulating hormones such as oestrogen, glucocorticoids and raloxifene, which influence their activities and survival. Recent data suggest that mechanical loading decreases the osteocytes' potential to regulate local osteoclastogenesis by direct cell–cell contact and/or via soluble signals. Quite possibly they also receive impulses from the muscles which they relay to the cells of the remodelling units at the surface of the bone. They also register the age of the bone and initiate its remodelling. Osteocytes also produce various factors, notably sclerostin, a molecule that regulates osteoblast activity, as well as DMP 1, and FGF 3, a factor also involved in the regulation of renal phosphate uptake. To summarize the function of the osteocytes: Osteocytes are actively involved in remodelling and in its control mechanisms. Osteocytes actively participate in ion exchange. Osteocytes are mechanosensory cells with a major part in the functional adaptation of bone. The number (density) of osteocytes determines bone mass both for cortical and trabecular bone. Disruption of the osteocyte network and decrease in osteocyte number with age

is inevitably accompanied by a decrease in bone mass, as well as by a decrease in bone quality by impairment of repair of microfractures. Although regulated by all the control mechanisms outlined above, in the final analysis it is the highly complex intercellular signalling between the osteoprogenitor cells and the mature osteoclasts, osteoblasts and osteocytes which balance their activities in growth and remodelling.

- *Endosteal lining cells* (bone "housekeepers"): these are flat cells that cover 80–95% of the internal surface of the bones. They are presumed to develop from inactive osteoblasts. They form a protective layer and constitute a surveillance system for the bones (Fig. 2.15). They are connected to a thin collagenous membrane covering the mineralized bone surface, the osteocytic lacunae and their canaliculi (Fig. 2.16). Recently, it has been shown that the endosteal lining cells may participate in activation of osteoclasts. Certain surface molecules expressed on lining cells and on osteoclast progenitors react with the receptor RANK (also found on osteoclast progenitors) and thereby set in motion a cycle of remodelling. Other important factors which participate in the remodelling cycle have also been analysed and these are: ODF (osteoclast differentiation factor), OPGL (osteoprotegerin ligand), TRANCE and RANKL (RANK ligand). PTH, PGE$_2$, IL1 and 1,25 (OH) vitamin D exercise a negative influence on osteoprotegerin production and thereby stimulate resorption. Osteoblast precursors produce M-CSF which can activate osteoclasts. The endosteal lining

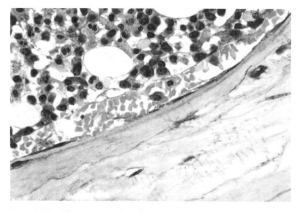

Fig. 2.15. Flat endosteal lining cells and paratrabecular sinusoid. Giemsa staining

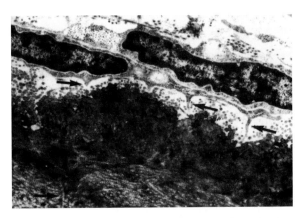

Fig. 2.16. At higher magnification, collagen in transverse section (thin collagenous membrane) under the flat endosteal lining cells, and in longitudinal section (mineralized bone) in the lower part of the micrograph. Note processes of endosteal lining cells (*arrows*) extending between collagen fibres, presumably to connect with processes of osteocytes within the canaliculi. EM × 11,300

cells also participate in bone remodelling. They remove fragments of bone collagen left by osteoclasts, thereby cleaning up resorption pits and initiating formation of new bone.

2.3 Remodelling Units

There are 2–5 million bone remodelling units (BRUs) in the skeleton (Fig. 2.17). These units, required for the maintenance and integrity of the skeleton, are of crucial importance for the development of osteoporosis (Table 2.2). The total quantity of bone decreases if more bone is resorbed than is produced over the years. It has been estimated that osteoporosis develops when for every 30 units of bone resorbed only 29 are produced. This negative "bone balance" has three possible causes:

- Increased osteoclastic activity without increased osteoblastic activity ("high turnover")
- Normal osteoclastic but decreased osteoblastic activity ("low turnover")
- Decreased osteoclastic and osteoblastic activity ("atrophic" or "adynamic" bone)

Consequently, an overall decrease in bone correlates primarily with the number of BRUs and with the lack of coordination between the cells of the BRU. The

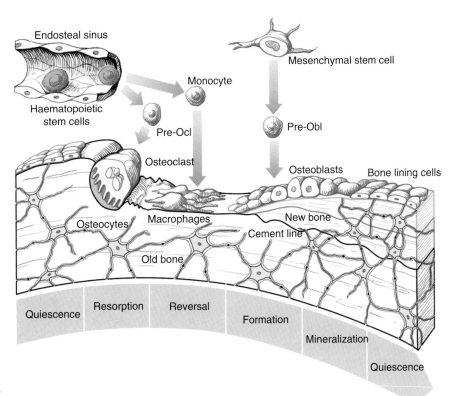

Fig. 2.17. Steps of bone remodelling in adult trabecular bone

Table 2.2. Bone remodelling and its clinical correlations

Phase of remodelling	Quiescence	Bone resorption by osteoclasts	Reversal	Bone formation by osteoblasts	Quiescence
Stimulating factors		Parathormone Vitamin D Thyroxine		Growth hormone Parathormone Oestrogen Testosterone Cytokines Prostaglandins Vitamin D	
Inhibiting factors		Oestrogen Calcitonin Testosterone Bisphosphonates Raloxifene		Corticosteroids Smoking Alcohol	
Bone markers		Pyridinoline NTX, CTX		Bone-specific alkaline phosphatase Osteocalcin	

level of excretion of calcium and collagen metabolites in the urine reflects the degree of resorption of bone. The process of bone remodelling is as yet incompletely understood. One remodelling cycle takes approximately 120 days, and it has been divided into six phases:

- Phase of quiescence: a layer of flat lining cells over a thin collagenous membrane covers the surface of the bone.
- Phase of activation: the quiescent bone surface is prepared for resorption. This involves retraction of the endosteal lining cells and removal of the thin collagenous membrane covering the bone surface. There is evidence that matrix metalloproteinases produced by osteoblasts are involved in this process. The site-specific activation may be achieved by mechanical stresses transmitted to the endosteal lining cells via the osteocytic-canalicular network.
- Phase of resorption: recruitment and fusion of osteoclastic precursors, preparation of osteoclasts for resorption, development of the ruffled membrane; osteoclasts resorb the bone, which leads to formation of lacunae or pits; osteoclasts migrate slowly or undergo apoptosis.
- Phase of reversal: osteoblast progenitors are attracted to the resorption pit, while monocytes and endosteal lining cells prepare the surface of the resorption pit for new bone production by removal of the debris left by the osteoclasts.
- Phase of early formation: production of osteoid by active osteoblasts.
- Phase of late formation: mineralization of osteoid.
- Phase of quiescence: the osteoblasts turn into the flat endosteal lining cells or into osteocytes if trapped in the newly formed bone.

The phase of resorption is completed within 2 weeks, while that of mineralization may take months and depends on the presence of active metabolites of vitamin D. On completion of a remodelling cycle a "structural bone unit" is formed; about 35 million are present in the whole skeleton. In total, 8% of the skeleton is replaced annually by the activity of the BRUs.

The following four stages of osteoclast activity are involved:

- Formation and differentiation of osteoclasts from their precursors (RANKL)
- Migration and attachment of osteoclasts to the osseous surface (β3 integrins)
- Osteoclastic secretion of factors for acidification and solution of minerals (V-H + -ATPase, chloride channels)
- Dissolution of matrix (cathepsin K).

Currently, the majority of treatments for osteoporosis tested so far target inhibition of bone resorption.

2.4
Some Biological Perspectives on the Mechanisms Involved in the Control and Regulation of Bone Remodelling

During the first few years of the 21st century, the complex mechanisms which characterize the control of bone remodelling were just beginning to be recognized and starting to be investigated. Results of the overwhelming amount of research subsequently published have illuminated the extreme complexity of the cellular and molecular interactions, as well as the network of interwoven highways and byways representing the numerous pathways that transport factors to stimulate or inhibit specific cellular activities. A highly significant aspect of the results of these investigations is the unequivocal demonstration of the participation of many of these pathways, not only in the control of bone remodelling, but also in numerous processes – both physiological and pathological – involving other organs and tissues, and as such are examples of systems biology.

One striking demonstration of this is *osteoimmunology* in which the participation of lymphocytes and various immunological cytokines (among other factors) in the processes of bone remodelling has now been unequivocally established. Inflammatory reactions, acute and especially long-lasting chronic reactions, are major causes of local and even systemic bone loss. One such cause, for example, is the tumour necrosis factor (TNF) in inflammatory arthritis. Another example is the induction of bone destruction by the activation of T-cells by means of RANKL. In complete contrast, CD44 acts as an inhibitor of the deleterious consequences of TNF on bones and joints, similar to the effect of selectin-9 (a growth hormone) which stimulates the production of regulatory T-cells. Moreover, additional studies have pointed out that various signalling molecules, transcription factors and membrane receptors are also shared by the immune and skeletal systems. For example, NF-kB is a vital component in inflammatory responses and also in osteoclast differentiation and osteolysis. Unhealthy lifestyles, including poor nutrition as well as overweight and morbid obesity, result in imbalances in the oxidation/redox systems, leading to inflammatory reactions and disorders of many organs including the bones and joints.

On the other hand, the localization of the osteoclastic resorption may affect haematopoiesis, such as the mobilization of haematopoietic progenitors when osteoclasts resorb an endosteal region of bone, with secretion and release of proteolytic enzymes, adjacent to stem cell niches. It has been speculated that this constitutes a link between bone remodelling and regulation of haematopoiesis.

Towards to end of the 19th century (in the 1890s) researchers developed the hypothesis that mechanical loads affect the architecture of bone in living organisms. However, the processes by which this occurs were only investigated much later in the 20th century when the weight-bearing and the load-bearing bones (not always the same), as well as various systems including "feedback systems", were identified and subsequently termed the "Mechanostat" and which was held responsible for the strength of the bones.

The Mechanostat hypothesis was then also applied in order to provide functional definitions of bone competence and bone quality in normal physiological conditions, as well as in pathological states, such as osteopenias and osteoporoses. Evidence was provided that:

- Muscle strength largely determines the strength of the load-bearing bones
- This in turn has implications for numerous aspects of bone physiology such as in Modelling and remodelling, and in interventions such as bone grafts, osteotomies, arthrodeses and possibly also in the actions of pharmaceutical agents.

Additional discoveries during the first half of the 20th century led to the formulation of the *Utah Paradigm of skeletal physiology*, according to which the skeletal effector cells (osteoblasts, osteoclasts, chondroblasts etc.) themselves determine the structure and function of bones, together with the fascia, ligaments and tendons. However, with the passage of time and a great deal of additional work, the results of studies on tissue-level mechanisms were added to the Utah Paradigm, which by then also encompassed determinants of skeletal architecture and strength. Moreover, with the accumulating information on skeletal physiology, the Utah Paradigm also came to include and integrate scientific evidence on anatomy and biochemistry – from histology to cellular and molecular biology – to pathologies of skeletal disorders and their clinical aspects.

Most significant for everyday medicine worldwide was, and still is, the bottom-line conclusion, which, simply expressed, states that strong muscles make and maintain strong bones throughout life!

The highly significant implications of this for diagnosis, the instigation of preventive measures and for therapeutic interventions are discussed later. Many studies have now been published on mechano-biology, i.e. the relationship between mechanical forces and biological processes, including the specific pathways involved in the transmission of signals elicited by mechanical loading and stress, also known as *mechanotransduction*, which is regulated by two structural combinations:

- Focal adhesions, linking cells to the extracellular matrix
- Junctional adhesions, linking adjacent cells to each other by means of adherins; and these, through the cellular circuits, co-ordinate tissue responses to mechanical loading; or, in simple terms, enable cells to translate the signals produced by mechanical loading into biochemical responses.

But these biomechanical stimuli are only a few of the numerous signals essential for an integrated osseous physiology, which are transported by the intra-osseous circulation formed by the dendritic extensions and gap junctions of the osteocytes, and possibly also the hemichannels which contain connexin 43 (CX 43). Immuno-reactive sites for CX 43 have already been identified in mature osteoclasts, as well as in marrow stromal cells.

It should also be remembered that the osteocytes, among their other responsibilities, function as sensors for mechanical stimuli and as regulators of mineralization in bone, which is part of their participation in overall mineral metabolism, particularly that of calcium. It is the gap junctions which enable adjacent cells to exchange second messengers, ions and cellular metabolites. The junctions also participate in development of bone cells, for example providing signalling pathways downstream of RANKL, for osteoclast differentiation.

To summarize with but one more example: as a response to mechanical stress, prostaglandins are released by osteocytes into the hemichannels. Among the actions of prostaglandin D2 is modulation of osteoprotegerin, RANKL and various receptors which, directly or indirectly, stimulate an anabolic response.

In addition, recent studies have shown that the prostaglandin D2 receptors expressed by osteoblasts participate in the control of osteoclastogenesis and in the activity of mature osteoclasts. Prostaglandin D2 itself has recently been shown to be chemotactic for mast cells, also by way of one of its receptors. The hemichannels (mentioned above) together with gap junctions constitute the intraosseous circulation for the transmission of signals required for maintenance and repair of the bones, and for implementation of the numerous skeletal functions including the effects of growth factors, hormones, cytokines and others, as demonstrated in the remodelling of bone by the BRUs. Clearly, these intercellular connections are crucial for the maintenance of the skeleton and therefore disruption of the communication between the bone cells themselves, and between bone cells and other cells (e.g. endosteal cells, endothelial and periosteal cells all active in osseous remodelling) is associated with many structural and functional disorders, localized and systemic, of the bones of the skeleton.

2.5
Minimodelling

"Minimodelling" is the term used to describe activity of bone cells, primarily of the osteoblasts, which is completely independent of the BRUs. First put forward about a decade ago, it was suggested that minimodelling is a mechanism for trabecular bone renewal that goes on throughout life. Minimodelling is accomplished by formation of bone on quiescent surfaces; it is not preceded by bone resorption and it leaves smooth cement lines, i.e. it is simply resumption of osteoblastic activity by the bone lining cells which results in increases in lamellar cancellous bone mass and possibly in trabecular connectivity.

An early study of bone biopsies from patients aged 38–81 years confirmed this hypothesis and the recommendation was made that the results of minimodelling should be taken into account when dealing with estimation of osteoid volume and mineralization. Shortly thereafter, an investigation was carried out on bone specimens taken from bone biopsies and from autopsy material of patients with adynamic bone disease. The results showed that in the absence of parathyroid hormone, and especially in bone from relatively younger patients (about 60–64 years), minimodelling correlated significantly with total bone volume. Another recent study of patients with hyperparathyroidism demonstrated minimodelling at the endocortical and intracortical surfaces, particularly in those specimens with narrow cortices and high porosity. Finally, results of the most recent study published to date demonstrated conclusively that bone formation by minimodelling accounts, in part, for the increase in bone volume which occurs after parathyroidectomy in patients with hyperparathyroidism. The mechanisms and stimuli involved in minimodelling have not yet been elucidated.

Additional investigations in the future will undoubtedly clarify the significance of minimodelling in the maintenance and repair of the bones.

2.6
Stimuli, Triggers and Mechanisms of Activation of Bone Remodelling

The elucidation of the mechanisms of maintenance of the size, structure and quality of the bones throughout life by means of the BRUs stimulated extensive research into the question of what activated these units. Moreover, it has been known for about half a century that the bones contain *cracks* caused by the physiological loading activities of daily life, and numerous studies have now been published on how cracks are formed and grow and how they can be detected and repaired. A large part of this research was carried out on animals – from rats to horses, in vivo and in vitro. These studies clarified many aspects of osseous reactions, what provoked them and what conclusions could be drawn; examples of these are briefly summarized below, in more or less chronological order. In the early 1990s, it was shown that remodelling repairs fatigue damage and thereby prevents fractures and it was deduced that microdamage itself evokes local bone remodelling.

At the start of the new century, investigations of bovine, equine and human long bones which had been loaded in vitro demonstrated that microcracks initiated at osteocytic lacunae, indicating that these functioned as stress concentrating organelles, thereby providing a potential mechanism for detection of strain and damage by osteocytes. Shortly thereafter,

studies on the effects of mechanical loading in sheep encompassed the timing, location, density and length of microcracks, as well as the stimulation of reactive resorption cavities. The conclusion drawn from these studies was that microdamage itself is a stimulus for initiation of bone remodelling. Subsequently, investigations were made on large bones from race horses, and from human autopsy material as well as biopsies. One of the results observed in the race horses is of special interest: namely that in the more exercised race horses, additional bone was deposited in the spaces previously occupied by adipocytic bone marrow and this was not preceded by resorption and not limited by hyper-mineralized cement lines. The conclusion was drawn that bone subjected to mechanical overload exercise, within normal limits, does not loose bone but makes more bone! Likewise, additional studies on the ulnae of rats during accumulation and coalescence of microcracks demonstrated that small increases in bone size and density substantially increased the resistance of the whole bone to microdamage. Nevertheless, the results of other studies led to the conclusion that the number of disrupted intracanalicular processes determines the osteocytic response and influences targeted remodelling. Similar data were obtained from an in vivo study on rats, which focused on microcrack formation, propagation, accumulation and disruption of osteocytic canalicular processes during increased, as well as normal, loading. Here also it was concluded that the effect on osteocytes participates in initiation of bone remodelling. However, an extensive evaluation of highly trained race horses led to the opposite conclusion, namely that in established athleticism bone turnover is influenced by pathways not involving microcracks and disrupted osteocytic processes. Moreover, the effects of a single period of cyclic fatigue on blood flow and interstitial fluid flow in the bone of the unilateral effected ulnae of rats, as well as changes in the contra-lateral unaffected ulnae of the same rats, suggested that functional adaptation to the cyclic fatigue included a more generalized neurovascular reaction.

Other recent studies have compared the response to loading, particularly that of the trabecular bone, in younger and older animals. The results indicated that in older animals the ability to initiate and repair microdamage is definitely reduced with age. Finally, the effects of microdamage on bone in both control and ovariectomized sheep, as examples of normal and osteoporotic bone, were investigated and the results demonstrated the differences between the two groups, as well as the unfavourable consequences for bone quality and bone fragility, of the osseous reactions in the ovariectomized group.

Many of the numerous investigations in animals have now been confirmed by studies in humans, both healthy and diseased. A brief summary follows. The mechanisms and pathways of bone remodelling were studied during the last decades of the previous century, and extensively at the beginning of the 21st century. Several reports dealt with hypotheses and results achieved so far have shown: that osteocyte apoptosis is induced by bone fatigue and is located in regions of bone containing microcracks as well as resorption cavities, indicating that the targeted removal and repair of microdamage is preceded by disruption of the osteocytic processes which then emit the appropriate signals to trigger repair. In addition, it was shown that the direction of crack growth, i.e. lengthening, is due to the local orientation of the fibres in the bone and also that the cracks were arrested by the vascular canals in the bone.

Various hypotheses were suggested and confirmed concerning remodelling in both compact as well as in trabecular bone. For example, in cortical bone the lamellar structure of osteons and the cement lines arrest the microcracks, changes are produced in the walls of the Haversian canals and repair is initiated, thus avoiding accumulation of microdamage and providing protection from fatigue fractures. However, some subsequent studies could not confirm the hypothesis that cracks always initiate resorption spaces, i.e. remodelling. Other investigations dealt with the density and length of microcracks and the number of resorption spaces as indicators of activated remodelling. Also demonstrated was a substantial increase in microcracks with age and this correlated with fracture incidence in the elderly.

Detailed investigation (of sections of bone from the ribs of women aged 50–60 years) demonstrated that both density and length of cracks were five times higher in interstitial than in cortical bone, while osteocytic lacunae were significantly fewer, indicating that accumulation of microdamage and osteocyte deficiency occurred in the same bone regions. Other investigations of age-related histologic changes, i.e. diffuse damage or linear microcracks, showed that the latter were longer in bones of older than younger

individuals, but that the opposite was true for microdamage, i.e. more in the younger bones. These results have recently been confirmed in the tibiae of humans (age 19–89 years) and the conclusion was drawn that age-related changes in bone microstructure play a key role in microcrack formation and repair. Recent reports have discussed the effects of microdamage as a stimulus for adaptation of bone as well as for bone biochemistry. It should be mentioned that targeted (activated) remodelling, as described above, also involves "steering", i.e. attracting or steering pre-existing BMUs towards areas of microdamage.

Other recent investigations have come to the conclusion that the BRUs are mechanically regulated: strain-induced osteocytic signals inhibit osteoblastic activity and stimulate osteoclastic activity. Consequently, cortical BRUs are attracted by apoptotic osteocytes and create load aligned osteons, while cancellous BRUs work on the trabecular surfaces, without piercing them, thus retaining the network. How these processes act on osteoporotic bone is dealt with later.

2.7
Control of Bone Remodelling: A Network of Complex Mechanisms

The skeleton possesses an efficient feedback-controlled system that continuously integrates both the signals and the responses which together maintain its function of delivering calcium into the circulation while preserving its own strength. The question arises: How do mesenchymal and haematopoietic cells, as well as the osteoclasts, osteoblasts and osteocytes cooperate to achieve such a perfect balance between resorption and formation of bone? This complex system is just starting to be unravelled (Table 2.3). There appear to be five groups of mechanisms regulating bone mass:

- *Systemic hormones*: The most important hormones are parathyroid hormone (PTH), calcitonin, thyroid hormone T 3, insulin, growth hormone (GH) and insulin-like growth factor-1 (IGF-1) which mediates many of the effects of GH on longitudinal growth and on bone mass: cortisone and sex hormones and, of these, oestrogens regulate mainly osteoclastic activity and thus bone resorption. PTH together with vitamin D is the principal regulator of calcium homeostasis (Fig. 2.18). PTH exerts its

Table 2.3. Hormonal and local regulators of bone remodelling

Hormones
  Polypeptide hormones
    Parathyroid hormone (PTH)
    Calcitonin
    Insulin
    Growth hormone
  Steroid hormones
    1,25-Dihydroxyvitamin D3
    Glucocorticoids
    Sex steroids
  Thyroid hormones

Local factors
  Synthesized by bone cells
    IGF-I and IGF-II
    Beta-2-microglobulin
    TGF-β
    BMPs
    FGFs
    PDGF
  Synthesized by bone-related tissue
    Cartilage-derived
      IGF-I
      FGFs
      TGF-β
    Blood cell derived
      G-CSF
      GM-CSF
      IL-1
      TNF
    Other factors
      Prostaglandins
      Binding proteins

tion in the mechanisms controlling bone turnover. Androgens are also important in bone formation. Osteoblasts and osteocytes as well as mononuclear and endothelial cells in the bone marrow possess receptors for androgen; the pattern and expression of the receptors is similar in men and women. Fat cells, the adipocytes, also have receptors for sex hormones which they are able to metabolize by means of the enzymes called the aromatases. Sex steroids also influence lipid metabolism in pre-adipocytes. Significant levels of both oestrogens and androgens are present in the blood in men and women and both hormones play important, but not necessarily identical, roles in bone metabolism. For example androgens may act on osteoblasts during mineralization while oestrogens more likely affect osteoblasts at an earlier stage during matrix formation. Moreover, the sex hormones may also act at different sites on the bones – for example androgens are important in the control of periosteal bone formation which contributes to the greater width of the cortex in men. There are receptors for oestrogen and testosterone on osteoblasts, osteoclasts and osteocytes, but one or other of the sex hormones may dominate at different stages of the remodelling cycle. Androgens in particular exercise a strong influence on bone formation and resorption by way of local enzymes, cytokines, adhesion molecules and growth factors. Androgens increase BMD in women as well as in men, in normal as well as in some pathologic conditions. Moreover, when given together therapeutically the two hormones increase BMD more than

effects by way of actions on the bone cells as well as on other organs such as the kidney and gut. On bone, PTH exerts its influence mainly by participa-

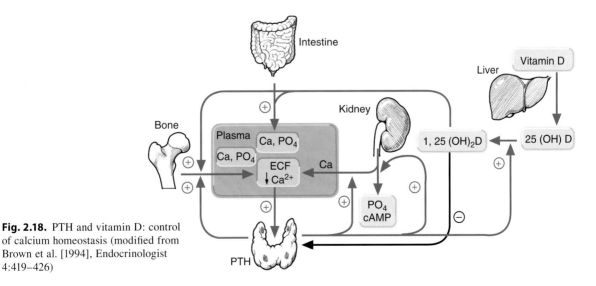

Fig. 2.18. PTH and vitamin D: control of calcium homeostasis (modified from Brown et al. [1994], Endocrinologist 4:419–426)

oestrogen given alone. Other influences such as muscular mass, strength, activity and mechanical strain may stimulate osteoanabolic activity – that is bone formation while inhibiting bone resorption. Put briefly, during growth the processes of modelling and remodelling optimize strength by deposition of bone where it is needed and decreasing bone mass where it is not. It is essential to stress that the highly complicated mechanisms controlling bone remodelling are only briefly outlined here and the elucidation of their pathways has already lead to disclosure of additional points of possible therapeutic intervention, and undoubtedly will continue to do so in the future.

- *Local cytokines and signals*: Also significant are local cytokines, electromagnetic potentials and, most importantly, signals transmitted over intercellular networks. Bone cells synthesize whole families of cytokines: for example IGF-I, IGF-II, Beta$_2$-microglobulin, interleukin (IL)-1, IL-6, TGF-β, BMPs, fibroblast growth factors (FGFs) and platelet derived growth factor (PDGF) (Fig. 2.19). Prostaglandins play a significant part in resorption of bone during immobilization. Osteoprotegerin (OPG), a member of the tumour necrosis factor receptor family produced by osteoblasts, blocks differentiation of os-

teoclasts from precursor cells and thereby prevents resorption. In fact, OPG could represent the long-sought-after molecular link between arterial calcification and bone resorption. This link underlies the clinical coincidence of vascular disease and osteoporosis, an association most frequent in postmenopausal women and in elderly people. OPG could represent a novel pathway for possible therapeutic manipulation of bone remodelling. Specific aspects of remodelling involve specific factors, as for example the impact of vascular endothelial growth factor (VEGF) in angiogenesis and endochondral bone formation, in ossification of mandibular condyles and in the growth of the long bones.

- *Vitamins and minerals*: The bone cells as well as the surrounding cell systems are also influenced by various vitamins, minerals and other factors. Vitamin D, K, C, B$_6$ and vitamin A are all required for the normal metabolism of collagen and for mineralization of osteoid.
- *Mechanical loading*: Exercise may improve bone mass and bone strength in children and adolescents. However, the osteogenic potential diminishes at the end of puberty and longitudinal growth of the bones. The adult skeleton is only moderately responsive to mechanical loading. A new way which might be use-

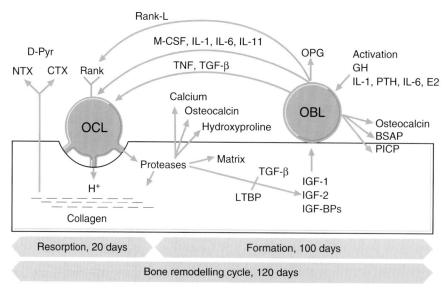

Fig. 2.19. Factors controlling bone resorption and formation. *OCL*, osteoclast; *OBL*, osteoblast. The osteoblast synthesizes cytokines and growth factors that activate osteoclasts. The two major ones essential for osteoclastogenesis are macrophage colony-stimulating factor (*M-CSF*) and osteoprote- gerin ligand (OPGL), also called Rank-L. Rank-L activates its receptor Rank on the osteoclast. Osteoprotegerin (*OPG*) is a dummy receptor for Rank-L and can suppress osteoclas- togenesis if it binds enough OPG (modified from Rosen and Bilezikian [2001])

ful to manipulate bone tissue is high-frequency, low-amplitude "vibration" exercise, combined with rest periods between loading events. Bone tissue cells must transduce an extracellular mechanical signal into an intracellular response. A mechanoreceptor is known to be a structure made up of extracellular and intracellular proteins linked to transmembrane channels. Touch sensation, proprioception and blood pressure regulation are mediated by ion channels. It has been proposed that osteocyte processes are tethered to the extracellular matrix and that these tethers amplify cell membrane strains. Presumably the extracellular fluid flow creates tension on the tethers which in turn stretches the cell membrane.

- *Transcriptional regulation and genes*: There are a number of transcriptional factors that control osteogenesis and differentiation of osteoblasts. These include runt-related transcription factor 2 (Runx2), Osterix (Osx) and sex determining region Y-box 9 (Sox9), "master" regulators of osteogenesis. New genes responsible for hereditary skeletal disorders could also provide new therapeutic opportunities. For example the identification of LRP5 as a key molecule in bone regulation was shown recently to promote osteoblastic differentiation. Finally, it should be noted that research is still ongoing concerning the cells involved, their origin and differentiation and the control mechanisms of remodelling, particularly at different sites, for example endosteal and periosteal, adjacent to haematopoietic (red) marrow, or to adipocytic (yellow) marrow, as well as the activities (if any) of the endothelial cells of the blood vessels connected to the active remodelling units. Results of these studies may reveal additional aspects of remodelling.

2.8
Osteoimmunology: A Representative of Systems Biology

It is important to emphasize that elucidation of the mechanisms underlying metabolism of bone has revealed that these mechanisms include elements of the immune system. This in turn has led to the establishment of a new interdisciplinary field. *Osteoimmunology*, originally triggered by the observation that the increased bone resorption in inflammatory disorders such as rheumatoid arthritis, is caused by increased expression of RANKL (receptor activator of nuclear factor kappaB ligand), which induced accelerated osteoclastic differentiation and activity. Moreover, such interplay/crosstalk also provides bridges for many factors – cytokines, signalling molecules, transduction factors, receptors etc. – which implement bone remodelling, are involved in the homeostasis of bone and are essential participants in the regulation of other organs and systems such as cardiology, nephrology, hepatology, gastroenterology as well as in cardiovascular, hormonal and endocrinological disorders. This multi-system participation provides a well-nigh irrefutable explanation for the fact that the skeleton is affected one way or another by disorders of practically all the other organs and systems in the body and why osteoporosis now constitutes a global epidemic.

2.9
The RANK/RANKL/Osteoprotegerin System

The *RANK/RANKL/Osteoprotegerin cytokine system* plays a key role in the regulation of and "coupling" within the processes of remodelling. The discovery of this cytokine system was a milestone for understanding osteoclastogenesis and the regulation of bone resorption as well as other processes involved in local bone remodelling. Osteoprotegerin is an important member of the TNF-receptor family which is produced by osteoblasts and which blocks the differentiation of osteoclasts from their precursor cells and thus inhibits bone resorption. RANKL (also known as osteoprotegerin ligand, OPGL) and its receptors RANK and osteoprotegerin (OPG) are the key components of the regulation of BRUs. RANKL, a member of the TNF family, is the main stimulus for osteoclast maturation and is essential for osteoclast survival. The processes of local remodelling are illustrated in Fig. 2.20.

An increase in the expression of RANKL leads directly to increased resorption and loss of bone. RANKL is produced by osteoblastic cells and by activated T-lymphocytes. Its specific receptor RANK is located on the surface membranes of osteoclasts, dendritic cells, smooth muscle cells and endothelial cells. The production of RANKL by T-lymphocytes and the consequent activation of dendritic cells represent

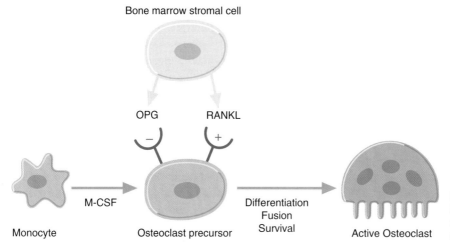

Fig. 2.20. The OPG/RANK/ RANKL system and its control of osteoclastic resorption of bone

a connection between the immunoregulatory system and osseous tissues. The close collaboration between bone and haematopoiesis is reflected by the fact that M-CSF is required for osteoclastic differentiation.

The effect of RANKL is regulated by OPG, which is secreted in various organs including: bone, skin, liver, stomach, intestine, lungs, kidneys and placenta. It also acts as a soluble endogenous receptor antagonist. Numerous cytokines, hormones and drugs may stimulate or inhibit the effects of RANKL or of OPG and thereby sway the results to the advantage or detriment of either of these two cytokines as follows:

- TGF-β increases production of OPG
- PTH increases RANKL/decreases OPG production
- Vitamin D3 increases production of RANKL
- Glucocorticoids increase RANKL/decrease OPG production
- Oestrogen increases production of OPG

Other stimulators of OPG production are vitamin K, leptin, genistein, raloxifene, statins, e.g. atorvastatin, bisphosphonates and mechanical forces. Moreover, new facets of these mechanisms are constantly being elucidated by ongoing research, for example the suppression of osteoclastogenesis by alpha-lipoic acid. In addition, it has become clear that the relationship between RANKL and OPG contributes to the preservation of the balance between resorption and formation in bone, i.e. "coupling" of these activities, and that the relative concentration of RANKL and OPG in bone is one of the main determinants of bone mass and strength.

Animal experiments have also demonstrated the important part played by OPG in the regulation of bone resorption. Genetically manipulated mice, which over-express OPG, develop osteopetrosis; while OPG knock-out mice develop severe osteoporosis. These experiments indicate that OPG functions as a "brake" for the effects triggered by RANKL. Quite possibly, in the not-so-distant future, OPG may well be introduced as a therapeutic agent in numerous disorders characterized by increased resorption, such as:

- Postmenopausal osteoporosis and osteoporosis of the elderly
- Disorders with locally increased resorption
- Paget's disease of bone
- Periodontitis
- Rheumatoid arthritis
- Bone marrow oedema syndrome
- Osteoporosis in various immunologic disorders
- Haematological disorders, e.g. multiple myeloma
- Carcinomatosis of bone
- Hypercalcaemic syndrome

During the last few years the significance of the OPG/ RANKL/RANK system has been elucidated, not only in primary disorders of bone but also in secondary skeletal-related and vascular conditions which include common diseases such as diabetes, atherosclerosis, rheumatoid arthritis and metastases (Table 2.4). This confirms that the RANKL/OPG system is a cytokine system with widespread, far-reaching systemic effects. In a recent study, a substantially increased risk of hip fracture in women was demonstrated after the onset of a cardiovascular disease (CVD), a finding compatible

Table 2.4. OPG/RANKL/RANK system in the pathogenesis of bone, immune and vascular diseases

Metabolic bone diseases
Postmenopausal osteoporosis
Glucocorticoid-induced osteoporosis
Hyperparathyroidism
Sporadic Paget disease of bone
Immune-mediated bone diseases
Rheumatic arthritis
Periodontal infection
Malignant diseases
Multiple myeloma
Bone metastases
Hypercalcaemia of malignancy
Inherited skeletal diseases
Familiar expansile osteolysis
Familial Paget disease of bone
Idiopathic hyperphosphatasia
Cardiovascular diseases
Atherosclerosis
Peripheral vascular disease
Coronary artery disease

with the concept of common pathologic pathways for osteoporotic fractures and CVD. The MINOS study, a long-term prospective trial, showed that aortic calcification is a considerable and independent risk factor for incident fractures in older men. Significantly, in all the conditions mentioned above, there are windows of opportunity for the inclusion of bisphosphonates in therapeutic interventions – some are already being explored and applied.

2.10
Leptin: Role of the Central Nervous System in Regulation of Bone

The observation that overweight individuals are less susceptible to osteoporosis implies a possible connection between obesity and the skeleton. It was first suggested that the effects of increased weight-bearing might protect bone mass (Fig. 2.21). However, experimental studies have implicated leptin: a hormone produced by fat cells and which interacts with neurons in the brain and thereby influences weight. It was then discovered that in mice leptin is also anti-osteogenic and it was speculated that increased bone mass in obese people may result from resistance to leptin's anti-osteogenic activity. The amount of leptin released

into the bloodstream is proportional to the amount of body fat. Leptin regulates the body´s energy balance as well as the bone mass by binding to certain receptor proteins of specific neurons in the hypothalamus, and these in turn activate sympathetic nerves. The nerves extend into the bones, where they stimulate release of the neurotransmitter noradrenaline, which then activates beta2-adrenergic receptors on osteoblasts, inhibiting osteoblastic activity. Leptin thus prevents bone formation through its action on already differentiated osteoblasts; it has no overt effect on osteoclast differentiation or function. These results seem to suggest that the millions of patients who have been treated with "beta blockers" such as propranolol for hypertension should have increased bone mass – an argument for re-assessing these clinical studies with respect to changes in bone density. Extreme changes in body weight and bone mass are also partly mediated by leptin, as well as the sex hormones. The identification of leptin as a powerful inhibitor of bone formation definitely has potential therapeutic implications in the future.

To summarize briefly: leptin has a circadian pattern of secretion with peak levels at midnight; it reflects total body adipose tissue mass. Many effects of leptin on energy metabolism are mediated by interaction with insulin. Leptin impacts skeletal metabolism and is also involved in pathological conditions such as obesity, atherosclerosis, oxidative stress and malignancies. Other neuropeptides such as neuromedin U are also involved in the control of bone remodelling, as are the endocannabinoids, synthesized by both osteoclasts and osteoblasts. Receptors for these substances are present in the sympathetic nerve terminals located near the bone cells and constitute a signalling pathway between brain and bone. The endocannabinoid receptors are also involved in the regulation of bone mass and osteoclast function such as, for example, enhancement of bone loss in ovariectomized animals. The endocannabinoids are involved in food intake and energy metabolism. These systems influence pathways from insulin signalling in the pancreas to oxidative processes in skeletal muscles. In summary, it should be stressed that the skeleton is equipped with numerous nerve fibres which participate in the regulation of skeletal metabolism by the CNS. More than 10 neuropeptides have already been identified in bone, including substance P (SP). Receptors for SP are located on osteoclasts and SP stimulates resorption.

2

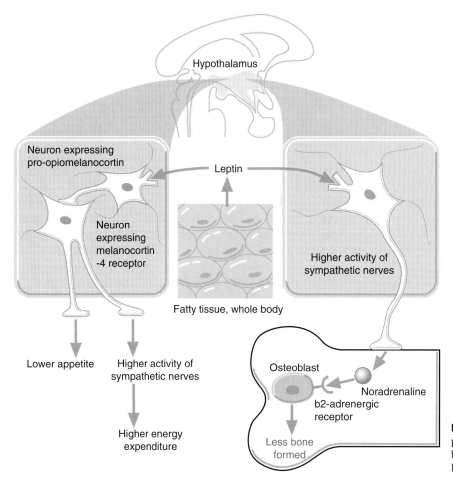

Fig. 2.21. Central nervous participation via leptin in bone turnover (modified from Harada and Rodan [2003])

Additional factors in bone metabolism are still being identified in current research projects, for example, prostaglandin E2, a notable lipid mediator of bone remodelling. It has also been shown that patients with hypercholesterolemia/dyslipidemia have increased bone remodelling associated with osteoporosis, as well as with atherosclerosis. Animal studies have recently demonstrated that haematopoietic stem cells in the niches adjoining the endosteum also participate in the production of BMP-2 and BMP-6 and participate in bone remodelling.

2.11
Growth of the Embryo in the Uterus

Genetic and environmental factors are involved in the normal growth and development of the embryo in the uterus, as well as in growth retardation. In ad-dition, recent studies that followed the trajectories of growth from birth to adulthood have demonstrated that size at birth and postnatal growth both effect the risk of, and are associated with, the development of a number of chronic diseases in adulthood. These include hypertension, coronary heart disease, stroke, diabetes and disturbances of renal function. Moreover, adverse maternal and other environmental factors are also involved. The most recent studies have shown that circumstances during the foetal period and early childhood may have life-long programming effects on different physical functions. This realization gave rise to the new concept of the developmental origins of health and disease (DOHaD). One characteristic example is the programming of the hypothalamic–pituitary–adrenal axis. Interestingly, not only physical, but also psychological aspects play a part, as shown by a Swedish study of 318,953 men, followed-up from date of birth (1973–1980) to date of attempted suicide, date of death, emigration or end of the study in 1999. The results showed that both short length at birth and short adult stature seemed to increase the risk of violent suicide attempts.

Intra-uterine growth restriction has now been positively associated with low bone mass in infancy and with increased risk of developing osteoporosis in adulthood. Importantly, in the context of this book, it is now believed that osteoporosis is, at least partly, programmed in utero and that nutritional and other environmental factors in the pre- and postnatal period exercise a profound influence on skeletal development, which, in turn, has considerable consequences in adulthood. In addition, there is no racial discrimination, since this applies equally to Blacks and Whites, as demonstrated in an investigation of bone size and bone mass in both black and white South African children. Moreover, not only organs such as the skeleton, but also cell systems may be modulated by the intrauterine metabolic environment as shown by intra-uterine epigenetic modification of beta pancreatic cells towards a pre-diabetic phenotype, but this could be corrected by early intervention, i.e. supplementation of the maternal diet. However, many other studies have now demonstrated that the adverse pre- and postnatal effects listed above can and should be modified by application of appropriate measures (nutrition, supplements, possibly medications, exercise and lifestyle) during childhood, adolescence and adulthood into old age.

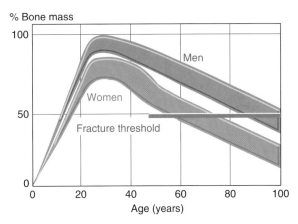

Fig. 2.22. Age-related changes in bone mass

programmed. Marked racial differences in peak bone mass occur, with higher values in American Blacks than in Caucasians, and the lowest values in Asians and Japanese. Some of the multiple pathogenic mechanisms and factors that contribute to subsequent loss of bone ("osteoporosis"), after the attainment of peak bone mass, include the following:
- Genetic factors
- Foetal and neonatal factors
- Factors during growth
- Inadequate peak bone density
- Nutritional and lifestyle factors
- Menopause and reduction of oestrogen in women
- Age and deficiency of testosterone in men
- Reduction of about 80% in adrenal steroids during ageing

2.12
Peak Bone Mass: An Investment for a Healthier Life

The skeleton acquires the maximal bone density – "peak bone mass" – at 25–30 years of age (Fig. 2.22). Consequently, the periods of growth before that age provide the maximal opportunities for building the peak bone mass, 60–80% of which is determined by genetic factors, the remaining 20–40% by other determinants such as nutrition and exercise. Thereafter, beginning at about 30 years, a negative bone balance sets in, so that on average 1% of bone is lost every year, independent of sex. Measurements of trabecular bone density between the ages of 20 and 80 years have shown reductions of approximately 50% in density (Fig. 2.23). This bone loss is apparently genetically

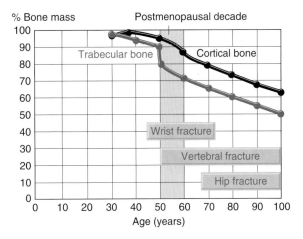

Fig. 2.23. Correlation between predominant trabecular bone loss and incidence of types of fractures

2

- Co-morbidities
- Other effects of ageing on the body and on the activities of daily life

Race and diet interactions are also involved in the attainment, maintenance and loss of bone. Some of the genes that may influence bone mass and rates of bone loss include the genes responsible for:
- Vitamin D receptor
- Oestrogen receptor
- Parathyroid hormone receptor
- IL-1 receptor antagonist
- TGF-β
- Sp1 site in α1 chain of type I collagen

The bones are like a bank savings account for calcium. If the calcium supply is adequate, savings deposits are made and the calcium bone bank account builds up. If the dietary calcium intake is too low, then withdrawals of calcium are made from the "bone bank" itself, i.e. the skeleton. The peak bone mass attained in early life is a major determinant of subsequent bone mass and of fracture risk in later life. Peak bone mass is greater in men than in women, although these differences are reduced or even reversed if bone mass is expressed as volumetric bone density.

Calcium tends to be stored in the osseous tissue during the day and slowly released during the night. A bone biopsy study has shown that the loss of bone occurs fairly equally in all regions of the skeleton, perhaps slightly more in the vertebral bodies and the proximal femur. In postmenopausal women, the decline in oestrogen is accompanied by an increase in the loss of bone of up to 4% annually. This implies that women may lose 40% of their bone mass from 40 to 70 years. During the same period men lose only about 12%.

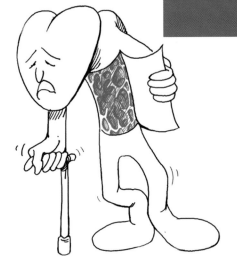

3.1
Factors in the Development of Osteoporosis

In women an age-related slow decrease is accelerated to an acute loss of bone in the menopausal and postmenopausal periods, and then followed by a gradual and progressive decline in bone mineral density (BMD) with age. In men, bone loss begins somewhat later, but it is due, as in women, to increased osteoclastic resorption, which is a direct consequence of *decreases in steroid hormones*, i.e. hypogonadism. The decrease in steroid hormones also directly impacts cells which have the oestrogen receptors alpha or beta such as the bone marrow mesenchymal progenitor cells responsible for the production of osteoblasts and adipocytes. Oestrogen promotes osteoblastogenic differentiation and inhibits adipogenesis. Therefore, with advancing age, bone formation is decreased as a direct consequence of a shift in the balance of production of the two cell lineages, in favour of adipocytes.

Many investigations have addressed the question of *additional factors* and pathways which regulate and control the differentiation of the mesenchymal progenitor cells in one direction or the other. The results of these investigations have implicated genomic, hormonal, for example intermittent parathyroid hormone (PTH), and various other pathways, including Wnt signalling as well as other ligands and receptors which influence mesenchymal stem cell differentiation and could tip the balance in favour of osteoblasts or adipocytes. For example, Wnt signalling favours osteoblastogenesis. It should be emphasized that the Wnt signalling pathway is involved in many biological processes from embryonic development to insulin secretion in adulthood. Some investigations have correlated the antagonism of oxidative stress to Wnt signalling in advancing age as a decisive contributing factor to the development of atherosclerosis, insulin resistance, hyperlipidaemia and involutional osteoporosis.

Earlier investigations implicated inhibition of *gap-junctional communications* between osteoblastic progenitors as responsible for the mesenchymal switch to adipogenesis. More recent studies have demonstrated that a ligand-activated transcription factor, known as PPAR gamma 2 in the mesenchymal stem cells participates in the control of adipogenic differentiation. Moreover, studies in animals have demonstrated that vitamin D3 inhibits *adipogenesis* and induces osteoblastogenesis, with a reduction in PPAR gamma 2. However, the net result of the activities of all the factors involved, after the decline in oestrogen levels, is production of adipocytes, not osteoblasts.

It is of interest that in animals, during periods of simulated microgravity, a mesenchymal switch from osteoblasts to adipocytes also occurs, due to changes in many factors and pathways. Returning to humans, it is postulated that similar changes may take place as a consequence of immobilization, disuse and in age-related osteoporosis. Many investigations into all the mechanisms of osteopenia/osteoporosis are ongoing, as well as into the possibilities for potential interventions in the future.

3.2
Definition of Osteoporosis

The word osteoporosis literally means porous bone, indicating that the bone density is low and the bones are thin. But bone does not fracture due to thinness alone. In the early 1990s a consensus meeting of the World Health Organisation (WHO) defined **osteoporosis** as:

"A systemic skeletal disorder characterized by a low bone mass and by microarchitectural deterioration of bone tissue, with a subsequent increase in bone fragility and susceptibility to fracture".

The first Consensus Conference on Osteoporosis of the new millennium proposed a new definition of osteoporosis as:

"A skeletal disorder characterized by compromised bone strength predisposing to an increased risk of fracture".

However, in order better to understand the aetiology of osteoporotic fractures and the effects of therapy

on the risk of occurrence of fractures, it is essential to recognize the factors that govern *bone strength*. The strength of an individual bone (and of the whole skeleton) depends on its mass, shape and the quality of the bone itself (Fig. 3.1).

Numerous large studies have already confirmed the connection between bone density, bone strength and fracture risk. Density is responsible for 60–90% of the strength of bone. From the outside, however, osteoporotic bones may even have the same size and look like normal bones, but inside they are brittle, with a thin cortex and a disrupted (or even localized lack of) trabecular network.

Low bone mass has proved to be the most important objective predictor of fracture risk. The lower the bone mass, the weaker the bone and the less force required to cause a fracture. Therefore, according to the WHO (The WHO Study Group 1994) osteoporosis in postmenopausal women was also defined in terms of bone density measurement and based on a comparison of the patients' measurement to the standard peak adult bone mass (PABM) as follows:

"Osteoporosis is present when the bone mass is more than 2.5 standard deviations (SD) below that of healthy premenopausal adult females, the T-score".

However, taking into consideration the multifactorial nature of bone fragility, an up-dated position paper was issued by the WHO and the International Osteoporosis Foundation (2007).

This proposed that "osteoporosis" is no longer diagnosed as such, but by a total individual 10-year

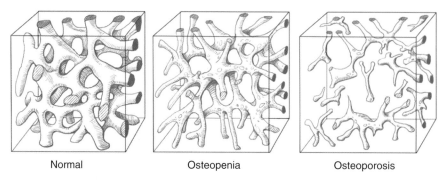

Normal　　　Osteopenia　　　Osteoporosis

Fig. 3.1. Progressive architectural deterioration of cancellous bone: increased osteoclastic resorption cavities and marked attenuation of cancellous bone (osteopenia); disconnected trabeculae, no longer a network (established osteoporosis)

fracture risk on the basis of independent and self-sufficient risk factors. Directions for diagnosis, differential diagnosis, methods of investigation and the sites for BMD measurements, fracture risk and prevention of falls, as well as possibilities of pharmacological therapy are outlined in the WHO position paper quoted above. Nevertheless, the T-score as obtained by measurements at the femoral neck is utilized internationally as an accepted criterion for osteoporosis. The hip and/or the lumbar spine are measured by the dual energy X-ray absorptiometry (DXA) method to obtain the T-score. The cutoff point of 2.5 SD below the PABM value is based on epidemiological data derived from a population of postmenopausal Caucasian women, 50% of whom had already suffered a fragility fracture. The WHO cutoff point of T –2.5 or lower used for the diagnosis of osteoporosis was based on a close association between prevalence at this cutoff point and lifetime fracture risk of hip fractures or all fractures (hip, vertebrae, forearm, humerus, and pelvis). These WHO criteria were not meant to be applied to healthy, oestrogen-replete premenopausal women, to women of other races, to young men or to children. Nevertheless, low bone mass in any individual is still the most important factor in the determination of fragility fractures. In the new European guidelines, from 2008 onwards, only measurements of DXA at the femoral neck are accepted as diagnostic criteria for osteoporosis.

> Osteopenia has now been defined by a T-score between -1.0 and -2.5.

As the emphasis on skeletal health shifts from treatment to prevention, the diagnostic term of osteopenia may take on increasing importance, especially in combination with the evaluation of the major risk factors. Hence, postmenopausal women with osteopenia should be targeted for prevention strategies to preserve their skeletal mass. Patients with osteopenia and relevant risk factors should be treated early with effective drugs to prevent fragility fractures! Obviously, this implies widespread screening to identify these groups in the population as a whole!

3.3
Osteoporosis – Which Bones are Vulnerable?

Where and how does bone resorption occur? The bone cells carry out their remodelling preferably on the inner surface of bone, the endosteum (Fig. 3.2). Bones with a large component of cancellous bone present the largest surface area to bone cells for remodelling: these bones include the vertebral bodies,

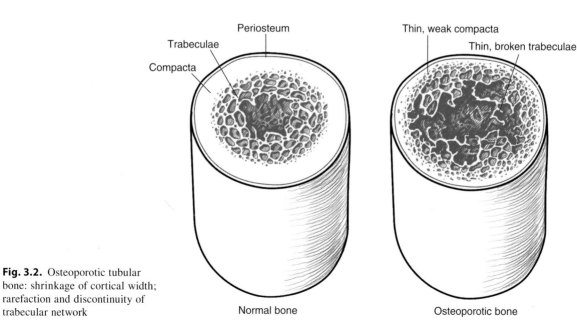

Fig. 3.2. Osteoporotic tubular bone: shrinkage of cortical width; rarefaction and discontinuity of trabecular network

Periosteum

Trabeculae

Compacta

Thin, weak compacta

Thin, broken trabeculae

Normal bone

Osteoporotic bone

3

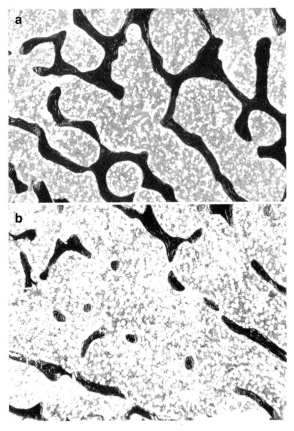

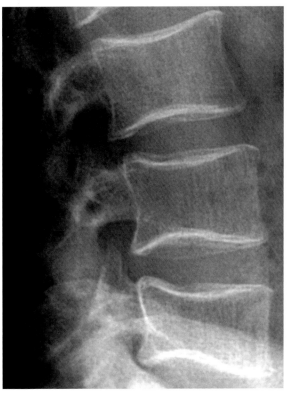

Fig. 3.4. Osteoporosis of the vertebrae: note relative preservation of the stress-bearing vertical trabeculae

Fig. 3.3. Normal (**a**) and osteoporotic (**b**) trabecular network. Note "button" phenomenon with disruption of the trabecular network in (**b**). Gomori staining

3.4
Osteoporosis – Also a Question of Quality!

the femoral neck, the ribs, the wrist and the heel. Due to their immense surface these cancellous bones are resorbed five times as fast as the cortical bone of the long bones (Fig. 3.3a,b). Considered sequentially the ossicles in the middle of the bone disappear first, especially those at the horizontal "stress" lines. The vertical "pillars" which carry greater loads remain intact for longer periods and are seen as vertical stripes on X-ray (Fig. 3.4). In vitro and in vivo studies have shown that bone density is indeed responsible for 50–80% of the strength of bone and therefore constitutes a very important risk factor, particularly in postmenopausal women. As numerous prospective studies have demonstrated, the risk of a fracture increases exponentially with the decrease in density: a reduction of 10–15% in bone density doubles the fracture risk.

Bone does not break only because it is thin – as indicated by the fact that half of all people with decreased bone density never sustain a fracture. The recognition that osteoporosis is far more complex than previously thought suggests that factors in addition to bone mineral density may contribute to bone fragility and therapeutic effectiveness. Recent studies have shown that osteoporosis is also a question of the quality of bone which, in many disorders, is adversely affected even more than the BMD (Fig. 3.5). This applies especially to conditions such as type-2 diabetes, in which bone remodelling is influenced by various metabolic mechanisms including insulin and angiopathies.

Perforations, "microfractures" of trabeculae, occur constantly throughout life and normal activity, and

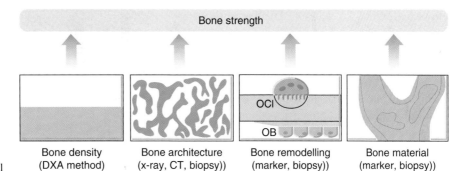

Fig. 3.5. The four main structural factors of bone strength are: bone density, bone architecture, bone remodelling and bone material

these lead to a decrease in bone strength and weight-bearing ability – and of course require immediate repair. Moreover, previous thinning of the trabeculae because of decreased osteoblastic activity accelerates the destruction of the microarchitecture. Disconnected trabeculae are functionally useless and are rapidly resorbed. Should a situation arise in which numerous microfractures are not completely repaired, a critical point will eventually be reached at which the bone will break. Should the bone structure be qualitatively inferior to begin with, bones of even normal thickness may break. This is an important point to take into account and has already been demonstrated in osteoporosis in hypogonadal men. Studies on mineral density by magnetic resonance microradiography have shown a marked deterioration in microarchitecture in the spine and hips of these patients – more than would be expected from the results of densitometry. Moreover, at the nano-scale level, it has been demonstrated that interactions between collagen fibres and mineral crystals can effect bone quality.

Combinations of up-to-date methods, as well as novel techniques, have now been applied to evaluate various aspects of bone quality, such as strength and density, biomechanical aspects, composition such as mobile and bound water and their relation to mechano-properties of bone, in particular the matrix content and its properties at the nano-level by micro-CT and biomechanical compression. It is worth noting that these methods can be – and some already have been – applied to assess effects of therapy in osteoporosis. Moreover, the WHO and the International Osteoporosis Foundation (2007) issued a position paper outlining the current understanding of osteoporosis, including the multifactorial nature of bone fragility and a number of risk factors.

An important (even crucial) aim of osteoanabolic therapy is to re-establish the microarchitecture. This goal could probably be achieved in the not-too-distant future by a combination of drugs: administration of basic fibroblast growth factor, which induces formation of new trabeculae and promotes restoration of connectivity, both of which could be maintained by antiresorptive agents and/or PTH. These results have been achieved in osteoporotic animal models. Many reports on trials in humans have now been published and the results have confirmed the efficacy of PTH therapy in both men and women, in moderate as well as severe osteoporosis, in responders as well as non-responders to antiresorptive therapy. Moreover, PTH has been shown to be effective in combination with, and either before or after antiresorptive agents. Teriparatide has now been given safely for over 5 years to both women and men with osteoporosis, in the US and in many European countries. Other forms of PTH such as 1–84 parathyroid hormone have been registered and are being tested.

Generally speaking, osteoporotic fractures are caused by *eight different abnormalities of bone*:

- Reduced thickness (density)
- Unequal proportions of compact and cancellous bone
- Decrease in number of "nodes" in the cancellous bone
- Transection of trabeculae caused by osteoclasts
- Inadequate bone formation
- Inadequate mineralization of bone matrix (osteoid)
- Anomalies of structure and binding of collagen molecules ("cross-linking")
- Faulty repair mechanisms

3

How can fragility be reduced? There are two ways to make bones stronger:

- Increase bone mineral density and distribute bone mass more effectively, i.e. increase bone tissue where the mechanical demands are greatest ("extrinsic biomechanical properties")
- Improve the material properties of bone tissue, from the microscopic to the molecular level ("intrinsic biochemical properties")

An effective treatment for bone fragility should improve the extrinsic biomechanical properties of bone, but at the same time should not substantially impair the intrinsic properties. Strong inhibitors of bone resorption such as bisphosphonates can reduce bone turnover by 80–90% causing a gain in bone mineral density. Due to reduced bone remodelling, the mean tissue age of bone is increased as is bone mineralization. Properly mineralized bone has the best combination of stiffness and brittleness, while poorly mineralized bone tends to be very weak with increased displacement, and hypermineralized bone is too brittle with decreased displacement. Consequently, in treating osteoporosis attention must be paid to bone density, improvement of the microarchitecture, mineralization and the repair mechanisms. With the modern bisphosphonates of today it is no longer a problem to fill up resorption lacunae, increase mineralization and thicken attenuated trabeculae. At present there is no evidence that microdamage accumulation occurs under treatment with bisphosphonates. But it is not yet possible – as far as we know from experimental studies – to completely restore the trabecular network (restitutio ad integrum) or the shape of bone that has been destroyed. The basic anatomic and structural properties of bone influence the load-carrying capacity and the changes in osteoporosis determine the fracture risk. New methods are needed to provide insight into the exact causes of bone fragility and the more detailed effects of drug therapies.

3.5
Definition of "Fracture"

A fracture has been defined as an "acute discontinuity" in a bone. When there *does not* appear to be adequate trauma, the terms "pathologic fracture", "*fragility fracture*" or "*low trauma fracture*" are used, and these of course need clarification. "Fatigue fractures" develop slowly due to the accumulation of numer-

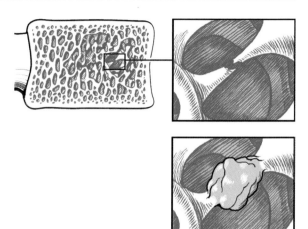

Fig. 3.6. Osteoclastic perforation of a horizontal trabecula (upper right) in the vertebral body (left), and formation of microcallus (early healing of microfracture) (lower right)

ous microfractures which were not properly repaired. Examples are *fatigue fractures* ("*bone bruise*") of the metatarsals in marathon runners or fractures of the pelvic girdle in patients with age-related osteoporosis. These microfractures ("micro cracks") (Fig. 3.6) should not be confused with "Looser's zones" in patients with osteomalacia (rickets). "*Infractions*" are partial fractures of the long bones when a localized unilateral break of the cortex occurs. "Vertebral compression fractures" often occur in stages and initially remain undetected until a total collapse of the vertebral body has taken place.

3.6
Vertebral (Spinal) Fractures

As mentioned above, a vertebral fracture rarely occurs in osteoporosis due to a sudden trauma, but rather develops in stages as a result of numerous microfractures. Moderate decrease in height of the vertebral bodies can only be detected by sequential X-rays or other imaging techniques. Three grades of vertebral deformities are recognized (Fig. 3.7):

- End-plate deformity
- Anterior wedge deformity
- Compression deformity

Biconcave deformities, with depression of the upper and lower cortices of the vertebral bodies are the first to appear (Fig. 3.8). Occasionally focal depression

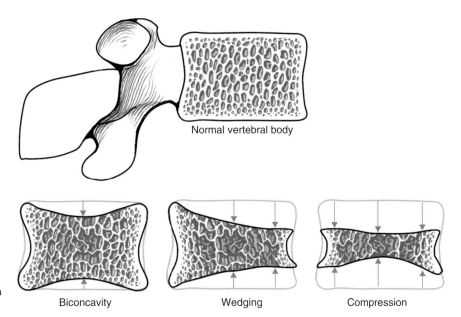

Normal vertebral body

Biconcavity   Wedging   Compression

Fig. 3.7. Effects of progressive compression fractures in the vertebrae

may be caused by material from an intervertebral disk ("Schmorl's knots"). Fractures of the vertebral bodies have been named according to the shape of the deformity:

- End-plate fracture
- Anterior wedging (Fig. 3.9)
- Posterior wedging
- Compression (crush)

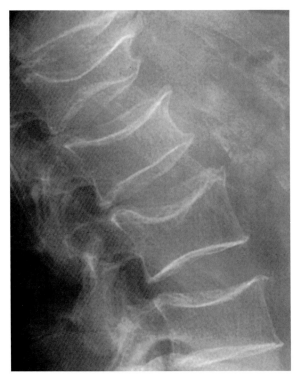

Fig. 3.8. The outlines of the vertebral bodies become a "picture frame" with compression of the roof and ground plates (biconcavities)

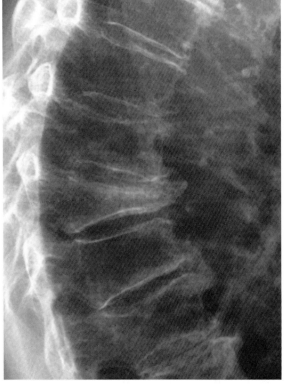

Fig. 3.9. Vertebral fracture with anterior wedge deformity

The last type involves the whole vertebral body. The deformity grading system in use comprises six degrees of severity and is based on a percentage reduction in vertebral height. Other types of deformities with various grades of severity also occur. An exact definition of vertebral body fractures has great practical significance because the number and extent of such fractures are used as significant parameters in therapeutic trials. Comparison and meta-analyzes of trials depend on a clear and reproducible definition of "fracture".

Recognition of vertebral fractures is also essential for consideration of treatment strategies, because such prevalent fractures are associated with a fivefold increased risk of sustaining new vertebral fractures, and the risk increases dramatically according to the number and severity of the prevalent fractures. The presence of morphologically defined vertebral fractures also predicts other non-vertebral fractures, including those of the hip. Therefore X-rays of the spine to identify prevalent vertebral fractures is a useful additional measurement in order to further assess a particular patient's risk of future fractures.

hip fracture. There are good correlations between fracture rates and the result of DXA measurements of the femoral neck, Ward's triangle and the trochanter. The *following parameters* have prognostic significance:
- Singh Index
- Femoral neck length
- Femoral neck width
- Upper neck region

The *Femur Strength Index* includes the patient's age, weight and height, the femoral neck BMD and several geometric parameters of the femur. The *Singh Index*, based only on X-ray examination, recognizes seven trabecular groups in the proximal femur which indicate pressure or traction according to their orientation. Between them lies an area which is relatively poor in ossicles called Ward's triangle. As osteoporosis progresses, the seven groups of trabeculae are steadily resorbed, so that *three types of fractures* could result:
- Medial
- Lateral
- Inter-trochanteric

3.7
Hip Fractures

Hip fractures are due to a slow but progressive loss of both cortical and trabecular bone. The bone loss is "silent" and manifests in fractures in individuals over 70 years of age (Fig. 3.10). There is only a weak correlation between vertebral fractures and future

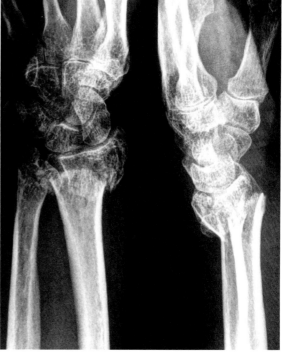

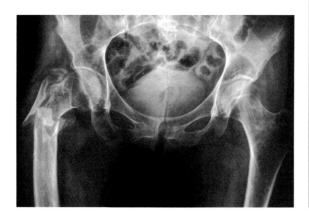

Fig. 3.10. Pertrochanteric fracture of the right femur

Fig. 3.11. Colles' fracture of the distal radius

3.8
Wrist Fractures

Fractures of the distal radius (Colles' and Smith's fractures) occur most commonly in women between 45 and 65 years of age (Fig. 3.11). These are nearly always caused by a direct fall forwards onto the outstretched arm, with distal dislocation of the hand.

3.9
Other Fractures

Other fractures associated with osteoporosis include those of the proximal humerus, the pelvis (Fig. 3.12), the distal tibia, the heel, the ankle, the clavicle and the ribs. All these bones contain large amounts of cancellous bone. In contrast, bones with a high content of cortical, compact bone such as the metatarsals, the phalanges and the proximal radius rarely fracture.

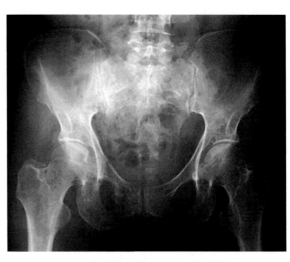

Fig. 3.12. Fracture of the right pubic bone in a patient with multiple myeloma and secondary osteoporosis. Note multiple small punched-out lesions in the right femur

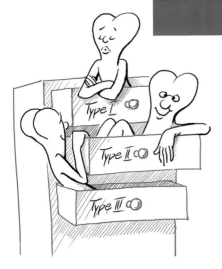

Osteoporosis has traditionally been categorized as primary or secondary. *Primary osteoporosis* occurs together with and as a result of the major physiological condition known as ageing (senescence) and its causes and consequences. *Secondary osteoporosis* develops as a consequence of the major physio-pathological effects on the bones of the skeleton of numerous disorders and diseases of other organs and tissues in the body.

The mechanisms involved in both categories have been extensively investigated and obviously depend on specific conditions and occurrences, such as for example the decrease in levels of ovarian and testicular hormones in primary, involutional osteoporoses. With respect to secondary osteoporoses, it is equally clear that these are correlated with the disorders with which they are associated, and possibly also with the mechanisms and corresponding pathways responsible for these disorders. These aspects are already being taken into consideration today when considering the treatment of osteoporosis required by patients with, for example, co-morbidities such as diabetes, AIDS or a cardiovascular disorder, all of which also affect the bones.

4.1
According to Spread

Osteoporosis may be *localized* to one or more skeletal regions, i.e. focal or regional osteoporosis, as distinct from the classic *generalized* osteoporosis (systemic, global). The most important causative factors responsible for bone loss are:

- *Inactivity* (immobilization osteoporosis): The classic example of this is regional osteoporosis which occurs when an extremity is immobilized either because of a fracture or a motor-neuron injury. The lack of use and movement results in increased osteoclastic resorption which, if sufficiently extensive, is also accompanied by hypercalciuria and hyperphosphaturia. On cessation of immobilization and resumption of activity the process can be reversed and the bones normalized, especially those in children and young people.

- *Complex regional pain syndrome* (CRPS, Sudeck's disease, algodystrophy, sympathetic reflex dystrophy): This affects mainly the hands, knees and ankles and is characterized by swelling, pain, hyperaesthesias and vasomotor reactions.

- *Transient (transitory) osteoporosis*: Transient osteoporosis is a regional process first described in the pelvic bones in pregnant women. Since then, it has also been observed in knee and ankle joints in both young men and young women. The pain appears to start spontaneously without apparent prior trauma. The diagnosis is established by means of magnetic resonance imaging (MRI), which shows extensive oedema of the bone marrow around the painful joint. Clinically, the process is self-limiting with

R. Bartl, B. Frisch, *Osteoporosis*, DOI 10.1007/978-3-540-79527-8_4,
© Springer-Verlag Berlin Heidelberg 2009

complete restitution within 1 year. Together with CRPS this disorder is now summarized under the heading of "bone marrow oedema syndrome" and can be treated effectively with intravenous bisphosphonates (complete remission in about 80% of cases) (see Chap. 31).

- *Gorham-Stout syndrome* ("vanishing bone disease"): The cause of this rare bone disease has not yet been elucidated, although a vascular and lymphatic connection has been suggested, mainly by way of activated endothelium. It begins with completely uncoupled osteoclastic resorption of a bone and spreads to adjoining bones. Progression is variable. Severe or life-threatening complications may occur when bones of the thorax or the vertebrae are involved. To date, the only effective therapy is administration of bisphosphonates as early as possible to prevent extensive loss of bone (see Chap. 31).

- *Other osteolytic syndromes*: These may be due to a variety of causes, including infections, tumours, trauma as well as metabolic, vascular, congenital and genetic aberrations.

- *Generalized* (*systemic*) *osteoporosis*: This is far more frequent than localized osteoporosis. In spite of its name, generalized osteoporosis is rarely manifested in the whole skeleton, but it does have a symmetrical distribution. Juvenile and postmenopausal osteoporoses generally affect the axial skeleton, while the age-related form also attacks the tubular bones, especially in men. Consequently, the presence of normal bone density in bones of the extremities does not rule out (possibly even severe) osteoporosis of the axial skeleton. This is important to bear in mind in the evaluation of local measurements of bone mineral density (BMD), which only represent the bone measured and cannot be extrapolated to the rest of the bones in the skeleton.

4.2
According to Age and Sex

- *Idiopathic juvenile osteoporosis*: This is a rare self-limiting disease in prepubertal children, usually occurring between 8 and 14 years of age. It generally manifests as compression fractures of the vertebrae accompanied by severe back pain. The differential diagnosis includes osteogenesis imperfecta, Cush-

ing syndrome and diseases of the bone marrow which are diagnosed by analysis of peripheral blood, bone marrow and bone biopsies.

- *Idiopathic osteoporosis in young adults*: This primarily affects men between the ages of 30 and 50 years and is also characterized by fractures of the vertebral bodies. Biochemical parameters and bone biopsy findings show increased resorption of bone. Frequently the patients are heavy smokers, smoking having been implicated as a possible contributory factor. A mild form of osteogenesis imperfecta, not previously diagnosed, must be excluded in these patients.

- *Postmenopausal* (*type 1*) *osteoporosis* (Fig. 4.1): This is the most common form of osteoporosis and occurs in women between 51 and 75 years of age as a consequence of cessation of ovarian function. The loss of bone actually starts years beforehand and increases at the time of the menopause (perimenopausal). About 30% of all women develop osteoporosis after the menopause. Cessation of oestrogen secretion leads to a decrease in IL-6 and other cytokines, which in turn leads to increased recruitment and activation of osteoclasts. In addition, bone becomes more sensitive to the resorption stimulating action of parathyroid hormones. As a consequence there is increased resorption of cancellous bone in the vertebrae and in the hip bones with a corresponding increase in fracture risk. Obviously this postmenopausal form of osteoporosis occurs only in women, but men are also subject to increased bone resorption as a consequence of testosterone deficiency, although at a later stage in life, from 50 to 60 years onwards. Intestinal absorption of calcium in some postmenopausal women has been associated with hypercalciuria and linked to bone loss in idiopathic osteoporosis as well as in calcium nephrolithiasis. The hypothesis was put forward that these might be two subtypes of the response to hypercalciuria of intestinal origin.

- *Involutional* (*age-related, type II*) *osteoporosis* (Fig. 4.1): In women, postmenopausal and in men postandropausal osteoporosis merges imperceptibly into the involutional, age-related type which represents part of the aging process and which can lead to frailty. This is characterized by many factors common to osteoporosis including sarcopenia, falls, decreased physical activity, cognitive decline, changes in many hormones, vitamins and cytokines.

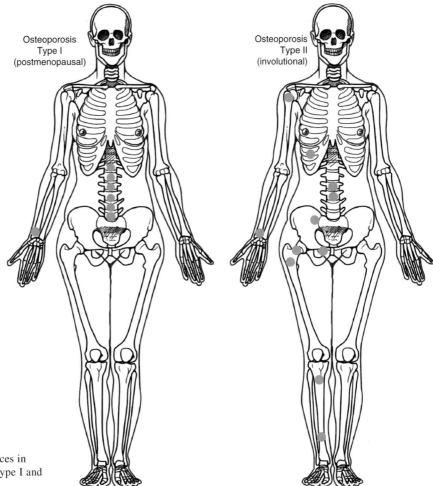

Fig. 4.1. Topographic differences in skeletal involvement between type I and type II osteoporosis

The bone is mainly affected by the increased osteoclastic activity. Clearly all these have a detrimental effect on quality of life such that today, in the first decade of the 21st century (the "Bone and Joint Decade"), efforts are now directed towards prevention of the frailty syndrome, which of course implies a decrease in all its consequences including osteoporosis. A study of bone biopsies taken from normal individuals (i.e. without any known metabolic, endocrine or osseous disorders) of different age groups has shown that the number of osteoclasts and osteoblasts increases from the age of 50 years. This indicates that bone, far from being a slow, inactive and atrophic tissue in the older age groups, presents the picture of increased osseous remodelling. Other causative factors for involutional osteoporosis include: decreased mobility, defective vitamin D metabolism, insufficient calcium and mild secondary hyperparathyroidism. Osteoporosis type II develops after 70 years of age and is now only twice as frequent in women as in men (however, they are catching up!). It has been postulated that a major factor in the mechanism of osteoporosis, especially severe osteoporosis in the elderly, in both men and women is the adipogenic shift, i.e. the predominance of adipogenesis over osteoblastogenesis in the bone marrow, due to the increased differentiation of mesenchymal stem cells into adipocytes. Studies have indicated that osteogenic and adipogenic differentiation in the mesenchymal stem cells is parallel until a late stage in the process. Cortical bone, especially that of the femoral neck, radius and pelvic bones, is then also involved in involutional osteoporosis, particularly in males. Approximately 80% of all osteoporotic fractures occur at this time, i.e. after 70 years of age. The

4

arbitrary separation of these osteoporoses – type I and type II – at this stage of the patients' lives (>70 years) is of little (if any) practical value. An investigation of the change in BMD at baseline and at 3- and 5-year follow-up visits in a cohort of 9423 participants, both men and women, demonstrated the decline in bone loss at different skeletal sites. The results were correlated to rates of fracture and recommendations were made for times and frequencies of BMD measurements. *Hypogonadism in men* – as mentioned above, the decline in testosterone levels – may begin earlier or later, the latter being known as *late onset hypogonadism* (LOH). When LOH is accompanied by detrimental physiological and mental effects it is designated as symptomatic LOH (SLOH). The many symptoms that may be present include reduced physical and mental activities and reduced muscle and bone mass, possibly even osteoporosis and anaemia. A randomized controlled trial of aromatase inhibition (1 mg anastrazole daily for 3–12 months) resulted in increased testosterone levels at 3 months, then declined by 12 months but remained significantly higher than at baseline. There was a modest decrease in levels of oestradiol, but no significant changes in body composition or strength. In view of the results of many population based studies which highlight the effects of low testosterone levels on the development of type 2 diabetes, metabolic syndrome and overall survival, testosterone replacement is the mainstay of therapy for symptomatic hypogonadism; however, it requires close monitoring.

4.3
According to Extent

In daily clinical practice the *degree of severity* of a bone disorder must be accurately determined before decisions are made on urgency and strategy of therapy. In women, osteoporosis can be diagnosed if the BMD is 2.5 SD below the mean of a young reference population. Kanis and coworkers commented on this definition and gave diagnostic categories that may be applied to white women:

- *Normal bone*: a BMD value that is higher than 1 SD below the young adult female reference mean (T-score greater than or equal to –1 SD).
- *Low bone mass (osteopenia)*: a BMD value more than 1 SD below the young female adult mean, but less than 2.5 SD below this value (T-score <–1 and >–2.5 SD).
- *(Preclinical) osteoporosis*: a BMD value 2.5 SD or more below the young female adult mean (T-score less than or equal to –2.5 SD).
- *Severe (manifest, established) osteoporosis*: a BMD value 2.5 SD or more below the young female adult mean value in the presence of one or more fragility fractures.

This definition uses the T-score of dual-energy X-ray absorptiometry (DXA) at the femoral neck as a diagnostic criterion, which in fact has already long been done in bone densitometry (Fig. 4.2). Bone density results are compared to those of age-, sex-, and race-matched controls. It is also evident that the T-score

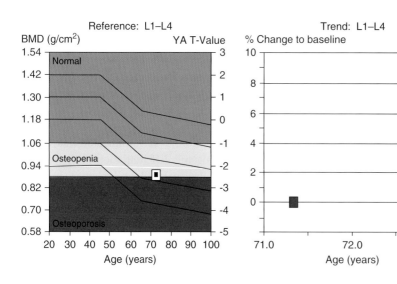

Fig. 4.2. DXA measurement of the lumbar spine with definition of the T-score

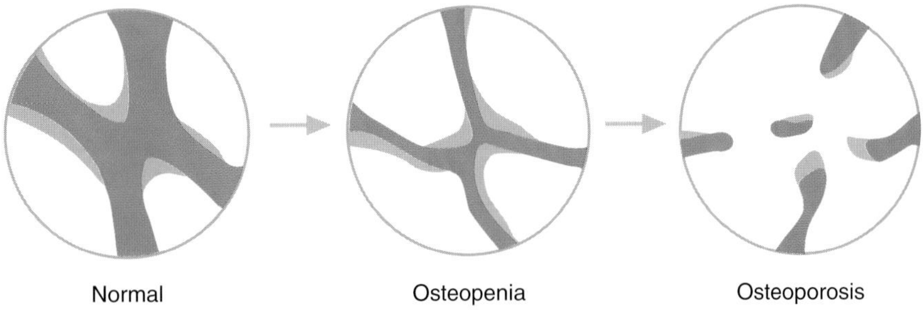

Fig. 4.3. Degrees of reduction in trabecular bone: osteopenia followed by osteoporosis with complete destruction of the trabecular network

Normal   Osteopenia   Osteoporosis

cannot be used interchangeably with different techniques and at different sites. Therefore, a reference standard must be adopted in terms of skeletal site and measurement technique, and measurements with DXA at the femoral neck have the highest predictive value for hip fracture, as established in many prospective studies. Data are also available for the total hip, but the evidence to date does not suggest any improvement in fracture prediction. In lumbar spine BMD, an important source of accuracy error is aortic calcification and osteoarthrosis that increase progressively with age. Moreover, the hip is the site of highest clinical relevance, since hip fracture is the dominant complication of osteoporosis in terms of morbidity, mortality and cost. The recommended reference range is that given in the *Third National Health and Nutrition Examination Survey (NHANES III) reference database for femoral neck measurements in white women aged 20–29 years*, as previously recommended by the International Osteoporosis Foundation and the International Society of Clinical Densitometry. These diagnostic criteria for osteoporosis are similar to those previously proposed by the WHO in 1994, but differ by specifying a reference site (the femoral neck) and by accommodating diagnostic criteria for non-white women as well as for men.

4.4
According to Histology

The trabecular bone volume in iliac crest biopsies of normal adults comprises approximately 20–25 vol% of the biopsy section. When this value drops to 16%, "rarefaction" of the trabeculae has occurred. Other histological parameters are also evaluated (Fig. 4.3):
- Cortical thickness and cortical porosity
- Disruption of trabecular network

- Trabecular width. Type A = long and thin, type B = short and stout
- Quantity and distribution of osteoid (degree of mineralization)
- Quantity and distribution of fat cells (atrophy in the endosteal region)
- Changes in the stromal elements (inflammatory reactions)
- Quantity and maturation of the haematopoietic cell lines
- Presence of foreign or malignant cells

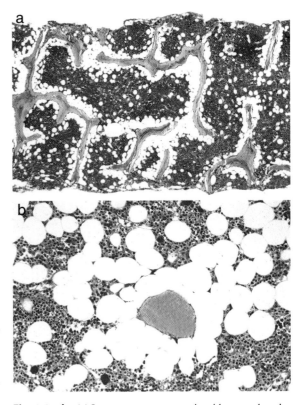

Fig. 4.4 a, b. (a) Low turnover osteopenia with paratrabecular localization of fat cells. (b) At higher magnification rim of fat cells around a button-like trabecula. Giemsa staining

When the trabeculae are surrounded by fat cells or layers of fatty tissue, osseous remodelling is then decreased and osteoid seams are absent (bone atrophy). This particular distribution of fat cells is a sign of incipient osteoporosis, the "low turnover" type as seen in sequential biopsies (Fig. 4.4a,b). Recent research has demonstrated that there is indeed a connection between fat cells and osteoblastic activity.

The volume, extent and width of osteoid seams are always noted in order to estimate the presence and degree of osteomalacia (Fig. 4.5). These data are required for estimating the therapeutic amounts of vitamin D required. The value for osteoid should not exceed 2 vol% of the trabecular volume. However, in older patients values of 2–5 vol% are frequently found, which indicate the presence of an "osteoporo-malacia", when a low trabecular vol% is also present. A *histologic diagnosis of osteomalacia* is based on three criteria:

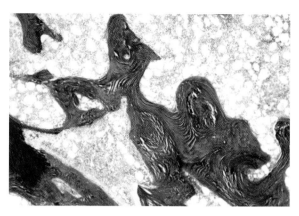

Fig. 4.5. Severe osteomalacia with irregular trabecular structure and increased trabecular volume due to increased amount of osteoid (*red*). Ladewig

- Periosteocytic demineralization (an early sign!)
- Osteoid occupies more than 50% of the trabecular surface
- Width of osteoid seams more than 10% of the total trabecular volume (vol%)

The *clinical diagnosis of osteomalacia* requires X-ray (Looser´s zones), serologic investigation and evidence of a basic disorder (usually of gastrointestinal, nutritional or renal origin).

Immunohistochemical evidence of bisphosphonates in bone biopsy sections is of particular interest (Fig. 4.6). A comprehensive description of the significance of bone biopsies in internal medicine can be found in the atlas *Biopsy of Bone in Internal Medicine* (Bartl and Frisch 1993). Moreover, with the introduction of improved biopsy needles and the latest immunohistological techniques as well as increasing interest

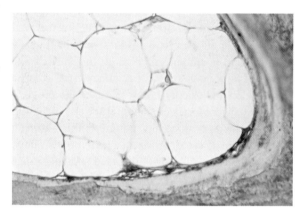

Fig. 4.6. Deposition of bisphosphonate (*red*) on the surface of a trabecula visualized by means of an antibody to ibandronate. Immunohistology

in bone and its cells, bone biopsies will also acquire greater significance in the investigation of bone disorders including osteoporoses, especially those of secondary and drug-induced nature.

Risk Factors for Fractures

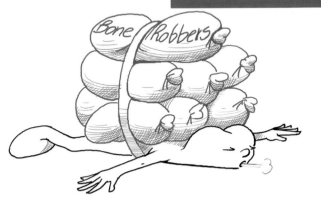

Until recently, the diagnosis of osteoporosis was made only when the patient presented with painful fractures. Today, with greater awareness of health and healthy living, we realize that recognition and avoidance of risk factors can prevent many chronic illnesses. A 50-year-old-postmenopausal woman who goes to her physician for a yearly "check up" expects to have her blood pressure taken, her cholesterol measured and

a mammography performed – that is good medical practice. Likewise, she should ask for a bone mineral density (BMD) measurement to investigate her risk for developing osteoporosis (Fig. 5.1). Results of studies even suggest that low bone mass density is a better predictor of fracture risk than increased cholesterol is of having a heart attack and high blood pressure of having a stroke (Fig. 5.2). We are now aware of many genetic and acquired factors which are responsible for and/or contribute to the development of osteoporoses. Furthermore, low BMD is associated with a lower risk of breast cancer: stimulating effects of oestrogen on both trabecular bone and mammary cells may be responsible for this correlation. Another study has shown that bone density changes might be related to the progression of atherosclerosis, or vice versa, in haemodialysis patients.

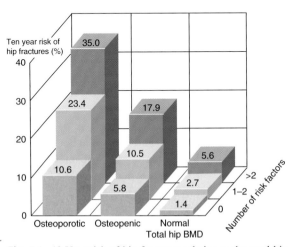

Fig. 5.1. 10-Year risk of hip fractures relative to the total hip bone mineral density (*BMD*) (normal, osteopenic and osteoporotic) and the number of risk factors (modified from Taylor B et al. [2004])

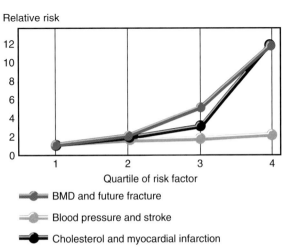

Fig. 5.2. Risk factors for three selected chronic disorders

5.1
Risk Factors Which Cannot (yet) be Influenced

Genetics: The saying "as mother so daughter" applies especially to osteoporosis. A family history of an osteoporotic fracture in a first-degree relative is a powerful indicator that genetic factors may play a role in the development of osteoporosis. We know that the "peak bone mass" and the subsequent later loss of bone are genetically programmed. Studies of twins have shown that genetic factors account for up to 80% of the variance in BMD, the best known predictor of the risk of osteoporosis. Some loci, such as for vitamin D and oestrogen receptor genes as well as the collagen type Iα1 locus are promising genetic determinants of bone mass, but the molecular basis of osteoporosis still remains largely undefined. Experts have also implicated gene–gene and gene–environment interactions as significant determinants of bone density and risk of osteoporosis. As yet there are no tests available to evaluate the genetic risk of osteoporosis. Nevertheless, a proper diet and exercise in childhood and youth can go a long way to ensure a peak bone mass in adulthood. Part of the heterogeneity of osteoporosis may be due to the presence of osteoporosis in a number of genetic syndromes ("syndromic osteoporosis"), or as a consequence of a congenital syndrome, such as Down's, in which skeletal changes including a low bone mass already occur in childhood. Information derived from genetic studies is being used to develop markers for the assessment of fracture risk and new drugs for osteoporosis. Genetic syndromes causing osteoporosis can be distinguished by careful physical examination (e.g. stature, as well as abnormalities of teeth, skin and eyes). These features are common to a number of the syndromes listed in Table 5.1. Although there is a genetic component to osteoporotic fractures, it is much smaller than that of BMD. As fracture is the end result of a number of factors including BMD, bone turnover, body size and shape, muscle function and the risk of falling, all of which are controlled by different genetic pathways, it is difficult to disentangle the underlying genetics of fracture. However, genetics also influence other aspects of the metabolism of the bones such as the parathyroid hormone (PTH) signalling pathways, by way of single nucleotide polymorphisms (SNPs) and various haplotypes, some of which are associated with risk of fractures, independently of BMD in certain populations.

Table 5.1. Genetic syndromes featuring osteoporosis

Syndrome	Clinical features
Turner (XO)	Short stature, primary amenorrhea
Klinefelter (XXY)	Tall stature, gynecoid features
Osteogenesis imperfecta	Blue sclerae, dental abnormalities
Ehlers-Danlos	Joint hypermobility, dislocations
Cutis laxa	Lax skin, premature aged appearance
Marfan	Tall stature, lens dislocation, aortic root dilation, "Floppy valve syndrome"
Homocystinuria	Tall stature, thrombosis, lens dislocation
Cleidocranial dysplasia	Sloped shoulders, dental abnormalities
Osteoporosis-pseudoglioma	Poor vision, early fractures
Werner	Short stature, premature ageing
Hereditary sensory neuropathies	Insensitivity to pain

Many factors control the development and growth of the skeleton, including the deposition, accrual and retention of mineral in bone from the embryonic stage onwards throughout life. Numerous epidemiological studies published towards the end of the last century demonstrated a relationship between weight and length at birth and during infancy and the bone mass, stature and height in adulthood. It soon became evident that heredity, i.e. genes, contribute to the control of physical traits such as bone mass and density, height and obesity, and this realization has stimulated a massive increase in research into the genes involved in these processes. It has been estimated that about 60–70% of the variability in bone mineral mass, or BMD, is due to genetic variation, while other environmental factors account for the remaining 30–40% of the phenotypical variation. Another hereditary factor, more strongly expressed in female than in male offspring, is paternal skeletal size. At the biochemical level, a cohort study of 966 men and women provided evidence of an interaction between an SNP in the calcium sensing receptor gene (CASR) and birthweight, and in the determination of bone mass in a female population. Correlations between the growth hormone gene, weight in infancy and adult bone mass have also been described. Numerous studies, and from various aspects, have addressed the question of bone growth in infancy and childhood and its effects on peak bone mass, bone strength and fracture risk later in life. To date, in the first decade of the new millennium, many large scale studies have been published on the genetics of both physiological and pathological aspects of skeletal development, modelling and growth, as well as on remodelling, repair and maintenance of the bones. In addition, linkages between mechanisms controlling metabolism of bone and a variety of chronic disorders prevalent in adulthood and in the elderly have also been elucidated, particularly with respect to osteoporosis. Polymorphisms have been identified in many genes active in different aspects of osseous metabolism and their associations with osteoporosis clarified. Moreover, the identification of specific genetic loci, for example loci connected to height, has revealed new biological pathways in human growth, and these could well indicate targets for the design of future drug therapies.

Additional large-scale analyses have now been reported on the effects on osteoporosis of the association of *genomic polymorphisms and other factors* in osseous metabolism. Examples include polymorphisms of the oestrogen receptor ESR1, vitamin D receptor variations, polymorphisms in the transforming growth factor (TGF) B1 gene, and in the LRP5 and LRP6. Today, one novel aspect of genetics is the ongoing investigation of genes in so-called causation, i.e. the relationships of genotypes to phenotypes, which are extremely complicated and conclusive observations are awaited. In addition, the patient's family history must also be taken into account, since it has been shown that family history is an important risk factor for osteoporosis in women in the US. Patients with developmental difficulties, congenital or acquired, are also liable to osteoporosis and fragility fractures. The passage of time sets in motion many processes such as mitochondrial dysfunction and apoptosis which, in various organs and tissues, gradually lead to reduction in mass as in the skeletal muscles: *sarcopenia*. This in turn leads to a decrease in BMD. It has been postulated that the detection of sarcopenia at the time of dual-energy X-ray absorptiometry (DXA) could be used as a screening test for women who require special exercises to restore muscles and BMD values. Another age-related pro-

cess that induces changes in bone cells and thereby promotes osteoporosis is *telomere shortening* with replicative ageing of osteoblast precursors.

Race: Caucasians tend to have the lowest bone mass, and hip fractures are far more common among Whites than non-Whites. Age-adjusted hip fracture incidence rates are higher among Scandinavian residents than other comparable populations. Afro-American women tend to have the highest bone density and lose bone less rapidly as they age.

Gender: Women have a greater risk for most fractures than men. In general, the rate of spine and hip fractures in women is two or three times greater than in men. These sex-related differences in osteoporosis-associated fractures have been attributed to higher BMD in men than in women, as well as to differences in body size, bone size and width, while differences in geometry of the bones and (possibly accumulated) microarchitectural damage may also be contributing factors. In addition, male and female hormones may differentially alter the mechanostat set points by which bone tissue is added to a particular location when and where it is mechanically needed.

Age: Between 30 and 35 years of age osseous remodelling, i.e. resorption and formation, are balanced. Thereafter, the genetically determined loss of bone sets in, to a somewhat greater extent in women than in men, at a rate of approximately 0.5–1% per year after the age of 30. With onset of the menopause and the drop in oestrogen secretion, the rate of osteoporosis and fractures in women increases steadily (Fig. 5.3). Early menopause is also an important risk factor for

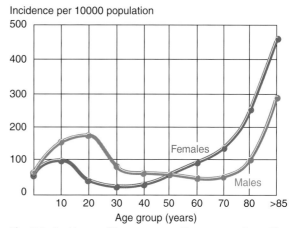

Fig. 5.3. Incidence of fractures according to sex and age. Notice the time lag of about 10 years in elderly men

osteoporosis. Moreover, it is worth remembering that now that hormone replacement therapy (HRT) is no longer acceptable, most of these women are subject to other hormone-dependent conditions affecting their general health and the bones. In men the risk of fractures increases steadily with the decline in testosterone secretion from about 60 years onwards. The risk increases even more with each decade of increasing age. The elderly also have an increased tendency to fall: one-third of individuals over 65 years of age will fall at least once a year. About 6% of falls for individuals over age 75 result in a fracture. Additional risks for developing osteoporosis are due to the following: increasing occurrence of co-morbidities together with the necessity to take various medications; deficiencies of calcium and vitamin D; decrease in physical activities that possibly potentiate the age-related decrease in muscle mass, i.e. sarcopenia; and unbalanced osseous remodelling due to the decline in osteoblastic activity.

Height and weight: Women with hip fractures have been reported to be taller than those without, whereas there was no effect of height on male hip fractures. Clearly, body weight and body mass index (BMI) are positively related to BMD and inversely related to osteoporosis and fracture rates. Investigations have demonstrated that low body weight and BMI are predictive of low BMD and increased fracture risk in women aged 40–59 years. It should be stressed that the maintenance of an appropriate weight is an important factor for the prevention of osteoporosis. Obese individuals need to lose weight to reduce the risk of co-morbid conditions. However, clinicians must be aware of the fact that marked weight loss can be detrimental to bone in the absence of appropriate precautionary measures. In addition, it is very important to take into account that osteoporosis in obese postmenopausal women is almost invariably associated with co-morbidities that may affect the bones. Moreover, there is a high prevalence of micronutrient deficiency (vitamin D included!) in morbidly obese people for which they should be checked and treated. This is also the case prior to and after bariatric surgery to avoid insufficiencies due to possible post-operative complications such as inadequate diet and malabsorption, including that of calcium and vitamin D.

Previous fractures: Even if the cause is unknown, the risk of sustaining another fracture is doubled when one has already occurred. Possibly individuals with one fracture tend to fall and develop subsequent fractures at a greater rate than individuals with no history of fractures. It has been estimated that a single spontaneous vertebral fracture raises the risk of further vertebral fractures by a factor of 5, while two or more fractures increase the risk by a factor of 12.

Family history: It has transpired from the comprehensive data on patients and their relatives, taken for the many trials on osteoporotic fractures, and which have now accumulated, that family history is also a significant and independent risk factor for osteoporosis.

Pregnancy and lactation: A woman nursing a baby secretes about 500 mg calcium daily into the milk. After nursing five babies, she will have secreted some 300 g of calcium – about a third of the amount of bound calcium incorporated in the skeleton. To some extent the high levels of sex hormones during pregnancy stimulate a greater absorption of calcium from the gastrointestinal tract and a greater uptake by the bones. However, there are additional risks for osteoporosis when several weeks' bed rest is required and also if muscle relaxants and sedation are administered during pregnancy. In some cases corticosteroids are also given. In these circumstances a massive excretion of calcium and loss of bone is the inevitable result, and the pregnant women must be given calcium and vitamin D to compensate for the loss. In general, there is a decrease in bone density during pregnancy and breastfeeding, but the bone density is restored to normal after birth and weaning. Only a few women suffer fractures during this temporary decrease in bone mass, mainly due to nutritional inadequacies.

5.2 Risk Factors Which *Can* be Influenced

Chronic inactivity: Insufficient physical movement is the single most important risk factor for osteoporosis. This applies also to younger, bed-ridden patients who may lose up to 30% of their bone mass in a few months,

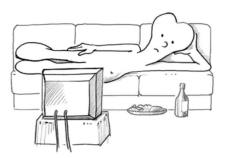

but may require years to regain their original bone density. When an arm is immobilized in plaster for 3 weeks because of a wrist fracture, the bones involved lose 6% of their density. A study of patients restricted to bed rest showed that trabecular bone was lost at the rate of about 1% per week! It has been suggested that trabecular bone increases at about 1% per month, so that restoration of bone mass is much slower than bone loss.

Examples of immobilization with rapid bone loss include:
- Paralysis after spinal injuries
- Hemiplegia after cerebrovascular events
- Paraplegia of the lower half of the body
- Immobilization after fractures of the lower extremities at any age
- Weightlessness in astronauts

Patients with osteoporosis who are confined to several weeks' bed rest after a fracture frequently sustain more fractures during the subsequent period of mobilization. A prolonged period of post-operative bed rest should therefore be avoided by implementation of new surgical techniques, early mobilization and the bones protected by administration of the appropriate drugs readily available today (e.g. aminobisphosphonates). In addition, there is a close relationship between muscle and bone mass. Moreover, with advancing age, many diseases could be avoided, or at least positively influenced, by regular exercise and physical activity. It is regrettable that the conveniences of civilization are exploited at the cost of our bones, and that we play a dangerous game in ignoring the increasing trends towards physical inactivity in our children, as witnessed by the well-nigh global epidemic of juvenile obesity!

Microgravity: Healthy astronauts must perform special exercises before and while they are in outer space due to the lack of gravity. Nevertheless they lose about 1% of their bone mass every month. Under spaceflight conditions astronauts experience a loss in bone density at a rate up to ten times faster than that of earth-bound patients with osteoporosis. Experimental studies have shown that weightlessness induces osteocytic apoptosis and this in turn attracts osteoclasts to bone during spaceflight has been extensively studied and used as a model for the decrease in BMD in osteoporosis on earth, for example in the case of mobilization due to fractures or paralysis, bone loss due to decline in hormones in the menopause, the andropause and in involutional osteoporosis. Two mechanisms observed in spaceflight under microgravity, i.e. the demineralization of bone and the inhibition of osteoblasts, also characterize bone loss here on earth.

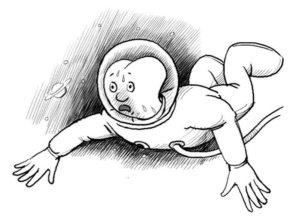

Excessive sport: Female athletes in particular are liable to osteoporosis later in life. Constant and lengthy training as well as strict control of diet and weight both lead to an extreme reduction in body fat and a drop in levels of oestrogen, with the result that menstrual periods become irregular or cease altogether; consequently, the risk of fractures is clearly increased.

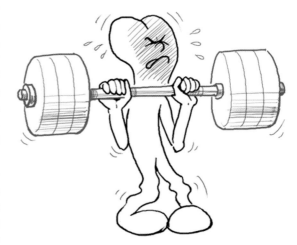

Low body weight (low body mass index): "Slim women, thin bones" – all large studies of risk factors for osteoporosis have confirmed this saying. Underweight women have a high risk of fractures, while overweight women are rarely affected by osteoporosis. This is because the increased weight strengthens the bones while the oestrogen metabolites produced by the fat cells further protects the bones from osteoporosis. After the menopause, the hormones produced by the adrenal cortex – androstenedione for example – are metabolized by the fat cells by means of their aromatases and converted to bone-protecting oestrogen. On the negative side, however, overweight has deleterious consequences such as deformities of the vertebrae and "wear and tear" of the joints, especially the knees and ankles. Low body weight with its decrease in bone density and increase in fracture risk affects both men and women equally. For decades our society has broadcast the message to women that to be thin is attractive, beautiful and desirable. Embroiled in this "thinness mania", millions of women still persist in following misguided attempts at attaining and maintaining thinness, at the cost of their bones. It is impossible to consume adequate amounts of the nutrients required for bone growth and bone maintenance on a low calorie diet alone. Patients with anorexia nervosa are particularly prone to the development of osteoporosis. In some countries 1–3% of women are subject to eating disorders, the consequences of which include osteoporosis. There are several potential mechanisms to explain the increased fracture risk in individuals with low body weight:

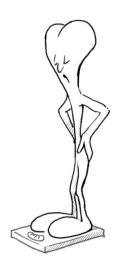

- Decreased mechanical loading of the skeleton
- Hypogonadism
- Reduced production of oestrogen by fat cells (adipocytes)
- Low insulin and IGF-I levels
- Less impact-absorbing fatty padding over the greater trochanter (hip fracture)

Obesity: It was previously believed that obesity and osteoporosis were two unrelated diseases, but recent studies have shown that both diseases share several common genetic and environmental factors. Normal ageing is associated with both a high incidence of osteoporosis and with bone marrow atrophy, i.e. reduction in haematopoietic tissue and a corresponding increase in fat cells (adipocytes). Bone remodelling and adiposity are both regulated via the hypothalamus and the sympathetic nervous system, and adipocytes and osteoblasts derive from a common mesenchymal precursor cell. But, based on the present state of knowledge, it is still unclear whether the fatty tissue has beneficial effects on bone. However, relationships have already been demonstrated between adiposity and adipocyte dysfunction and adverse effects on many systems, which in turn can also adversely affect the bones. Obesity is also closely related to insulin and diabetes, which in turn are part and parcel of the metabolic syndrome which also affects the metabolism of bone. The increased risk of osteoporosis posed by morbid obesity has now been demonstrated by the results of measurements of BMD, BMI and other parameters, such as bone turnover markers taken before and after bariatric surgery. Risk factors for osteoporosis, if not already present, are increased after bariatric surgery due to various factors including difficulties with nutrition, absorption and periods of decreased physical activity. A comprehensive program for a change in lifestyle is required, including nutrition, physical exercise and appropriate medication, possibly i.v. bisphosphonates to avoid gastrointestinal problems and vitamin supplements as required.

From a practical point of view, the adverse metabolic consequences of obesity can best be avoided, or managed if already present, by scrupulous attention to lifestyle factors! Moreover, as recently pointed out, not only during the work days of the week, but especially during the weekends, the temptation to indulge must be resisted!

Low lifelong calcium intake: The average adult ingests about 500 mg of calcium daily. If there is a decreased calcium intake over years, increased parathyroid hormone levels stimulate bone to release calcium from its stores, and this causes osteoporosis. The greater the calcium intake in childhood and adolescent years, the higher the peak bone mass, making the bone less susceptible to fracture with normal ageing in women as well as in men.

State of depression: Depression by itself is most probably not a main cause of osteoporosis, but the accompanying circumstances are. Studies have shown that women with severe longstanding depression have 6% less bone mass than matched controls without depression. The main contributory factors linking depression, low BMD and fracture risk include:

• High levels of stress hormones
• Low levels of gonadal steroids
• Various anti-depressant drugs
• Lack of appetite and inadequate nutrition
• Increased alcohol abuse
• Co-morbid medical conditions, and most importantly
• Reduced physical activity
• Lack of motivation

Cigarette smoking – "bone terrorist number one": Cigarette smoking has a negative influence on BMD independent of differences in weight and physical activity. Smoking doubles the risk of osteoporosis and therefore constitutes an important risk factor. Women who smoke one pack a day during adulthood have 5–10% less BMD at the age of menopause than do non-smokers. Swedish studies report that the BMD of a 70-year-old woman who smokes is equivalent to an 80-year-old non-smoker. According to the results of recent studies, it is estimated that smoking increases the lifetime risk of vertebral fractures by 13% in women and 32% in men. The figures for hip fractures are: 31% for women and 40% for men. It is suggested that 10–20% of all hip fractures in women are attributable to smoking. Although the exact mechanism is not known, various chemical substances in cigarettes are probably responsible. Nicotine inhibits oestrogen secretion, stimulates oestrogen breakdown in the liver and accelerates the onset of menopause. Smoking also depletes the body of certain nutrients, such as vitamin C, which are essential for bone building. Smoking seems to impair the bone protective effects of nutritional calcium in postmenopausal women, more clearly in the lumbar spine than in the femoral neck. In addition, smoking increases the body's toxic burden of cadmium, lead and many other toxic substances which interfere with calcium absorption and mineralization. It has been demonstrated that smoking impairs the

protective effects of nutritional calcium on bone. Finally, smoking also inhibits osteoblasts and diminishes blood circulation in bone. Cigarette smokers also tend to be thinner than their non-smoking counterparts, which may also play a role. No BMD differences were found between former and never-smokers. Reducing current smoking would help prevent many fractures, including hip and spine fractures, and may also improve the healing of fractures.

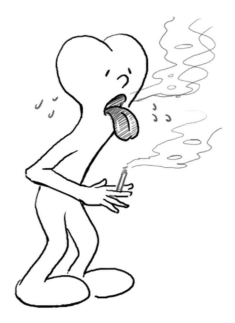

Excessive alcohol intake: Many physicians believe that alcohol intake is bad for bone. However, studies have shown that modest intake is associated with increased oestradiol concentration and therefore with higher bone density and a lower risk of fractures. Consequently, there is no reason to advise individuals who drink alcohol in moderate amounts to stop for reasons of preventing osteoporosis. However, no study published to date has given the definition of "moderate amounts" in measured quantities of alcohol; the amount is usually given as "0.5–1.0 drinks per day". Genuine alcoholism, however, increases the risk of osteoporosis and fractures and substantially delays fracture healing. However, in an assessment of patients with chronic alcoholism, it should be noted that decisive factors are the accompanying poor nutrition, lower weight, hepatic damage, lower calcium absorption and decreased levels of oestrogen. Chronic alcoholism induces cardio-, hepato- and splenomegaly, which contribute to the adverse consequences and poorer outcome of patients with chronic alcoholism. Chronic alcoholism may be five to ten times more frequent among patients with fractures than among those without fractures. The negative effects of excessive alcohol on bone are seen in women as well as in men.

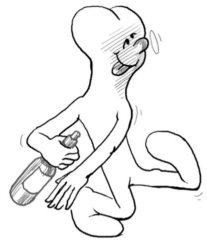

Excessive lipid intake: Hyperlipidaemia and an increased susceptibility to lipid oxidation may also constitute risk factors for osteoporosis. In addition, dietary lipids have now been implicated in calcium exclusion, fatty acid metabolism and osteoblast function.

Nutritional deficiency: Nutrition is an essential factor in the maintenance of bone health and the following factors are known to be important:

- Minerals: calcium, phosphorus, magnesium, zinc, manganese, copper, boron, silica
- Vitamins: D, C, K, B_6, B_{12}, folic acid
- Proteins
- Essential fatty acids

A number of articles published in 2008 have stated clearly that hypovitaminosis D is widespread, regardless of geographic location. The far-reaching consequences include osteoporosis, falls, altered glucose and lipid metabolism and increased risk of cancer on an international scale.

We frequently under-consume most of these key bone-building nutrients. In a recent survey, not a single person consumed 100% of the Recommended Daily Allowance (RDA) for the nutrients listed above. As mentioned previously, when insufficient calcium is absorbed from food, it is mobilized from the bones by

PTHs, causing a negative bone balance with respect to remodelling (i.e. more resorption than formation). In childhood, youth and pregnancy, it is particularly important to meet the needs of the growing bones by strict attention to appropriate nutrition. On the other hand, too much of certain substances should also be avoided; to give but one example: daily consumption of chocolate by 70- to 85-year-old women resulted in a reduction in BMD and in bone strength.

Hormones: For women, an early menopause (natural or surgical) is an important risk factor. Likewise insufficient *testosterone* in men also leads to osteoporosis. Moreover, alcoholism and anorexia nervosa can both contribute to testosterone deficiency. Therefore, testosterone levels in the serum should always be investigated in young men with osteoporosis of unknown aetiology to detect hypogonadism or testosterone deficiency. Oral *contraceptives* contain a combination of oestrogen and progesterone, and both may increase bone mass. Indeed there is some evidence that women who have used birth control pills for a long time have stronger bones than those who have not. Oral contraceptives may especially protect some women athletes against the risk of stress fractures.

Medications: Many drugs weaken the bones and the most important are *cortisone* and its derivates, the glucocorticoids. These are used systemically in many diseases: bronchial asthma, allergies, rheumatic, haematologic, intestinal and immunologic diseases, as well as after transplantations. Adult and elderly patients with co-morbidities are very likely to be at risk for medication-induced osteoporosis. Patients who are treated with cortisone (or its derivates) for more than a year develop osteoporosis with a high risk of fractures. There is another long list of medications which weaken the bones on long-term use including lithium, isoniazid, carbamazepine and other antiepileptic drugs, heparin, warfarin and other anticoagulants, antacids containing aluminium and, in particular, immunosuppressive drugs such as cyclosporin A. However, thyroid hormone when given in daily doses of 75–125 µg probably does not harm the bones. Warfarin competitively inhibits vitamin K, but concern about osteoporosis should not deter the use of anticoagulants for the prevention of thromboembolic disorders. In contrast, thiazide diuretics and beta-blockers, however, both appear to exert some skeletal benefit as indicated by higher BMD values, less bone loss and lower fracture rates. A recent study has demonstrated that the use of beta-blockers is associated with a reduced risk of fracture in middle-aged and older subjects. It should also be noted that occasionally therapy of a co-morbidity has a beneficial effect on bone, as observed in patients treated with ultraviolet light B for psoriasis. On the other hand, patients treated with radiotherapy localized to one particular site in the body may develop osteoporosis in adjoining skeletal areas.

Homocysteine: Increased plasma homocysteine levels have been suggested as an independent risk factor for osteoporosis, bone loss and fragility fractures, perhaps by interfering with collagen cross-linking and stimulating osteoclast activity. Although some of the risk may be related to low serum levels of folate and vitamin B12, it is now acceptable to consider an elevated level of homocysteine as a marker of elevated fracture risk.

Imbalance, tendency to fall and obstacles: Almost a third of elderly people fall at least once a year but only 10% break a bone. Obviously, in addition to the degree of severity of osteoporosis, the type of fall also determines whether or not a fracture is likely to occur. Protective reflexes – such as stretching out the arms to break a fall – are reduced in older people who also have less energy-absorbing soft tissue around the hip joints, resulting in an increased tendency to break the hip bone on falling. Similar considerations apply to lateral or forward falls. Moreover, cognitive or visual impairment, dizziness and syncopal events, as well as various rheumatic disorders may further diminish the capacity to prevent and/or mitigate a fall. A very simple test can be used to evaluate a patient's coordination and thereby the risk of falling and of fracture: the *"rise and walk" test*. The patient gets up from a chair, walks to a wall 3 m away, touches it and returns to sit on the chair again. If this takes longer than 10 s, then there is an increased risk of fracture. Examples of physiologic changes found in frequent fallers include impaired proprioception and motility, impaired visual acuity, impaired ankle dorsiflexion, decreased reaction time and increased body sway. Protection against blows to the hip is afforded by *pads* sewn into the underwear or worn beneath it. The pads disperse the impact of the fall and thus protect the hip joint (Fig. 5.4a,b). When osteoporosis is already established, various other factors – either health-related as listed above, or in the environment – increase the fracture risk. These include muscular weakness, poor coordination, awkward movements and inadequate protective reactions, excitement, dizziness, brief fainting attacks, Parkinson's disease and alcoholism, fatigue, including drug-induced, possibly due to antidepressive or antihypertensive medication as well as a variety of sleeping tablets which entail a high risk of falling while simultaneously decreasing the body's protective mechanisms. Cardiac medications and analgetics have also been implicated as risk factors. Other culprits are obstacles in the home such as telephone and other wires and cables, stairs, loose carpets, slippery bathroom mats, lack of grab-bars and poor lighting.

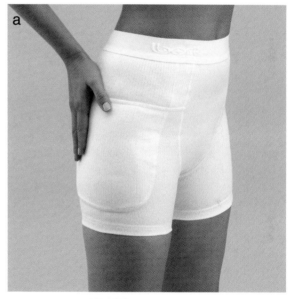

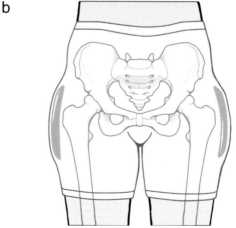

Fig. 5.4a,b. Hip protectors to absorb the energy of a fall and redistribute the load to the surrounding tissues

A previous fracture: Patients who have already sustained a fracture in the past are at increased risk of another fracture in the future; therefore, preventive care is especially important and all the considerations outlined above apply equally to these patients.

Education and knowledge: Many of the risk factors listed above could be avoided by proper information and emphasis on how the patients themselves could contribute to a reduction in risk factors. The emphasis should be on aspects of daily living, especially in the elderly, who could probably also benefit from a device such as a picture, sketch or other graphic reminder which would be constantly displayed in their rooms (homes). Finally, it should be remembered that, even in the absence of osteoporosis, falls and fractures may occur. One such example is fracture of the ankle, which may occur as a consequence of a heavy fall, or an accident which caused multiple injuries. Results of the National Osteoporosis Risk Assessment (NORA) study of 158,940 postmenopausal, 50- to 98-year-old women showed a positive association between a previous wrist fracture and future osteoporosis-related fractures within the subsequent 3 years. Consequently, a previous wrist fracture can be considered as an independent risk factor for postmenopausal women, regardless of the presence or absence of other risk factors.

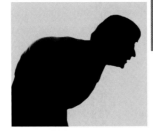

Clinical Evaluation of Osteoporosis

Early and correct diagnosis is essential for effective therapy. Reliable information concerning the state of bones is absolutely crucial, especially if risk factors are already present. The following key questions must be accurately answered:

- What is the present bone mass? [Results of recent (and previous) measurements]
- What is the present rate of bone loss? (Markers of remodelling in blood and urine)
- Has physical damage already occurred? (Evidence of previous fractures on X-rays)
- Are the changes (if present) reversible?

The aims of clinical investigations are to:

- Exclude a disease that can mimic osteoporosis (e.g. osteomalacia, myeloma)
- Elucidate the causes of osteoporosis
- Define the severity and topography of osteoporosis and determine the risk of subsequent fractures
- Select the most appropriate form of treatment
- Perform the baseline measurements required for the subsequent monitoring of any treatment given

6.1
Indicative Symptoms

Back pain is one of the most frequent reasons for seeking medical advice, and every case of acute or chronic back pain must be thoroughly investigated. Since osteoporosis may be dormant and symptomless for extended periods, the onset of pain may indicate collapse or fracture of a vertebra. On the other hand, osteomalacia is characterized by widespread, early, systemic and severe bone pain – an important factor in differential diagnosis, which includes numerous other disorders:

- Vertebral diseases: inflammatory, degenerative, myelogenous and neoplastic
- Extravertebral diseases: visceral, neurological, muscular, psychosomatic and neoplastic (e.g. carcinoma of the pancreas)

A detailed *evaluation of back pain* comprises localization, onset, duration, continuous, intermittent, extent, type, intensity, sensory/motoric disturbances and responsiveness to various stimuli and drugs. Possible underlying causes include:

- Muscular contractions and tension
- Vertebral collapse
- Disc protrusion
- Ankylosing spondylitis
- Bone metastases
- Pancreatic tumours
- Myocardial infarction.

Clinical history and a careful physical examination (Table 6.1) must include the following:

- Loss of height
- Posture and bearing
- Pain on percussion of spinal processes
- Mobility of the vertebral column
- Presence of thoracic kyphosis or lumbar scoliosis
- Muscle tone and contractions
- Signs of congenital osteoporosis (e.g. blue sclerae)

R. Bartl, B. Frisch, *Osteoporosis,* DOI 10.1007/978-3-540-79527-8_6,
© Springer-Verlag Berlin Heidelberg 2009

6

Table 6.1. Medical history and physical examination in osteoporosis

Skeletal history	Fractures, pain, deformity, reduced mobility, height loss
Risk factor assessment	
Family history	Osteoporosis, fractures, renal stones Age, ethnicity, weight
Medical history	
Reproductive	Menarche > age 15 years, oligo/amenorrhea, menopause
Diseases	Renal, GI, endocrine, rheumatic, neurologic, eating, depression
Surgery	Gastrectomy, organ transplant, intestinal resection or bypass
Drugs	Glucocorticoids, anticonvulsants, cytotoxic agents, heparin, warfarin, GnRH agonists, lithium
Lifestyle and exercise	Smoking, poor nutrition and exercise, alcohol
Diet and supplements	Frequent dieting, calcium, vitamin D, caffeine, protein
Current medications	Hormones, sedatives, hypertensives, diuretics, non-prescription drugs
Physical examination	
Weight loss, diarrhea	Malabsorption, thyrotoxicosis
Weight gain, hirsutism	Cushing's syndrome
Muscle weakness	Osteomalacia, Cushing's syndrome
Bone pain	Osteomalacia, fracture, malignancy, hyperparathyroidism
Tooth loss	Hypophosphatasia
Joint and lens dislocation	Collagen disorders
Skin pigmentation, stria	Mastocytosis, Cushing's syndrome
Nephrolithiasis	Hypercalcuria, primary hyperparathyroidism

Acute back pain in osteoporosis is caused by sudden collapse or fracture of a vertebra. Patients often report having heard a snapping or cracking sound in the back. In contrast, chronic pain in osteoporosis is due to inability of the axial skeleton to match up to the demand made on it by muscles, joints and extremities. The following questions should be answered to make the most comprehensive diagnosis of the pain

syndrome: location, nature, timing, radiation and severity of the pain, as well as factors that make the pain worse. Neurological features such a persistent nerve root pain or spinal cord syndromes are rare. The massive spinal shrinkage in osteoporosis (>4 cm) is mostly a consequence of the collapse of one or more of the thoracic vertebrae, but the distance from foot to hip remains constant. Other reasons for moderate decrease in height are poor posture, disk deterioration and muscle weakness. *Loss of height* can be approximated from the difference between the standing height and the arm span; loss of height occurs only in the spine, with hip-to-heel length remaining constant (Fig. 6.1). When the height of the lumbar spine is reduced, the ribs may come to rest painfully on the bones of the pelvic girdle. A distinctly longer arm span indicates the degree of vertebral bone damage. Loss of height also entails characteristic folds in the skin of the back

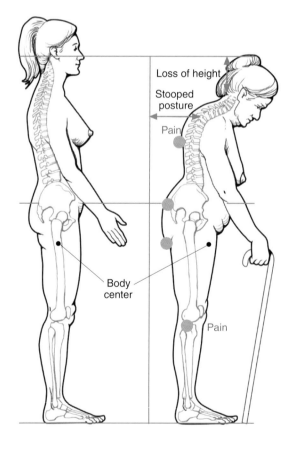

Fig. 6.1. Changes in stature and posture due to generalized osteoporosis

("*Christmas tree phenomenon*"), as well as a forward-bulge of the abdomen ("*osteoporosis tummy*"). Moreover, the decrease in height of the vertebral bodies results in painful contact between the spinal processes ("*Baastrup syndrome*" or "kissing spine"). The body's centre of gravity is displaced forward, so that movements during walking become slow and unsure, with small steps to avoid transmitting shocks to the vertebral column. The resulting faulty weight-bearing in turn gives rise to arthroses of the knee joints (*gonarthrosis*). Moreover, the unsure gait carries with it an increased risk for falls and fractures. The collapse of the thoracic vertebra produces the typical "round" back ("*dowager's hump*"). A good way to estimate the degree of "hump" is to measure the distance between the back of the head and the wall when the patient is standing straight up against it. When thoracic kyphosis is marked, the thoracic capacity may be reduced, impairing total lung volume, respiratory efficiency and exercise tolerance: and the patient's chin may come to rest on the sternum.

6.2
Osteoporosis and Teeth, Skin and Hair – What are the Connections?

Metabolic osteopathies involve the whole skeleton, and that includes the alveolar bone supporting the teeth. Consequently, patients with osteoporosis frequently experience problems with teeth which loosen and fall out due to widening of the alveoli – the canals in which they are situated and loosening of the collagen which holds them in place. There is indeed evidence that loss of teeth may be related to skeletal bone mass. As shown in various studies, women with severe osteoporosis are three times as likely as their controls to experience edentulism. It is tempting to discuss a relationship between systemic osteoporosis and residual ridge resorption. Alveolar bone loss is also caused by periodontitis. Studies have shown that alveolar bone loss and collagen breakdown may be inhibited by the administration of aminobisphosphonates. But attention must of course be paid to the state of the gums. The findings of recent studies in patients with osteoporosis indicate that there is benefit in oral bisphosphonate therapy as it protects against periodontal bone loss and osteoporosis. The very small risk of developing osteonecrosis should be

considered with due regard for the benefit in preventing alveolar bone loss. Almost all cases of osteonecrosis of the jaw bones have been reported in cancer patients treated with high-dose intravenous bisphosphonates, and in the presence of additional risk factors such as chemotherapy, glucocorticoids and prior dental interventions. Poor oral hygiene might also play a part.

There is a connection between "thin, transparent" skin and osteoporosis. Thin skin can be a sign of corticosteroid drug excess or of Cushing syndrome. Thin skin can best be recognized on the back of the hand, especially when the veins are visible. However, reliable conclusions about bone density cannot be drawn from ultrasound measurements of skin thickness.

It is well established that greying and loss of hair is associated with the ageing process, as is involutional osteoporosis, although some studies in the 1990s also showed that patients with premature greying were more likely to have osteopenia. Moreover, if the patients were young (in their 20s), they were very likely to have a family history of osteoporosis. A case control study confirmed this association in patients from 20 to 40 years of age by bone density measurements; but the numbers of these patients within the population of osteoporosis patients are very low. However, the more recent Rancho Bernardo study of greying and balding patterns and results of bone density measurements in 1207 older men and women did not find a significant correlation. Nevertheless, it is of interest in this connection that the reports in the literature on Werner's syndrome, a congenital disorder characterized by premature ageing (progeria), include greying and alopecia as well as osteoporosis in the symptomatology of very young patients.

6.3
Role of Conventional X-Rays in Osteoporosis

Skeletal X-rays indicate bone loss only when the density has been reduced by 30–40%; therefore, X-rays are not appropriate for early diagnosis. But they are very useful to reveal previous fractures or compressions (Fig. 6.2). The *vertebral bodies* exhibit various changes in shape which occur when the cancellous bone is resorbed while the cortex remains intact. Loss of trabecular bone occurs in a predictable pattern. The non-weight-bearing trabeculae are resorbed first and

6

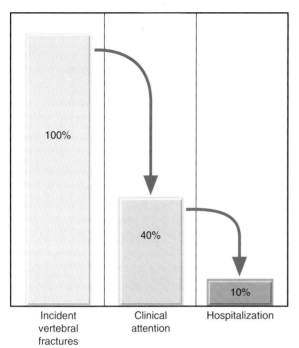

Fig. 6.2. Overall outcome of vertebral fractures. (Data from Cooper C, Atkinson E, O'Fallon W et al. [1992] Incidence of clinically diagnosed vertebral fractures: a population-based study in Rochester, Minnesota, 1985–1989. J Bone Miner Res 7:221–227)

therefore the vertebral bodies typically show a rarefaction of the horizontal trabeculae accompanied by a relative accentuation of the vertical trabeculae ("*verticalization*", "*vertical striation*") (Fig. 6.3) and the presence of reinforcement lines. Furthermore, the cortical rim of the vertebral bodies are accentuated, while the vertebral bodies demonstrate a "*picture frame*", "*empty box*", "*ghost-like*" appearance. Another use-

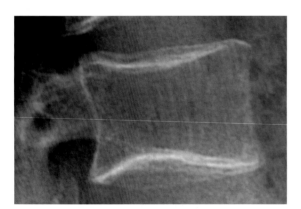

Fig. 6.3. Vertical striation of a vertebral body in osteoporosis

ful criterion is the *ballooning* of the intervertebral spaces, an indication of the incipient compression of the roof and ground plates (biconcavity of the vertebrae). Schmorl's nodes, which are caused by protrusions of the intervertebral disk into the vertebral body, are common in osteoporosis, although not pathognomonic. The *criteria* used to suggest the presence of osteoporosis on lateral X-rays of the spine include:
- Increased radiolucency
- Prominence of vertical trabeculae
- Presence of reinforcement lines
- Thinning of the vertebral endplates
- Presence of compression fractures

For a semiquantitative evaluation of vertebral deformities, Genant has published a grading scheme based on reductions of the anterior, middle or posterior height of vertebral bodies (Fig. 6.4):

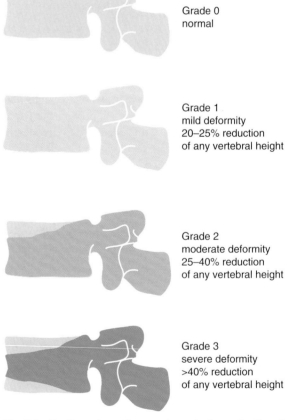

Grade 0
normal

Grade 1
mild deformity
20–25% reduction
of any vertebral height

Grade 2
moderate deformity
25–40% reduction
of any vertebral height

Grade 3
severe deformity
>40% reduction
of any vertebral height

Fig. 6.4. Grading scheme for a semiquantitative evaluation of vertebral deformities, according to Genant

- Grade 0: normal
- Grade 1: mild deformity, 20–25% reduction of any vertebral height
- Grade 2: moderate deformity, 25–40% reduction of any vertebral height
- Grade 3: severe deformity, >40% reduction of any vertebral height

From this semiquantitative assessment a *"spinal fracture index"* (SFI) can be calculated as the sum of all grades assigned to the vertebrae divided by the number of the evaluated vertebral bodies.

Roentgenograms of the thoracolumbar region in lateral projection serve two other useful clinical purposes:

- Identification of disk degeneration and osteoarthritis (Fig. 6.5), which often cause back pain and thus indicate a different treatment.
- Clarification as to why some patients with known severe osteoporosis may have relatively "normal" bone mineral density. Callous formation, degenerative disks, osteoarthritis and calcification of the overlying abdominal aorta (Fig. 6.6) may artificially increase bone density measurement.

It should be emphasized that conventional X-rays of the vertebral column are indispensible in the *investigation of secondary osteoporoses*. Characteristic findings are observed in the following conditions:

- *Degenerative-inflammatory conditions of the joints*: Subchondral scleroses with osteophytes or even more extensive ossifications are typical for spondylarthrosis and spondylitises.
- *Osteomalacia*: "Stout" trabeculae and "Looser's zones" at painful weight-bearing parts of the extremities are characteristic (Fig. 6.7). However, these must be differentiated from osteoporotic fatigue fractures. A bone biopsy in these circumstances provides an unequivocal demonstration of osteomalacia.
- *Malignant bone lesions*: Even a slight possibility that a bone lesion is due to a malignant process requires immediate clarification by imaging techniques. Magnetic resonance imaging (MRI) is the method of choice in many cases – for example in multiple myeloma or suspected metastases in mammary cancer.

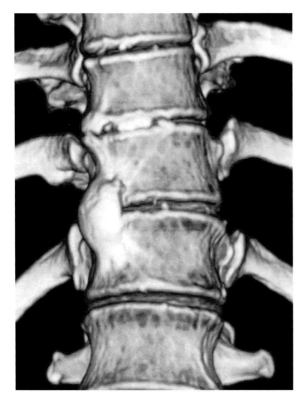

Fig. 6.5. Degenerative disk with spondylarthritis

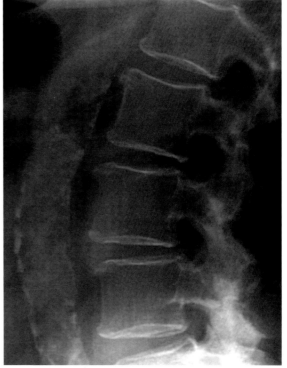

Fig. 6.6. Calcification of the abdominal aorta with "picture frame" appearance of the vertebral bodies

6

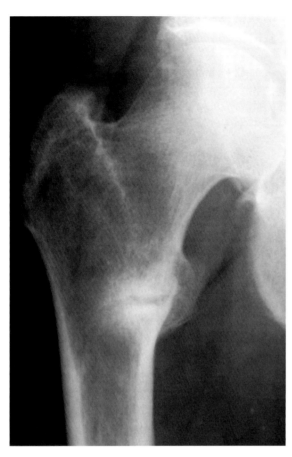

Fig. 6.7. Looser's zone in the weight-bearing part of the right femur, in osteomalacia

- *Hyperparathyroidism (HPT)*: Primary and secondary HPT show similar features on radiology, with the addition of a disturbance of mineralization in many cases of renal osteodystrophy. In advanced stages there are also pseudocystic clarifications, but the cancellous bone is thicker than in osteoporosis. The vertebra shows a "rugger-jersey-spine" caused by attenuation of the central areas and thickening of the end plates of the vertebral bodies.
- *Fluorosis*: The vertebral bodies become completely sclerotic (like marble) with osteophytes and ossification of the vertical bands in the later stages of fluorosis. This is rarely seen today in the US and Europe, as other therapies are now given, but may still be seen in Asian and other countries, such as India where many people were previously treated with fluoride and where it is still in use in some parts of the country today. In general, lateral radiographs of the thoracic and lumbar spine should be taken in

any patient in whom a vertebral fracture is suspected clinically. Clinical suspicion is heightened by new or worsening back pain, height loss of more than 4 cm and by prominent thoracic kyphosis. A vertebral fracture causes approximately 1 cm loss of height. However, after about the age of 50, women and men tend to lose height slowly as a result of thinner intervertebral discs and loss of muscle tone in the back. The chance of detecting a vertebral fracture increases with the increase in the degree of height loss. Moreover, radiographs are also significant in evaluation of bone and joint disorders in many other skeletal sites, for example the wrist and hand.

6.4
Other Useful Imaging Techniques

Morphometry (morphometric X-ray absorptiometry, MXA) of the vertebral bodies: X-rays of the thoracic and lumbar spine are taken and the size and contours of the vertebral bodies are measured by means of an automated computer programme. All similar techniques in use measure the following parameters: the height of the anterior (Ha), medial (Hm) and posterior (Hp) sides of the vertebral body. A 15% or 4-mm reduction in height signifies compression of the vertebral body. Two examples of evaluation of the vertebrae are:
- *"Vertebral Deformation Score"* (VDS) according to Kleerekoper: This programme also provides the fracture angle, projected surface area of the vertebral bodies and intervertebral space. Six points are utilized to calculate the deformities of the vertebral bodies. A simple definition of a fracture is the 25% definition: a difference in height of 25% from one measurement to the next. The VDS score is calculated according to the extent of the compression, i.e. VDS 0–3, where VDS 3 for example signifies a compression fracture effecting Ha, Hm and Hp.
- *"Spine Deformity Index"* according to Minne: This correlates the shape of the vertebral bodies with that of the 4th thoracic vertebra of the same vertebral column.

"Singh Index": The degree of rarefaction of the tensile groups in the proximal femur corresponds to the fracture risk in this area. Five anatomical groups of trabeculae can be defined which form the basis of the

Singh Score. It consists of three normal stages and between three and four stages of increasingly severe osteoporosis (grades 1–7).

Other parameters of the proximal femur: The *length of the femoral neck* (hip axial length) correlates with the fracture risk at this site independently of the cancellous and compact bone of the proximal femur. Each centimetre of increase in length doubles the fracture risk. The following radiological parameters are useful to calculate the fracture risk in the proximal femur:
- Thickness of the medial femoral shaft 3 cm below the trochanter minor
- Thickness of the medial cortex at the centre of the femoral neck
- Femoral head width
- Intertrochanteric region width
- Acetabular bone width

Vertebral fracture assessment (VFA): Dual-energy X-ray absorptiometry (DXA) can also be used to visualize lateral images of the whole spine to detect deformities and fractures of the vertebral bodies. This technique involves less radiation and is less expensive than a conventional X-ray examination. VFA has a sensitivity and specificity of about 90% for the detection of grade 2 and 3 fractures, according to the semiquantitative method of Genant.

Three-dimensional X-ray absorptiometry (3D-XA) allows 3D reconstruction of bones from DXA scans and the direct measurement of geometric parameters of the vertebrae with accuracy and precision; these parameters include the heights, depths and volumes of the vertebral bodies. This technique has the advantage of a lower radiation dose and of greater availability than CT scanners. Such a technique also enables direct measurement of the bone density and bone size with minimal radiation, and therefore is most suitable for the follow-up and monitoring of children.

Microradioscopy: To detect relatively early radiographic signs of osteoporosis, methods such as magnification radiography and radiogrammetry have been developed for application to the appendicular skeleton. Magnification radiography is a technique used to obtain finely detailed radiographs of the hands. Radiogrammetry of the metacarpals is a reproducible method used to determine the cortical thickness of a bone. This method is inexpensive and readily carried out, but does not detect early osteoporosis.

Bone scan: ^{99m}Tc-Labelled bisphosphonate is used to detect focal bone lesions (Fig. 6.8) and fractures. The whole skeleton can be scanned quickly by this method. Foci of increased uptake in the spine indicate fractures as well as degenerative, inflammatory or neoplastic lesions. At 2 days after a fracture, an increased uptake at the site can be expected. However, because of the limited structural details, additional imaging techniques are required for further identification.

Computed tomography (CT): This technique is particularly good for the analysis of bones (Fig. 6.9), and therefore it is now also applied for the demonstration of the cancellous bone. However, this can only be done with modern high resolution instruments using sections 0.5-mm thick, together with special picture

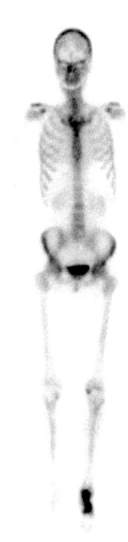

Fig. 6.8. Bone scan with focus of increased intake in one foot in a patient with Paget's disease of bone

6

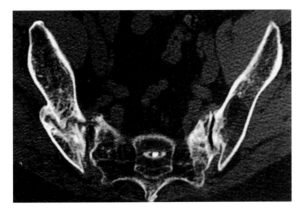

Fig. 6.9. Fractures of the pelvic girdle demonstrated on CT

enhancing facilities, but at the cost of higher exposure to radiation. The value of CT lies in the quantitative CT (QCT), which will be discussed later.

Magnetic resonance imaging (MRI): This method involves no exposure to radiation and is especially suited to the demonstration of the bone marrow. It offers the possibility of identifying both haematopoietic and fatty bone marrow, as well as inflammatory and neoplastic infiltrates (Figs. 6.10 and 6.11). It is the method

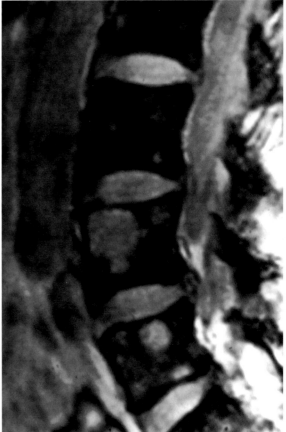

Fig. 6.11. Nodular metastatic process in the spine in a patient with breast cancer and secondary osteoporosis, MRI

of choice for demonstrating myeloma, lymphoma and metastases, as well as localized oedematous processes (transient osteoporosis and early stages of Sudeck's disease). It is the ideal method to distinguish between an osteoporotic fracture and one due to spinal metastases. In addition, the diagnostic capability is greatly enhanced by the application of special gradient echo-sequences and the use of contrast media.

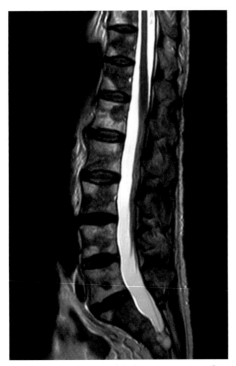

Fig. 6.10. Spondylarthritis with bone marrow oedema syndrome of the whole spine, MRI

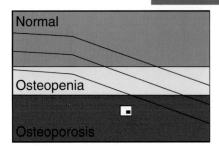

7.1
Why Measure Bone Mineral Density?

The early diagnosis of osteoporosis, before the occurrence of fractures, can only be made by means of bone density measurements [bone mineral density(BMD) tests] (Table 7.1). These measure bone density at various skeletal sites and thereby enable a prediction of risk of later fracture. A 10% decrease in bone density doubles the fracture risk for the vertebral body and trebles it for the hip joint. If a fracture has already occurred, this test is used to confirm the diagnosis of osteoporosis and determine its degree of severity. BMD provides the following information:

- Detects osteopenia and/or osteoporosis before occurrence of a fracture
- Predicts risk for later development of osteoporosis
- Indicates the rate of bone loss – progression – in sequential measurements
- Documents the efficacy or failure of therapy
- Increases compliance of both doctor and patient

The relation between BMD and fracture risk is well established (Fig. 7.1). The association between bone density (measured at hip and lumbar spine) and hip fracture is three times stronger than that between cholesterol levels and heart disease. Currently, a bone density measurement remains the best and most readily quantifiable method for assessing fracture risk and skeletal response to different treatments.

7.2
Which Instruments to Use?

The *bone mineral content* (BMC) is measured in grams (g), and the BMD in g/cm^2 (area) or g/cm^3 (volumetric). The precision and accuracy of a measurement depend on:

- Type of instrument (pencil or fan beam techniques)
- Regular (daily) check and setting of the instrument
- Cooperation of the patient (must keep still)
- Exact adjustment of the instrument by the investigator
- Degree of osteoporosis: the lower the bone mass, the more inaccurate the measurement!

Dual energy X-ray absorptiometry (DXA, DEXA, rarely also called QDR, DPX, DER): Today DXA is the most completely developed, reliable and popular bone densitometric technique in use, the "gold standard" and the "reference standard" (Figs. 7.2 and 7.3a,b). It is versatile and can be used to assess bone mineral content of the whole skeleton as well as of specific sites, especially those most vulnerable to fractures. DEXA was developed in the 1980s and its widespread use began in 1988. The skeletal site is exposed to two X-ray beams of different intensity, and the mineral content of the bone is calculated by means of computer programs from the amount of radiation. The technique therefore measures an areal density (g/cm^2) rather than a true volumetric density (g/cm^3) since the scan is two-dimensional. A real BMD accounts for about two-thirds of the variance of bone strength. By using the results of the two measurements, the contributions of the soft

7

Table 7.1. Techniques for measuring bone mineral density (BMD)

Method	Precision (%)	Accuracy (%)	Scan time (min)	Radiation dose (mrems)
Dual-energy X-ray absorptiometry (DXA) • Lumbar spine AP • Lumbar spine lateral • Proximal radius • Distal radius • Proximal femur • Total body	1–2	3–5	2–8	1–3
Quantitative computed tomography (QCT) • Lumbar spine • Radius	2–10	5–20	10–15	100–1000
Quantitative ultrasound (QUS) • Calcaneus • Phalanges • Patella	–	2–8	5–10	0

tissue components (different quantities of muscle and fatty tissue) can be calculated and discarded. DXA can measure individual central (hip and spine) and peripheral (forearm) sites, and can even perform a total body scan ("full body DXA scanner").

The hip joint and the lumbar spine are routinely measured from the front (AP) or the side (lateral). The combined evaluation of these two measurements improves the assessment of a patient's bone mineral status and the fracture prediction, especially in cases with anatomic variations, severe degenerative changes

or fractures (Fig. 7.4). The measurements of the lumbar spine are not confined to the vertebral bodies; they also include the arches and spinous processes which have a considerable quantity of compact bone. The International Society of Clinical Densitometry (ISCD) suggests measurement of at least two sites if possible and recommends that diagnosis be based on the lowest T-score. It suggests using the L2–L4 average measurement rather than a single vertebra if possible (Fig. 7.5). This has recently been revised by the recommendation that the total spine T-score should be used for the di-

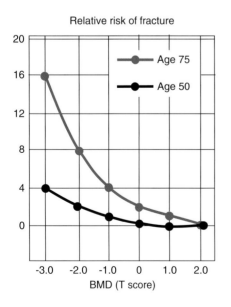

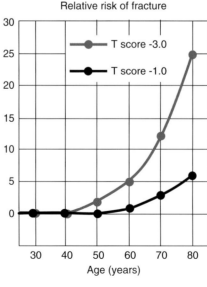

Fig. 7.1. Relative risk of fracture according to bone mineral density (*BMD*) and age

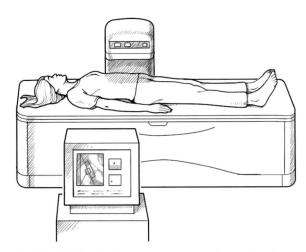

Fig. 7.2. DXA unit for the measurement of bone density in the lumbar spine and hips. Note posture of patient required for accurate measurement

agnosis of osteoporosis. In measurements of the hip, either the total hip or the femoral neck measurement is used, whichever is the lowest standard deviation (Fig. 7.6). To summarize, important advantages of DXA include that:

- It is not invasive, the patient remains clothed and it is therefore not a burden to the patient.
- It is very quickly carried out (5–10 min).
- It is cost-effective.
- It has a very low radiation dose (1–3 mrem equivalent to 1/10–1/100th of a normal X-ray film).
- It measures those skeletal areas most vulnerable to osteoporosis and to fractures – the lumbar spine and the hips.
- It has a documented strong gradient of risk for fracture prediction. The risk of hip fracture increases 2.6-fold for each standard deviation decrease in BMD at the femoral neck.
- The measurements are accurate and therefore ideal for follow-up and control investigations (accuracy error 1–10%, precision 1%).
- It is recognized by the WHO as the standard method for diagnostic definition of osteoporosis.
- It is recognized by the ESCEO and the IOF as the "reference standard" in the diagnosis of osteoporosis (2008).

The results of the measurement of the lumbar vertebral bodies 1–4 are expressed separately as well as in combination, by means of which single, possibly defective vertebrae can be excluded. Many factors dealing mainly with variations in density in the spine and/or in neighbouring soft tissues can give misleading values and must be considered in the results. In really difficult cases, measurement of the lumbar spine may have to be abandoned and only the bones of the hip joint measured. But there may also be variations in density in the proximal femur so that great care must be taken to measure the same areas in sequential investigations. The only real disadvantage of DXA is that everything in the selected area is included. Sometimes it may be difficult to decide what an ossification is due to (for example aorta, calcified lymph nodes or muscles, spondylophytes etc.). Other X-ray dense substances such as metal fasteners on clothes, X-ray dense contrast media or calcium tablets may also be included in the overall measurement. These "pitfalls" can be recognized and subsequently avoided by a prior X-ray of the skeletal area to be measured. An important limitation in the general application of DXA for diagnosis should be recognized: the presence of osteomalacia will underestimate total bone mass because of decreased mineralization of bone.

Recent developments in instrumentation enable lateral measurement, and by means of picture enhancement the vertebral bodies and the hip are clearly displayed (Fig. 7.7). Because of its high precision, it is wise for premenopausal women to get a baseline DXA scan that can serve as a reference value to determine loss of bone density after the menopause.

Guidelines for application and interpretation of the results of BMD measurements have just been published. Various review articles have also outlined the fundamentals of positioning, scan analysis and interpretation in clinical practice.

Two terms, T-score and Z-score are commonly used to report DXA results and both of these rely on a *standard deviation* (SD) for the measurement. SD represents the normal variability in a measurement in a population: the difference between the 5th and the 95th percentile of a group covers about 4 SDs. One SD of the hip or spine BMD corresponds to about 10–15% of the mean value.

- *Z-score* is the number of SDs below (minus) or above (plus) the mean BMD value for people of the same age ("age- and sex-matched" controls).
- *T-score* is the number of SDs below or above the mean value of BMD for young (20- to 30-year-old) adults ("peak bone density").

7

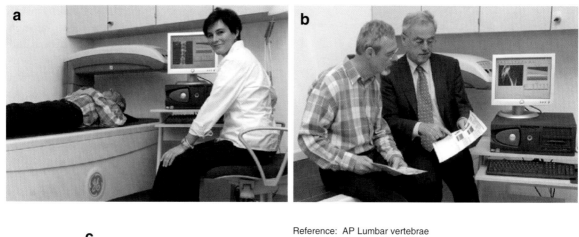

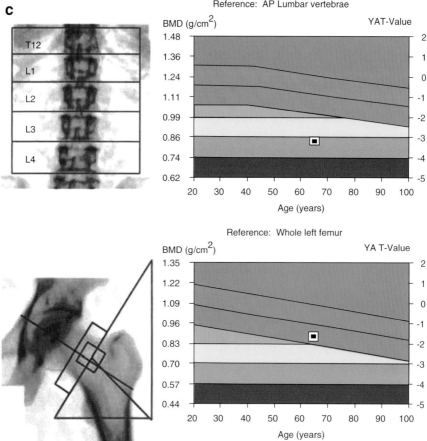

Fig. 7.3 a, b, c. Measurement of bone density of the hip and lumbar vertebrae using the DXA method (**a**), subsequent discussion of the results with the patient (**b**), and DXA of the lumbar spine (L1-L4) and left hip of a male patient showing different BMD values in the two skeletal areas measured (**c**)

Because BMD declines with age at all sites, after age 30 the T-scores are lower than the Z-scores, and the differences increase with age. By definition, diagnosis of osteoporosis is based on a T-score of <−2.5 SD. Geo-graphic variations in results of BMD measurements in young people from different European countries have been noted [Network in Europe on Male Osteoporosis (NEMO) study]. This is obviously important for a com-

BMD hip (T-score)

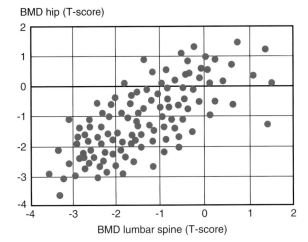

Fig. 7.4. Plot of the T-scores of total hip and lumbar spine (L2–L4)

parison of results in international trials; so recommendations have been made, such as the use of the NHANES III-based hip scores to equalize the differences.

Single energy X-ray absorptiometry (SXA): This method is still used today to measure the bones of the ankle because of the paucity of surrounding soft tissue.

The peripheral assessment of bone densitometry has been used for many years and recommendations for its use, quality control and reporting were published by the International Society for Clinical Densitometry in 2008 (see references).

Quantitative computed tomography (QCT): This is an established technique to measure BMD of the lumbar spine and appendicular skeleton. Moreover, it provides cross-sectional images and therefore separate measurements of trabecular and cortical bone, as well as true volumetric mineral density in g/cm³. In clinical studies, QCT has been used for the assessment of vertebral fracture risk. The method is usually applied to the spine to measure trabecular bone in consecutive vertebrae (Th L2–L4). The measurement takes about 20 min and has a relatively high radiation exposure of about 100–1000 mSv. The region of interest

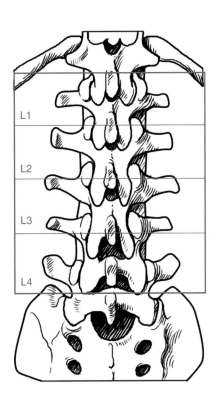

Fig. 7.5. DXA of the lumbar spine (L1–L4). *Upper right*: note T-score of –2.5, a borderline value between osteopenia and osteoporosis. *Lower right*: positive effect of alendronate on bone density with 15% increase after 1-year of therapy

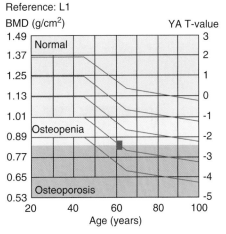

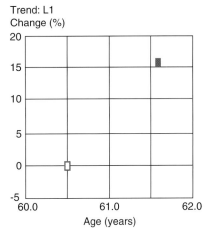

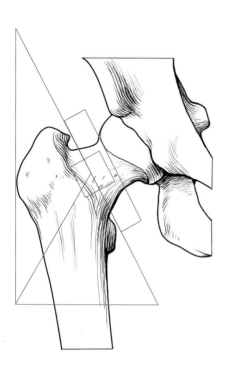

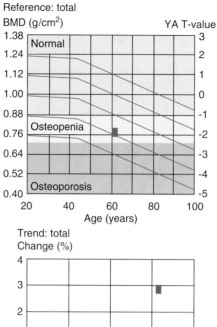

Fig. 7.6. DXA of right hip showing femoral neck, Ward's triangle, trochanter and shaft. *Upper right*: note T-score of –2.0, within osteopenic range. *Lower right*: positive effect of raloxifene on bone density with 3% increase after 1-year of therapy

(ROI) is either manually or automatically positioned. QCT can be performed in single-energy (SEQCT) or dual-energy (DEQCT) modes, which differ in precision, accuracy and radiation exposure. The presence of marrow fat in the vertebral bodies may cause an underestimation of BMD by 10–15%. The values obtained by direct measurement and by means of a "calibration phantom" should not be reported as T-scores, but they are calculated as hydroxyapatite mass per volume:

- Normal >120 HA/cm^3
- Osteopenia 120–80 HA/cm^3
- Osteoporosis <80 HA/cm^3

Special, small instruments are used to measure bone density in the fingers and wrist (*pQCT*). The values obtained, however, cannot be considered as representative of the skeleton as a whole, even though they do give accurate values for the bones measured. For example, cancellous bone in the radius may show osteoporosis in density measurements, but may be nowhere near that of the lumbar vertebrae or the hips. The

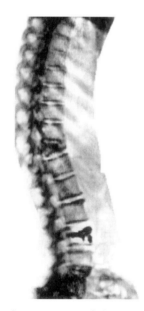

Fig. 7.7. Lateral measurement of the whole spine using a modern DXA machine (Lunar Prodigy Advance), in order to document or exclude any vertebral fractures. Note proof of a wedge-shaped vertebral fracture and a further fracture in the lumbar spine treated by kyphoplasty

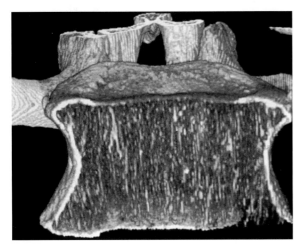

Fig. 7.8. High resolution and three-dimensional imaging CT for direct visualization of trabecular bone architecture

future of computed tomography (CT) lies in the field of direct visualization of trabecular bone architecture by high-resolution and by 3D (volumetric) imaging (3D-CT) (Fig. 7.8). However, this development does entail a greater amount of radiation.

Radiographic absorptiometry (RA): This technique determines BMD through computed analysis of hand radiographs. RA has proved to be a practical, inexpensive and rapid way to evaluate BMD:

- Two posteroanterior radiographs are taken of the hand, one at 50 kVp and the other at 60 kVp using nonscreen film.
- The films are sent to a central laboratory where they are digitized by a high-resolution imaging system.
- BMD is calculated in arbitrary units using the aluminium reference wedge as a calibration material.
- RA measures both trabecular and cortical bone.
- RA has high precision and accuracy.
- The radiation exposure of about 100 mrems is lower than that of QCT but higher than that of DXA.
- RA has high sensitivity in predicting low bone mass of the lumbar spine and femoral neck (90 and 82%, respectively).
- Dental panoramic radiographs have also been utilized for the recognition of osteoporosis.

RA plays an important role in paediatric osteology as radiographs of the hand are taken routinely in paediatric individuals for the purpose of determining skeletal age and development.

Quantitative ultrasound (QUS): This is already used successfully in many different conditions. The FDA has approved QUS of bone for its diagnostic value in osteoporosis and in related fractures. The behaviour of these ultrasound waves in bone differs greatly from that of X-rays. Absorption, speed, reflection in bone and from its surface are all measured. Two major parameters are used in measuring bone by QUS:

- Speed of sound through bone (transit velocity, SOS)
- Attenuation of sound as it passes through bone (broadband ultrasound attenuation, BUA dB/MHz)

Some instruments combine SOS and BUA to formulate a clinical index (quantitative ultrasound index, QUI). The skeletal part to be measured is placed between the ultrasound transmitter and receiver. Consequently, this method is very suitable for easily accessible bones: calcaneus, radius, tibia and phalanges. It is currently accepted that the QUS results are influenced mainly by three parameters:

- Microarchitecture of bone
- Mineral constituents of bone matrix
- Elastic modulus

Recent studies have shown that QUS of the calcaneus is a predictor of hip fracture risk, independent of femoral BMD, and that this technology can discriminate between normal and osteoporotic subjects. For every SD decrease in BUA of the calcaneus, the risk of hip fracture increases 2-fold, comparable with the results of DXA. QUS is becoming increasingly popular because of the absence of exposure to radiation and the simplicity of application. An additional advantage is that the cortical and cancellous bones are described separately. These advantages account for the fact that QUS is now widely applied as a screening test, although it cannot yet replace DXA measurements of the spine and hips. It must be emphasized that normal values for the fingers using QUS do not rule out the possibility of a severe osteoporosis elsewhere, for example of the spine or hips. Conversely, if the phalanges show osteoporotic values, then this should be regarded as a manifestation of generalized osteoporosis and DXA of the lumbar spine and/or hips should be carried out for clarification and WHO classification. Measurements of the fingers are especially indicated in patients with rheumatic disorders involving the hands. At present, QUS is not recommended for the monitoring of treatment.

7.3
Which Bones to Measure?

A fundamental rule states that "the result of a bone density measurement applies only to the particular site measured". Osteoporosis does not affect the bones of the skeleton to the same degree. Bones with a high proportion of cancellous (trabecular) bone, such as the vertebrae and hip bones, are the first victims and these bones are also the first to suffer fractures. Concordance of bone mass between different skeletal sites in individual patients increases in the elderly population. However, even in the elderly female population, measuring only the hip to make a diagnosis of osteoporosis (<–2.5 SD) will detect slightly less than 50% of the affected people, whereas measuring multiple skeletal sites in this population will detect nearly 80% of the affected people. Therefore, the lumbar vertebrae and hip bones are always measured according to a precise, topographical plan. The more sites measured, the higher the likelihood that a diagnosis of osteoporosis will be made. Of course, the reverse is also true: if only one peripheral site is measured, there is a much higher probability of missing osteoporosis. The peripheral techniques are quick and easy to use, but they are not appropriate for initial diagnosis or to measure response to therapy.

Lumbar vertebrae are measured individually and together, but fractured or otherwise deformed vertebrae are excluded.

Five areas are measured in the *hip joint*:
- Femoral neck
- Trochanter
- Intertrochanteric region
- Ward´s triangle
- Total

Subsequently, when bone density is checked to monitor therapy or disease progression, it is crucial that exactly the same areas are measured again.

The *ankle* is also a good site to measure, because of its content of trabecular bone and its accessibility. When performed using QUS, differences in rarefaction of the trabecular network along stress lines must be taken into account, and exactly the same area must be measured for subsequent monitoring. DXA does not have this drawback since the whole ankle is measured and the exact area is illustrated.

Although in the past the *radius* was frequently measured, the significance of the results is reduced because of the variable amounts of cancellous and cortical bone and because of the surrounding soft tissues. The same applies to pQCT and QUS of the radius. However, one advantage of pQCT is that the architecture of the distal radius is displayed.

Worried patients frequently come into the out-patient clinic and produce the results of density measurements of the fingers together with the diagnosis "severe osteoporosis with very high risk of fractures". Subsequent density measurement of spine and hip may reveal normal values. The opposite may also occur – normal bone density in the fingers with severe osteoporosis in the axial skeleton and multiple fractures of the vertebral bodies. Such situations simply indicate different bone density in different parts of the skeleton! The lesson to be drawn from this is that the diagnosis of generalized osteoporosis must never be based on the result of a peripheral bone density measurement. In addition, DXA density measurements to monitor therapy must always be made on the same skeletal site, preferably by the same instrument (DXA) at yearly intervals.

Investigations of the *whole skeleton* to determine bone mineral content are only made in clinical trials.

7.4
Who is Due or Overdue for a BMD Test?

Until recently, the diagnosis of osteoporosis was largely based on history, X-rays and clinical symptoms, especially fractures. The clinical relevance of quantitative bone density measurements are based upon two important assumptions:
- That bone density is related to fracture risk
- That treatment to increase bone mass can be administered.

And indeed, with the introduction of quantitative techniques of bone densitometry, the diagnosis of osteoporosis can now already be established in the early asymptomatic phase of the disease. Low bone density is accepted as the most important predictor of fragility fractures, comparable with blood pressure and cholesterol as reliable predictors of subsequent cardiovascular disease. Nevertheless, density measurements are not yet recommended as a screening procedure. However, for health-conscious individuals, this test is just as important as other generally established investigations. It is cheap, simple to perform and facilitates subsequent diagnosis and monitoring. Furthermore, BMD has also been demonstrated to be an independent predictor of increased mortality – and this appears unrelated to the occurrence of fractures. This *increased mortality with BMD loss* was most evident with death due to coronary heart disease (atherosclerosis) and pulmonary heart disease (HR 1.3 and 1.6, respectively, per SD decrease in BMD, $p < 0.05$ for both).

Indications for bone density measurements: The simplest way to determine who should have a bone density test is to decide in each case whether the results will influence a clinical decision (Fig. 7.9). Any individual with risk factors should have a bone density measurement, for example a postmenopausal woman who does not take HRT or its equivalent, a woman with early menopause, a woman with a family history of osteoporosis or men with decreased levels of androgens. According to the *National Osteoporosis Foundation (NOF)*, a BMD measurement is recommended for:

- All women >65 years regardless of additional risk factors
- All women <65 years with one or more risk factors
- All postmenopausal women with fractures
- All women contemplating osteoporosis therapy and whose decision depends on the result of BMD
- All women undergoing protracted hormone therapy (Fig. 7.10).

Additional indications: Anyone who has a disease or condition or is taking certain drugs with the potential to induce bone loss is a candidate for a bone density measurement (DXA preferred):

- Age-related decrease in height
- Back pain of obscure origin
- Slim smokers
- Previous fractures
- Diseases of joints which limit movement
- Long-term use (>6 months) of drugs such as cortisone, warfarin, heparin or anti-epileptic drugs
- Hyperthyroidism and hyperparathyroidism
- Post-transplantation, especially of kidney, liver, heart and lungs
- Chronic diseases and operations which can lead to bone loss, e.g. gastric and intestinal resections
- Anorexia nervosa
- Chronic renal insufficiency
- Neoplasias, pre and post therapy

Measurements in children are problematic for a number of reasons:
- There are inadequate reference data for children.
- There is a broad variability in developmental age at any given chronological age.
- DXA has inherent limitations for paediatric use because of its inability to measure the bone size in three dimensions.

To ameliorate this problem, whole-body bone mineral content (BMC) is sometimes recommended for paediatric measurements. Also, the Z-score rather than the T-score is the appropriate criterion for assessing the bone mineral status. One appropriate use of bone densitometry in paediatric populations is serial measurement for the detection of change in bone mineral status. BMC is preferable to BMD because of the problems posed by changing bone size and shape during growth.

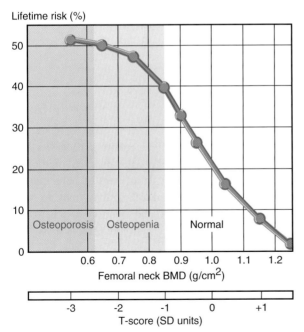

Fig. 7.9. Lifetime risk of hip fracture in 50-year-old Swedish women (modified from Kanis [2002])

7

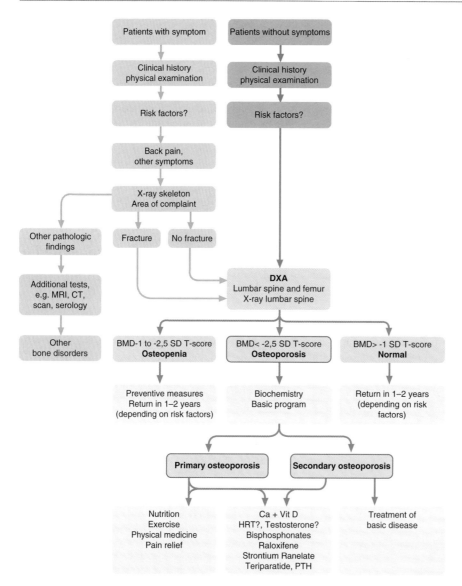

Fig. 7.10. Algorithm for diagnostic investigation and treatment of osteoporosis

Bone density measurement by DXA is currently the only reliable method to document the effects of therapy on osteoporosis ("*monitoring*"). Decrease in the incidence of fractures is another. Moreover, annual BMD measurements increase the patient's compliance (although this is now less of a problem). Clinical trials have documented significant increases in bone density under therapy with bisphosphonates after 3 months in the vertebrae and 1-year in the hips. Bi-annual measurements should be carried out in high-risk patients, for example those on corticoid therapy or patients with rapid bone loss (as indicated by biochemical parameters).

It should be noted that combinations of risk factors with an imaging technique have also yielded good results, as shown by a study on clinical risk factors

and heel bone ultrasound in a cohort of 12,958 elderly women. Results of initial studies on early prediction of fracture risk by using parameters of bone quality including micro-computed tomography (muCT) were more effective than DXA, and therefore also better as indicators for primary prevention of osteoporosis.

7.5
Bone Densitometry in Children – Now Readily Available!

So far little attention has been paid to the analysis of bone mass during growth. Four current techniques are now employed in paediatrics:

- The most widely used: DXA
- The most versatile: QCT
- The newest: QUS
- Under investigation: high-resolution magnetic resonance (hrMR)

The preferred sites for scanning include the lumbar spine, hip, and whole body as well as peripheral sites such as the forearm and hand. The radiation dose is extremely low, approximately 1 μSv for lumbar spine and 4 μSv for whole skeleton scans. In children, the precision ranges from 1–2.5% in most studies. Although various manufacturers have developed special software to be used in paediatrics, this software requires longer scanning time, making cooperation from children difficult. Correct positioning is also of the utmost importance in scanning children. Recently, leading manufacturers have proposed standardized software for measurements of the lumbar spine. The low costs, availability and ease of use are the main advantages of DXA. With respect to QUS, SOS values have been obtained at the calcaneus, patella and phalanges of the thumb, whereas BUA values in children are mainly obtained at the calcaneus. These measurements seem to be correlated more with bone size than with changes in the amount, density or geometry of bone. Local applications of these methods have also been used to assess bone strength in relation to muscle function in

teenagers. Another combination is the investigation of bone mineral density distribution (BMD) together with an imaging technique which can give insights into the structure–function relation of the bone matrix and is used for fracture risk assessment as well as for monitoring after therapy. This technique is also informative in osteogenesis imperfecta.

7.6
BMD Measurement – Not a Scary Procedure, Nothing to be Afraid of!

Low bone mass is the most important objective predictor of fracture risk and BMD measurement is simple to perform for the patient. Considering that the "natural" exposure to radiation is about 2400 μSv, for example 100 μSv during a transatlantic flight, then the 10 μSv of a DXA measurement is so low that it is the most suitable for monitoring. For comparison, the radiation doses of currently used techniques are listed:
- X-ray, lateral lumbar spine 1000 μSv
- QCT 100 μSv
- DXA PA pencil beam 10 μSv
- DXA PA fan beam 1 μSv
- pQCT 1 μSv
- QUS 0 μSv

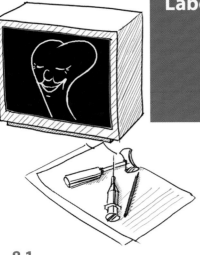

Laboratory Evaluation of Osteoporosis

8

8.1
Recommended Tests

The parameters usually tested in blood and urine are within normal limits in primary osteoporosis in the absence of co-morbidities. The significance of laboratory tests therefore lies mainly in recognizing secondary osteoporoses (Table 8.1). Consequently, the following "basic" laboratory screening tests should be carried out at diagnosis and regularly thereafter:
- Erythrocyte sedimentation rate
- Complete blood count
- Calcium and phosphate (serum)
- Alkaline phosphatase (serum)
- Glucose (serum/urine)
- Transaminases and gamma GT (serum)
- Creatinine (serum)

When the appropriate indications are present:
- T3, T4 and TSH.
- Oestrogen and/or testosterone levels.
- Vitamin D metabolites.
- Vitamin K has recently been introduced as a new biochemical marker.
- Parathormone.
- Protein electrophoresis and immunoelectrophoresis.

It is important to note that 20% of women and up to 64% of men with osteoporosis also suffer from diseases linked to osteoporosis (co-morbidities), hence the importance of the analyses listed above.

In summary, every patient should be investigated according to their personal risk profile as indicated by medical history and lifestyle factors, which determine the appropriate tests and examinations. Subsequent management will depend on the results, i.e. whether or not there is osteopenia/osteoporosis, presence of co-morbidities, current medications etc.

8.2
Significance of Markers of Bone Turnover

The measurements of collagen metabolism (Fig. 8.1) and bone turnover in daily practice are essential for the diagnosis and monitoring of progressive bone diseases such as skeletal metastases or Paget's disease of bone (Table 8.2). However, bone markers cannot be used to diagnose osteoporosis, although they may help to answer some important clinical questions:
- Predicting the future rate of bone loss (high or low bone turnover)
- Predicting the risk of osteoporotic fractures
- Monitoring response to therapy

The metabolites of bone remodelling i.e. of resorption and formation, as well as the products of bone matrix metabolism such as collagen type 1 pass into the blood stream and from there into the urine. These products can be identified biochemically and their levels in blood and urine indicate "high turnover" or "low turnover" osteoporoses (Fig. 8.2). But it should be noted that bone markers do not replace bone density

R. Bartl, B. Frisch, *Osteoporosis*, DOI 10.1007/978-3-540-79527-8_8,
© Springer-Verlag Berlin Heidelberg 2009

Table 8.1. Laboratory tests for the evaluation of secondary osteoporoses

Basic tests	Diseases	Additional tests to include
Complete blood count	Malabsorption	PTH, vitamin D, calcium (S)
		Ferritin, vitamin B12
	Multiple myeloma	Bone marrow biopsy
		Protein electrophoresis (S,U)
	Leukaemia	Blood smear
	Bone metastases	PSA, Ca15-3, CEA
Thyroid-stimulating Hormone (TSH)	Hyperthyroidism	Thyroxine (T4), T3
Glucose (S,U)	Diabetes mellitus	Oral glucose tolerance test
Cortisol (S)	Cushing's syndrome	ACTH, dexamethasone test
	Addison's disease	ACTH
HIV-antibody	AIDS	Infection diagnosis
HLA B-27	Ankylosing spondylitis	CRP
Testosterone in men	Hypogonadism	SHBG, LH, FSH, Prolactin
Calcium (S)	Hyperparathyroidism	PTH
	Malabsorption	Complete blood count
	Morbus Crohn	PTH, vitamin D
	Celiac disease	Alkaline phosphatase, gliadin
	Osteomalacia	PTH, vitamin D
		Alkaline phosphatase
Alkaline phosphatase	Chronic renal failure	PTH, calcium, phosphate (S)
	Osteomalacia	PTH, vitamin D
		Calcium (S)
Protein electrophoresis	Multiple myeloma	Complete blood count
		Bone marrow biopsy
Liver enzymes	Haemochromatosis	Iron, ferritin (S)
	Alcoholic liver disease	
	Primary biliary cirrhosis	Antibodies
Creatinine	Chronic renal failure	PTH, calcium, phosphate (S)
Histamine 24-h U	Mastocytosis	Bone marrow biopsy

measurements for the diagnosis of osteoporosis. However, these markers do provide information about the future risk for bone loss and fragility fractures. Changes in bone formation in response to therapy are relatively slow, starting after some weeks and reaching a plateau after several months, in contrast to bone resorption which decreases rapidly a few days after initiation of antiresorptive therapy with for example a bisphosphonate, and reaches a nadir a few weeks later. These characteristics of bone remodelling must be taken into consideration when evaluating the sig-nificance of the levels of markers of bone remodelling in blood and urine. However, large scale studies have shown that serial evaluation of markers of bone turnover in the serum do identify people at highest risk of bone loss and osteoporosis.

Parameters of bone formation are bone-specific alkaline phosphatase (bone ALP), osteocalcin and osteonectin. These are produced by osteoblasts (possibly also by endothelial cells) and their levels in the peripheral blood reflect osteoblastic activity. ALP is also produced in various tissues including liver and kidney;

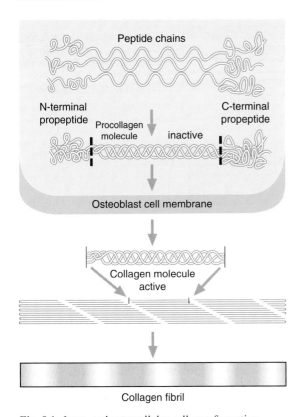

Fig. 8.1. Intra- and extracellular collagen formation

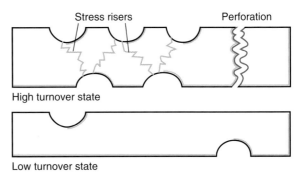

Fig. 8.2. Osteoporotic trabeculae in high- and in low-turnover osteoporosis

however, bone-specific ALP can be distinguished by immunoassays with high specificity. Osteocalcin (OC) shows a diurnal rhythm and only about 50% is released into the circulation, while the remaining 50% is incorporated into hydroxyapatite. OC reflects total bone turnover, i.e. the sum of both resorption and formation. The serum concentrations of the C- and N-terminal propeptides of type I procollagen (PICP and PINC) reflect changes in the synthesis of new collagen, produced by osteoblasts in bone and fibroblasts in other connective tissues. All the PICP and PINC produced are secreted into the circulation.

Parameters of bone resorption: these consist primarily of collagen degradation products such as "cross links" which are released into the blood stream and then excreted into the urine (Fig. 8.3). They appear to predict the risk of hip fracture in elderly women independently of bone density. Studies have shown that women with high levels of markers of bone resorption have about a 1.5- to 3-fold increased risk of hip or non-vertebral fractures. Desoxypyridinoline and cross-link telopeptides of type I collagen are the two markers of resorption most frequently investigated. Telopeptides are distinguished by their terminals: amino- (NTX, Osteomark) and carboxy- (CTX, Crosslaps). Variations in diurnal rhythm and the effect of meals must be taken into account when results of these tests are evalu-

Table 8.2. Biochemical markers of bone turnover

Bone resorption	Bone formation
Blood:	**Blood:**
Tartrate-resistant acid phosphatase (TRAP)	Total or bone-specific alkaline phosphatase
Free pyridinoline or deoxypyridinoline	Osteocalcin
N- or C-telopeptide of type I collagen	Procollagen I C-and N-terminal extension peptides
Cross-links	Osteocalcin
Urine:	
Fasting urine calcium-to-creatinine ratio	
Pyridinoline and Deoxypyridinoline	
Glycosides of hydroxylysine	
Pyridinoline and deoxypyridinoline	
N- and C-telopeptides of type I collagen	

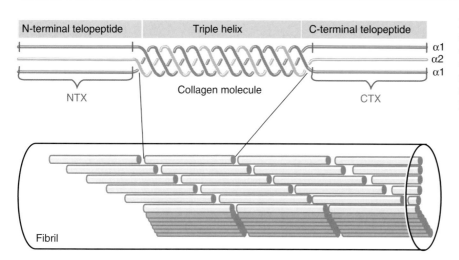

Fig. 8.3. Molecular structure and organisation of collagen into fibrils. Note position of end terminals CTX and NTX, used as biochemical markers of collagen break-down products in the serum

ated. Both NTX and CTX show a significant response to antiresorptive therapy and are currently considered to be the most reliable parameters of bone resorption. However, serum NTX concentrations are elevated in chronic renal failure and, of course, this must be taken into account, i.e. by investigation of renal function.

Bone sialoprotein (BSP) also appears to be a sensitive marker of bone turnover. Furthermore, BSP is thought to play an important role in attraction and growth of tumour cells in the bone marrow, e.g. in multiple myeloma and breast cancer metastases.

Hydroxyproline should no longer be used as a marker of bone metabolism because of its lack of specificity. Its level in the urine is influenced by the breakdown of collagen in sites other than the skeleton, as well as by dietary intake of collagen.

Excretion of *calcium* in a 24-h urinary specimen is also not an accurate reflection of bone resorption, since it depends on the renal threshold for calcium reabsorption and dietary calcium intake.

Results of bone markers prior to starting a treatment are not useful predictors of treatment response. It is also not clear whether patients with high bone turnover are more likely to gain bone under therapy. Some studies have demonstrated that patients with the largest decreases in markers of bone resorption during treatment with alendronate tend to have the greatest increases in bone mineral density (BMD). Nevertheless, changes in markers during treatment must be interpreted with caution. The results of each patient must be compared with the *"least significant change"* (LSC) (Fig. 8.4). The LSC is the minimum change that must be seen in an individual patient to be at least 95% sure that

the change is "real" and not caused by biological or laboratory variations. The LSC is about 25% for most formation markers and 40–65% for most resorption markers. About 65% of patients treated with oestrogen or bisphosphonates have changes in bone resorption markers that are greater than the LSC. In contrast, raloxifene and calcitonin are associated with smaller changes in these markers. However, patients may benefit from a decrease in risk of fractures even if they do not have reductions in bone markers or improvements in bone density. In these cases with little or no change while on antiresorptive medication, it is important to check carefully whether:

- The patient is taking the medication
- The patient is taking the drug as prescribed
- There are secondary causes of osteoporosis

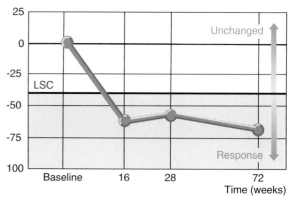

Fig. 8.4. Response of bone markers to antiresorptive agents. A decrease below the least significant change (*LSC*) is regarded as statistically significant

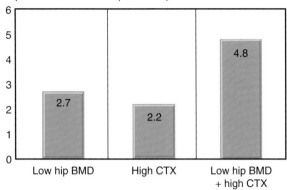

Hip fracture relative risk (odds ratio)

Fig. 8.5. The combination of a low hip bone mineral density (*BMD*) and a high serum CTX have a greater predictive value than either low hip BMD or high serum CTX alone (modified from Garnero et al. [1996])

The advantage of monitoring treatment with markers is that changes in levels can be observed within weeks of starting therapy, and evidence of its efficacy is psychologically important at a time when patients are most likely to discontinue their medications (Fig. 8.5). It is necessary to emphasize that the specimens for investigation should always be taken at about the same time of day and with the patient fasting. Furthermore, indices of bone turnover may show seasonal and circadian variations.

8.3
Recommendations for Practical Use of Bone Markers

When using bone markers one should keep in mind that:
- They are not unique to bone
- They may reflect both formation and resorption
- They are influenced also by non-skeletal diseases

When using bone markers in the monitoring of anti-resorptive therapy:
- Always compare the same marker
- Use only markers validated for assessing bone resorption/formation
- Collect the samples at the same time (8.00–10.00), if necessary after an overnight fast
- Keep reasonable intervals between the controls (about 3–6 months)

- Use cutoff values to identify responders (-30% for urinary DPD, -65% for urinary NTX and CTX, -40% for serum bone-specific AP).

8.4
Potential of Bone Biopsy in Clinical Practice

Many clinicians still maintain that clinical history and examination combined with a biochemical profile, radiology and a bone scan provide sufficient information in most cases to make the diagnosis of osteoporosis. However, the limitations of the radiologic and densitometric examinations in this disorder have been described in detail above and are well known and apply to both primary and secondary osteoporoses. It is therefore reasonable to take a bone biopsy (Fig. 8.6) under the following circumstances:
- When the diagnosis is in doubt
- When confirmation of a specific process is sought, for example metastases (Fig. 8.7), multiple myeloma, systemic mastocytosis, among other possibilities
- When further categorization is required for therapeutic decisions (e.g. different subtypes of renal osteopathy)
- When follow-up of a specific process is necessary, as after therapy for osteomalacia or metastases

Moreover, the unique attraction of a bone biopsy is that it allows direct visualization of both cortical and

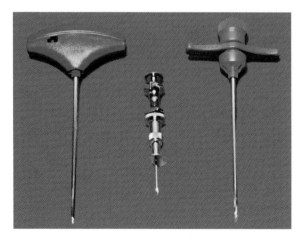

Fig. 8.6. Different manual trephines for bone biopsy and aspiration of bone marrow

8

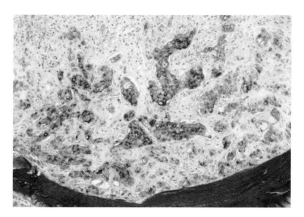

Fig. 8.7. Extensive metastatic invasion of bone/marrow in a patient with metastatic breast cancer. Immunohistology

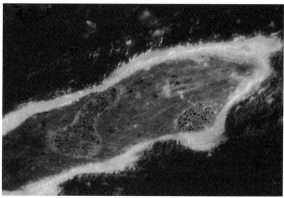

Fig. 8.9. Tetracycline labeling of mineralization in osteoid layer. Plastic section

trabecular bone and the bone cells, as well as the bone marrow and its constituents: haematopoiesis, mesenchyme and adipose tissue. In addition, when the biopsy has been embedded in plastic, the histologic sections permit reliable identification of both calcified bone and osteoid (Fig. 8.8), enabling quantification of various morphologic parameters, i.e. "histomorphometry". These measurements reflect the amount and "metabolic state" of the bone and its cells by providing information on both osteoclastic resorption and osteoblastic formation of bone. Finally the dynamics of the formation of osteoid and its calcification can be studied by double-labeling with tetracycline (Fig. 8.9).

To summarise: although bone histomorphometry has contributed little to the diagnosis of osteoporosis, it has provided unique information on the heterogeneity of bone cell behaviour in osteoporosis, i.e. low turnover versus high turnover states. In addition, analysis at the level of the basic bone remodelling unit, and possibly minimodelling of the trabecular bone, permits a more critical choice of therapeutic regimens in individual cases. In the future, there may well be more

widespread use of bone biopsies for the immunohistochemical demonstration of osteotropic factors and their receptors on bone cells.

8.5 When is a Bone Biopsy Indicated?

Before dealing with this question, it should be clearly stated that the diagnosis of osteoporosis is based on clinical findings and bone density measurements. In addition, it should be pointed out that normal bone histology in an iliac crest biopsy does not exclude osteoporosis elsewhere, for example in the axial skeleton. Nevertheless, a bone biopsy is sometimes required for the investigation of other bone disorders.

Obtaining a bone biopsy nowadays is a relatively simple procedure and nearly always without complications. The vast majority of bone biopsies are taken from the posterior iliac crest with an 8-gauge manual trephine (3-mm width). This needle technique is less invasive, can be performed relatively easily and is particularly suitable for outpatients. Manual anterior transilial trephines are recommended when detailed histomorphometric measurements of bone are necessary, but at the cost of greater invasiveness and rate of complications. There are a number of new improved biopsy needles available, as well as up-to-date techniques for processing bone biopsies from fixation and embedding to histology and immunohistology. These methods provide optimal biopsy sections for evaluation of the overall structure of the cortex and the trabecular network, demonstration of the bone cells and

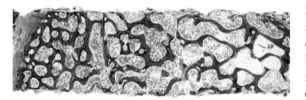

Fig. 8.8. Semi-thin section of a biopsy revealing increased extent of osteoid and dissecting osteoclasia in a patient with renal osteopathy. Ladewig

their activities in remodelling, distinction between and quantification of osteoid and calcified bone and, last but not least, state of the bone marrow – from the proportion of adipose tissue to haematopoiesis and mesenchyme, to the visualization of all the stages of differentiation of the haematopoietic cell lineages. In clinical trials any of these parameters can be evaluated quantitatively by histomorphometry. Quantitative histology of bone comprises four main types of primary measurement: surface, volume, thickness and number. Other more sophisticated parameters can be derived from combinations of these primary variables.

Bone biopsies are indicated in the investigation of secondary osteoporoses; in these conditions they frequently provide essential information. When a disturbance of mineralization is suspected, histologic evidence of undecalcified bone can be obtained by means of bone biopsies. In renal osteodystrophy (ROD) bone biopsies provide essential information required to determine the type and severity of ROD. Parathyroid hormone (PTH) levels in serum, though widely used, are not necessarily predictive of the underlying bone disease, which can, however, be readily assessed by bone biopsy. In addition, an estimation of the histologic aspects of bone and its cells enables a correlation with the measurable parameters of bone remodelling and age. Disorders of the bone marrow and suspected metastatic processes are additional indications.

To summarise, a bone biopsy is no longer necessary for the demonstration of uncomplicated bone loss in primary osteoporosis; it has been replaced by the non-invasive BMD measurements. However, when other underlying causes are suspected or established, a bone biopsy may provide essential information. Finally, in trials on the therapeutic efficacy of specific, possibly newly developed drugs, the data in a bone biopsy may be necessary for comprehensive evaluation. In this connection, a novel method of tetracycline labelling allows longitudinal (i.e. sequential) evaluation of short-term effects of hPTH therapy, for example over 1-month, on bone formation in a single bone biopsy. It has also been postulated that improvements in trabecular micro-architecture, as seen in iliac crest biopsies, can be correlated with increases in BMD in patients on teriparatide therapy. In contrast, a comprehensive histological analysis can also be applied to analyse adverse effects of, for example alcohol or drugs as well as beneficial effects of antiresorptive and osteo-anabolic therapies.

8.6
Up-to-Date Methods

The first decade of the 21st century has witnessed an out-pouring of results from investigations on osteoporosis, in all its different forms, using the latest technologies. In addition, various combinations of methods have been applied to address specific questions, aims and hypotheses in the investigation of pathogenic mechanisms, physiological processes, and diagnostic aspects of both primary and secondary osteoporoses.

Refinements in methodology have contributed to investigation of undecalcified bone, immunocytochemical characterization of bone cells, as well as fluorescent in situ hybridization (FISH) for cytogenetic anomalies, demonstration of the composition of bone and bone matrix, as well as the structure and micro-architecture of both cortical bone and networks of trabecular bone from the macroscopic and microscopic to the nanoscale, at which level interactions of mineral crystals and collagen fibrils and their influence on bone quality are investigated. Importantly, non-invasive in vivo assessment of the micro-architecture of bone is now possible and available. These techniques include *high resolution magnetic resonance imaging* (MRI), which involves no contrast or ionizing radiation and can be carried out at various anatomic sites. *Quantitative micro-MRI* (muMRI) is particularly informative with regard to trabecular structure, for example demonstration of the conversion of trabecular plates to rods and their subsequent disconnection from the nodules.

Micro-damage in bone can now also be detected by *micro-computed tomography* (micro-CT). The latest non-invasive technique for the in vivo estimation of induced damage accumulation in bone is *non-linear resonant ultrasound spectroscopy* (NRUS). In contrast, a combination utilizing bulk staining together with *confocal laser scanning microscopy* (CLSM) has been used for distinguishing newly formed bone around ceramic implant material.

Briefly stated, application of such techniques is contributing to the assessment of risk for fracture, efficacy of interventions, and preventive therapy. Methods for the assessment of precision in BMD measurements and monitoring have also been recommended. It should also be mentioned that various techniques have now been developed and applied to address specific questions, aims and hypotheses, improve understanding and detection of specific aspects of bone fragility and fracture-healing. To give a few examples:

- Application of large panels of *immunocytochemical markers* to detect antigenic determinants of target cells.
- Various *biochemical markers of bone turnover* to clarify pre-clinical models of osteoporosis.
- Development of *non-linear ultrasound techniques* for characterization of in vivo bone damage in cortical and trabecular bone.
- *Micro-CT* of trabecular architecture to assess role of microdamage formation such as the length and density of micro-cracks. Also, micro-CT of fatigue micro-damage in cortical bone, using a barium sulphate contrast agent to investigate the role of micro-damage in bone fragility.
- Utilization of *scanning transmission microscopy*, conventional and high resolution electron microscopy (TEM & HRTEM), as well as X-ray dispersive spectroscopy to evaluate bone composition and processes of dissolution, formation and remineralization of bone, as well as comparison of normal bones with abnormal ones.
- Sequential application of *quantitative ultrasound "Speed of Sound"* (SOS) to clarify biological mechanisms in skeletal structure, development and function.
- Phalangeal quantitative ultrasound can also be used for screening of postmenopausal women with a high risk of fracture.

- Use of recently clarified *biochemical markers* for diagnostic evaluation of osteoporosis, i.e. value of IGF-1 as an early marker for osteopenia or osteoporosis, and serum levels of free RANKL and total RANKL/osteoprotegerin complexes in relation to age and gender.
- Preparation of *osteocytic RNA* from frozen bone for the characterization of the in vivo physiology of osteocytes by functional genomics.
- In vitro studies of bone strength such as effects of bending to assess the part played by elastic and material properties in bone strength.
- Serum levels of IGF-1 to identify young women at risk for osteopenia/osteoporosis.
- Investigation of bone quality by nano-indentation, a technique that evaluates the mechanical properties of the matrix and can be carried out on very small samples of tissue.
- Comparison of levels of aromatase-RNA in bone samples of patients with hip fractures and with osteoarthritis, and possibly other disorders of bone.
- Detailed method for RNA extraction and analysis after therapy with teriparatide.
- 18F-fluoride PET demonstration of regional changes in parameters of bone metabolism in response to therapy.
- Finally, an example from a practical therapeutic point of view, application of *conebeam CT imaging* (CBCT) for the detection and treatment of spinal metastases.

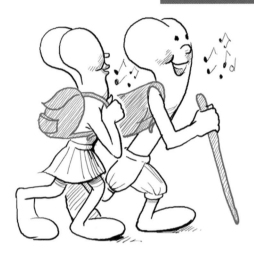

Maintaining healthy bones and thereby avoiding osteoporotic fractures can be achieved by the institution of, and adherence to, a specific *plan of action*, a programme of ten specific steps for the prevention of loss and maintenance of the structural and functional integrity of the bones. These *self-help measures* are specifically intended for people who do not have osteoporosis, because their implementation unequivocally reduces the risk of developing the disease. But there is one absolute condition for success of the plan (a sine qua non!): the individual person must have the willpower to start and the perseverance to continue!

Two goals for the 21st century:

- For the whole population – the quality of life must go up!
- For the authorities – the cost of health care must go down!

Note that the second is the consequence of the implementation of the first!

9.1
Step 1: First of all a Calcium-Rich Diet!

Calcium is the most important mineral for the prevention and treatment of osteoporosis (Table 9.1). An adult has over 1 kg of calcium in the body, 99% of which is in the skeleton. A fifth of total bone mass is calcium.

- Prevention of osteoporosis begins in *childhood*. M. Drugay defined osteoporosis as a "paediatric disease with geriatric consequences". As the skeleton develops and grows, a calcium-rich diet provides the building blocks required to attain a peak bone mass at about 25 years. During this period, children and young people need about four times as much calcium as adults per kilogram of body weight, which means that 500–5000 mg of calcium should be ingested daily, depending on age.
- Even weight conscious *teenagers* can achieve this goal by means of a calcium-rich, fat-poor diet composed mainly of low-fat milk, cheese and yogurt, bread and calcium-rich drinks such as fruit juice. Just one large cup of yogurt provides nearly a third of their daily calcium requirement. The early to mid teens are a critical time in bone formation, as demonstrated in one clinical trial which found that by the age of 16 young women had already reached about 95% of their mothers' premenopausal bone density.
- The requirement for calcium is particularly high during *pregnancy* and *lactation*, totalling about 1200–1500 mg a day.

R. Bartl, B. Frisch, *Osteoporosis*, DOI 10.1007/978-3-540-79527-8_9,
© Springer-Verlag Berlin Heidelberg 2009

9

Table 9.1. Suggested calcium intakes

Age groups		Amount mg/day
Infants		
	0–6 months	210
	6–12 months	270
Children		
	1–3 years	500
	4–8 years	800
	9–18 years	1500
Adults		
	19–50 years	1200
	51 years and older	1500
	Pregnant and lactating women	1500

Table 9.2. Major dietary sources of calcium (approximate values)

Nutrient	Calcium mg/100g
Primary food sources of calcium	
Milk, whole	111
Milk, skimmed	124
Yoghurt	134
Cheese	600–1000
Ice cream	120
Secondary food sources of calcium	
Beans	65
Nuts	75
Almonds	250
Salmon, canned with bones	200
Sardines, canned with bones	300
Broccoli, cooked	130
Spinach, cooked	160
Rhubarb, cooked	300
Kale, cooked	200
Parsley	100

- It is not too late to start a bone-conscious diet even after the *menopause*, especially since there is a dramatic increase in bone loss at this time. Clinical trials have demonstrated that 80% of postmenopausal women require more than 800 mg calcium daily in food, but during the perimenopausal period of increased resorption, the daily intake should be 1500 mg to prevent the drastic increase in bone loss. In other words, preventive measures should be instituted before cessation of ovarian function and continued thereafter.
- Likewise, calcium intake should be adjusted to the decline in male sex hormones – the andropause – and continued indefinitely, as one of the preventive measures for involutional osteoporosis.
- Recommendations for appropriate amounts of calcium, vitamin D and the other nutrients required for healthy bones are frequently included in overall dietary protocols (see for example the WHO report in 2003 for prevention of osteoporosis, as well as national reports published by official agencies of various countries).

Sufficient calcium can be obtained by means of a "*bone-friendly*" diet (Table 9.2):
- *Milk and milk products* are rich in calcium, especially low-fat milk and hard cheeses. The harder the cheese, the more calcium it contains. Soft cheeses also frequently have supplementary calcium. Low fat cheeses are especially recommended. Moreover, lactose in milk facilitates absorption of calcium by the gut. Some people avoid milk and dairy products because of several misconceptions, for example: Milk makes you fat! It weakens bone! It causes allergies! It is full of antibiotics and hormones! Unfortunately, these people are depriving themselves of foods that provide important nutrients, especially calcium.
- *Fresh green vegetables, fruits and wheat products* are important sources of calcium. However, it should be pointed out that oxalate in some vegetables inhibits its absorption. Wheat products are also good sources of calcium except for white bread and some other processed varieties. Likewise, addition of sugar, salt, phosphate, fat and protein can substantially decrease calcium absorption (see below).
- *Mineral water*: This can contribute to a positive calcium balance when the water is enriched with calcium. But the amount in each type of mineral water varies and may range from 10 to 650 mg/l. The exact amount is always stated in the label on the bottle.
- *Fruit juices*: These are particularly useful for patients with allergies to milk or milk products, especially if the juices have been fortified by the addition

of calcium. Moreover, the vitamin D in the fruit juice increases absorption of calcium from 30 % (milk and milk products) to 40 %. The addition of vitamin D to various food products may further increase intestinal absorption of calcium.

Calcium tablets: Additional calcium in the form of tablets should only be taken on medical advice. There are some dangers if excessive amounts of calcium are taken, including the possibility of kidney stones and adverse cardiovascular events; the results of studies published so far have not reached definitive conclusions but do flag cardiac health as an area of concern in relation to excessive calcium intake. Calcium carbonate is the least expensive and most commonly used compound, but only some 200 mg calcium is absorbed when a tablet containing 500 mg calcium carbonate is taken. Calcium citrate has been found to dissolve more easily than carbonate, phosphate, lactate or gluconate, and has about 60 % more bioavailability in the body. While calcium carbonate and calcium phosphate must be taken with food, because gastric acid is required for absorption, calcium citrate can be taken with or without food. It also has the advantage of not producing gas or causing constipation but it is more expensive. The following hints may help to get the maximum benefit from calcium tablets:

- A single dose should not exceed 500 mg, so the daily amount should be taken in divided doses as necessary, with sufficient fluid.
- One dose before bedtime makes up for withdrawal of calcium from bone during the night.
- Calcium should be taken with meals. Absorption in the gut is also improved by vitamin C as well as a little fat and protein together with the tablets.
- Absorption is inhibited by foods rich in fibre and fat.
- Calcium should not be taken together with iron as these combine to form insoluble compounds and so are lost to the body. This is important for patients taking iron supplements.

Other useful minerals: Numerous minerals necessary for the absorption of calcium and other activities include magnesium, boron, copper, manganese, zinc, silicon, strontium, fluoride and phosphorus. They are also essential for normal growth of bones and play an important role in bone metabolism and turnover. The best way to ensure the correct balance is through a variety of foods, as these minerals may be dangerous if taken in excessively large amounts. *Magnesium* in particular is essential for bone health; below is a summary of its actions:

- Activates osteoblasts
- Increases mineralization density
- Activates vitamin D
- Enhances sensitivity of bone tissue to PTH and active vitamin D
- Facilitates the transport of calcium in and out of bone
- Is highly effective for the prevention of painful muscle cramps

About 60 % of magnesium is stored in bone, the rest in muscles and other tissues. The recommended dosages are 300–500 mg daily, with an appropriate calcium/magnesium ratio of 2:1. Since high single doses of magnesium may cause diarrhoea, it is best to distribute the total amount throughout the day. However, there is little evidence that magnesium is needed to prevent osteoporosis in the general population.

Taking the above recommendations into consideration must be done with adequate attention to age, especially the young and the old, because of their different physiological functions and therefore also nutrient requirements. Moreover, interactions between race/ethnicity and diet have also been demonstrated in studies of areal bone density in different populations, e.g. African, Hispanic and Asian Americans, as well as American White populations and Chinese Americans. However, there are still ongoing studies regarding interactions between race and diet and results are awaited.

9.2
Step 2: Ensure an Adequate Supply of Vitamins!

Vitamin D promotes bone formation by improving intestinal absorption of calcium and phosphate and by stimulating maturation and mineralization of osteoid – the ground substance of bone. A daily allowance of 400–800 IU is required for healthy bone. A daily 15-min sunbath would be required for an individual to produce an equal quantity of vitamin D by way of the skin. But this is not a practical option for the

9

majority of people under today's living conditions. In addition, there is the fear of skin cancer caused by over-exposure to the sun. Moreover, the conversion of sunlight into vitamin D in older people is only half that of younger people. Consequently, a daily intake of 800–1000 IU of vitamin D in the form of tablets with meals is reasonable and cost-effective. Different segments in any population may have inadequate intakes of vitamin D and recent investigations have emphasized that hypovitaminosis D can be considered a widespread epidemic, regardless of geographical location at all ages and in both sexes. Therefore, take heed and take the supplements, and don't join the deprived populations!

Vitamin C, another relatively new player in bone health, is required for maturation of collagen (cross-linking), it stimulates the osteoblasts and improves absorption of calcium. An intake of 60 mg vitamin C is the minimal daily requirement – enough to prevent scurvy – but not enough to reap all the possible benefits. The best sources are citrus fruits. Ideally, 1000 mg should be taken daily as calcium ascorbate. Epidemiologic studies have shown a positive association between vitamin C and bone mass. There is also a connection between vitamin C and immunology, as shown by its beneficial effects in infections such as the common cold.

Vitamin K is now recognized as a "new" bone-building vitamin. Though better known for its part in co-agulation, it plays a significant role in the synthesis of osteocalcin, one of the building blocks of bone. Vitamin K mediates the attachment of calcium to proteins for their incorporation into hydroxyapatite crystals in bone matrix formation. Vitamin K is also required for fracture healing. Observational studies have shown that women with high intake and serum levels of vitamin K tend to have high bone densities, and patients who sustain fractures have been reported to have low serum vitamin K levels. Between 100 and 300 μg of vitamin K are required daily, taken with meals. It is produced by bacteria normally found in the intestinal tract (mena-quinone). Dark green vegetables (e.g. spinach or broccoli) also contain large amounts of vitamin K (phyllo-quinone). Since this is a fat-soluble vitamin, it is helpful to consume vitamin K-rich foods with a little fat or oil.

Vitamin A is a fat-soluble vitamin and so can be stored by the body. It influences the development of bone cells. The recommended daily allowance is 5000 IU.

Vitamin B$_{12}$ and folic acid are necessary for formation as well as maintenance of healthy bones. Vitamin B$_{12}$ protects the bones against the effects of homocysteine, the levels of which decrease with age. The recommended daily dose of vitamin B$_{12}$ is 1 mg.

Other elements, such as boron, are also important for bone health, and they require a well balanced diet, rich in fruits and vegetables.

The significance of proteins and the quality of the proteins ingested should also not be overlooked, as these are essential for good quality bones.

9.3
Step 3: Protect the Spine in Everyday Life!

Thoracic and lumbar vertebrae are composed largely of cancellous bone and are therefore highly susceptible to fracture – caused by the combined effects of a reduction in trabecular bone without a decrease in weight-bearing. Osteoporosis usually induces collapse of the upper and lower plates of the vertebrae and their protrusion into the vertebral bodies. When the bone mineral density (BMD) shows osteoporotic values, everyday life should be adapted to ensure protection for the spine and hip joints (Figs. 9.1 and 9.2; Table 9.3):

- *Activity while upright*: upright posture in front of a working surface adapted to the height of the worker.
- *Activity while sitting*: The back of the chair should provide support for the spine from 15 to 12 cm above the seat of the chair. The spine should not be curved (danger of wedge fractures!). One should never stay in the sitting position for long, but rather get up, stretch and move around every now and then.
- *Load lifting and carrying*: Do not bend down with a curved back and straight legs! This may damage the lumbar discs and cause vertebral body compression. Instead, bend the knees, lift up the load and rise up keeping the spine straight. This applies especially to heavy objects such as crates of drinks.
- *Housework*: During the daily performance of household activities, bending or curving the spine should be avoided; it is better to go down on one's knees or to crouch.
- *Lying down and sleeping*: Soft mattresses should be avoided, but a flexible mattress on a hard frame is

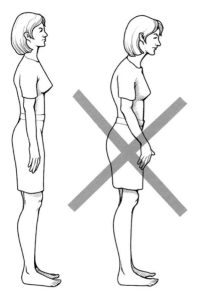

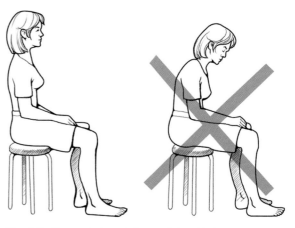

Fig. 9.2. Proper sitting: sitting upright with feet on the floor reduces stress on the spine

Fig. 9.1. Upright posture: head held high, shoulders back and tummy pulled in, together assure proper alignment and good posture

recommended as it gives equal support to the whole body. Also recommended is a small flat pillow, just to provide support for the head and neck.

9.4
Step 4: Regular Physical Activity – for the Preservation of Strong Bones!

With ageing there is a continuous and significant reduction in axial muscle strength. Men lose as much as 64% and women as much as 50% of the peak muscle strength in the fourth decade to the lowest muscle strength in the ninth decade. Bone, muscles and joints are all strengthened by movement. Exercise also has the benefit of improving flexibility and balance, and therefore has a positive effect, i.e. a decrease in the number of falls and fractures in the elderly.

The theory that putting stress or forces of gravity onto the skeletal system causes it to form more bone is known as *Wolff's law*. Physical fitness ensures confidence both in locomotion and coordination. Physical activity stimulates blood flow and stabilizes blood pressure which in turn decreases attacks of dizziness in older people, a common cause of falling. In the event of a fracture, anybody who exercises regularly will have shorter periods of pain and recovery. Training and ex-

ercise should be regular rather than irregular and then exaggerated. Comparative studies have shown that women who walk daily for half an hour have stronger bones than those who do not. The relationship between mechanical loading and bone strength is curvilinear, with a much steeper slope at very low levels of loading (complete immobility, weightlessness or spinal cord injury). Immobilized patients may lose 40% of their initial bone mass within a year. Studies have shown that standing upright for as little as 30 min each day prevents bone loss. However, increasing the level of exercise of active people results in very small gains in bone (about 1% per year) (Fig. 9.3). In postmenopausal women, the lumbar spine BMD increased by 1.3% per year for impact programs and 1% per year for non-impact programs. Femoral neck BMD increased 0.5% per year to 1.4% per year in the impact and non-impact groups. In premenopausal women, there was no difference in femoral neck BMD between exercise and control groups. A meta-analysis of fall prevention trials found a modest but significant reduction in the risk of falling (10%) associated with general exercise. It is worth stressing that the age-related decrease in muscle mass and strength (sarcopenia) can be modified by exercise and calorie restriction (if the intake is above the recommended amount).

The optimal exercise regimen for preventing osteoporosis and related fractures is not known. A recent Swedish study of randomly selected elderly women could not confirm an effect of previous and present everyday physical activity on bone mass. However, any exercise is better than none, and consistent

Table 9.3. Guidelines for safe movement for osteoporotic patients

- Proper posture and alignment when standing, sitting or walking: lift breastbone, keep head erect, look forward, keep shoulders back, gently tighten abdominal muscles, maintain small hollow in the lower back
- Standing for a long time: point feet straight ahead, periodically switch from one foot to the other
- Sitting: use a pillow at the small of the back, maintain upright alignment, rest feet flat on the floor or on a small footstool. Sit on chairs with backs, not on stools
- Standing from a chair: move hips forward to front of the chair, shift weight over the feet leading with a lifted chest, stand by pushing down into the floor using leg muscles, the arm muscles can assist by pushing down on arm rests of the chair
- Walking: hold chin in and head upright, point feet straight ahead
- Bending: keep feet shoulder width apart, maintain straight back, bend at the hips and knees (not at the waist), avoid twisting and bending together, use one hand on a stable support devise
- Lifting: keep object close to the body, first kneel on one knee and stand with the object close to the waist, use lightly packed plastic grocery packages with handles and carry one in each hand. Following acute vertebral fracture, limit weight to 4.5 kg
- Tying shoes: first, sit in a chair, cross one foot over the opposite knee or rest one foot on a stool
- Getting in and out of bed: in – sit on the edge of the bed, lean trunk towards head of bed and lower body down with the help of one arm, while lowering trunk to the bed, bring legs and feet on to the bed, roll on to the back with knees bent; reverse for getting out of bed
- Coughing and sneezing: gently tighten abdominal muscles to support back, and place one hand on the back, or press back into chair or wall for support

From "Boning up on osteoporosis: a guide to prevention and treatment". National Osteoporosis Foundation 2003, Washington DC

activity is associated with the greatest long-term benefit. Indeed, current or past activity is associated with a 20–60 % reduction in the rate of hip fractures in both women and men. Weight-bearing exercises, those which counteract the force of gravity, such as climbing mountains or stairs (instead of taking the elevator) and walking, running and jumping are the most effective in strengthening the bones. Take the car or the bus only when absolutely necessary! More-

over, regular sport – in one form or another – improves quality of life. But it must be stated that if the person concerned does not enjoy a particular activity it will not be carried out regularly – if at all – and therefore the exercise, sport or activity chosen must be in tune with the patients' wishes and abilities. In addition, it is advisable to choose a sport or activity which involves as many muscle groups as possible, as well as not causing physical complaints and pain. Today sport-oriented institutions and clubs offer a whole variety of activities in a friendly and social environment. There are no age limits. For the sedentary or frail elderly, a program of walking, low-impact aerobics or possibly light gardening, in addition to muscle strengthening programs are recommended. Training-induced gains in strength are initially rapid but tend to plateau after more than 12 weeks, even with progressive increases in training loads. When correlating mechanical load with bone mass, there is greater gain in bone mass when starting at the lowest levels of activity (complete immobility to sedentary) than at the higher levels from moderately active to walking with high impact loading. Tai chi may have beneficial effects on balance, prevention of falls and non-vertebral fractures, but there is no convincing evidence for any influence on the prevention or treatment of osteoporosis.

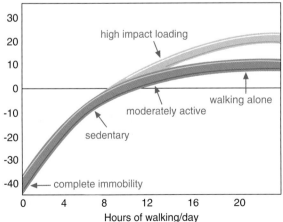

Fig. 9.3. Relationship between mechanical loading and bone mass. There is a greater gain in bone density at the lowest levels of activity than at the highest

Although exercise is usually considered with respect to muscles and bones, it also has a beneficial effect on a wide range of diseases associated with increased reactive oxygen species (ROS), which in turn may be related to osteoporosis. The diseases include: cardiac conditions, type 2 diabetes, rheumatoid arthritis, Alzheimer's and Parkinson's diseases, and various cancers. It would appear that exercise strengthens the body's resistance to certain types of diseases.

It has been shown that in *childhood and adolescence* bone responds more favourably to mechanical loading than at other ages, presumably because this is part of the period in which active growth takes place. A study of female tennis players showed that when training was started before the menarche, differences in bone mineral density in the humerus ranged from 17 to 24 % compared to 8–14 % when training began after menarche. In 15- to 20-year-old Olympic weightlifters, the mean distal and proximal forearm BMD was 51 and 41 % above that of the age-matched controls, respectively. Swimming, on the other hand, did not increase bone mass as measured by dual energy X-ray absorptiometry (DXA). Although elite swimmers undertake intense training programs, their BMD is similar to that of control subjects; clearly this is because the water supports the weight of the body. There is some evidence that higher levels of bone mass and density attained in childhood are maintained in gymnasts, but whether childhood physical activity influences the rate or timing of adult bone loss is not known. It should be pointed out that there is a peak fracture incidence in young people: 10–14 years in girls and 15–19 years in boys. These fractures are not related to osteoporosis, but are the result of falls or trauma sustained during intense physical activity – possibly "extreme sports" and the fractures occur in completely healthy, well-nourished young people with no deficiencies whatsoever. With the right therapeutic care and management, healing and "restitutio ad integrum" are also rapid.

More attention must be devoted to the role of exercise for *osteoporotic patients* or those who have already sustained fractures. Studies have shown that the rehabilitation of patients after hip fractures, for example, is frequently inadequate. Usually these patients show reluctance to participate in an exercise program because they may have pain or fear of additional fractures. This attitude must be overcome, in order to facilitate the patient's recovery and to prevent additional complications. Moreover, avoidance of any activity

will further aggravate bone loss. Bed-bound bones rapidly lose bone mass, and a bed-rest study showed that trabecular bone was lost at a rate of about 1 % per week and cortical bone at a rate of about 1 % per month. Restoration of bone mass is much slower than bone loss: about 1 % per month for trabecular bone. An exercise program should increase the ability to carry out routine daily activities while minimizing the risk of falls or subsequent fractures. Patients with vertebral fractures should avoid activities that place an anterior load on vertebral bodies, such as back flexion exercise. However, studies have shown that significantly fewer refractures occur in patients who practice back-extensor strengthening exercises. When advising patients with osteoarthritis or associated conditions, patients who have been previously sedentary and frail elderly patients, physicians should consider referring the patients to physical therapists to start with a moderate exercise program and for instruction in proper exercise techniques. Patients with cardiovascular diseases require cardiologic consultation for risk evaluation before starting an exercise program.

To summarize, exercise is potentially crucial for the prevention and reduction of osseous fragility in later life. The favourable effects of physical activity and exercise on bone strength, and on muscular strength and balance, apparently contribute to the 20–70 % reduced risk of hip fracture among people who engage in regular physical activity, compared to their sedentary counterparts. The positive effects of exercise on falls and fractures have been demonstrated even in osteopenic women, who are already in a high-risk category. Primary prevention of fragility fractures focuses on regular weight-bearing (high impact) activity, starting in childhood and continued throughout life. Management of an elderly individual with low bone mass and increased risk for falling includes lower-impact exercises designed to improve balance, lower limb strength, posture and gait. In this respect, brisk walking, Nordic pole walking, climbing up and down stairs, dancing, modified tennis and adult-age gymnastics can be recommended. Among elderly persons with a high risk for falling, gait-stabilizing devices and external hip protectors are useful additions to the list of measures for the prevention of falls and fractures. Additionally, one should not forget that exercise training has general beneficial effects on health, as demonstrated by the reduction in oxidative stress levels in postmenopausal women. Exercise training also has a positive

9

effect on the actions of hormone replacement therapy (HRT) (even in the small doses given today) in post-menopausal women.

9.5
Step 5: No Smoking, Please!

Every smoker has the power – in the truest sense of the word – to stop smoking and thereby reduce by half the risk of osteoporosis. Smokers have almost double the risk of hip fractures compared to non-smokers. Up to 20% of all hip fractures are attributed to cigarette smoking. Women who smoke a pack a day have 10% less mineral bone density at menopause than non-smokers. Studies have shown that smokers sustain fractures of the vertebral bodies earlier and more frequently than non-smokers, while fracture healing is delayed or prolonged (or both). Smokers also experience menopause 1–2 years earlier than non-smokers.

Smoking produces a number of *effects* harmful to bone:

- Decreases production of oestrogen in women
- Increases breakdown of oestrogen in the liver
- Decreases production of testosterone in men
- Reduces conversion of adrenal androgens to oestrogens
- Damages bone and bone cells by means of many toxic substances
- Decreases blood flow through bone and bone marrow circulations
- Effects pulmonary function and causes decreased uptake of oxygen
- Creates free radicals

Some experts are convinced that the anti-oestrogen effects of smoking are enough to cancel the effects of oestrogen therapy in the menopause. In men, smoking causes a significant reduction in testosterone levels which (as in women) results in decreased mineral bone density, i.e. accelerated loss of bone. This loss occurs primarily in trabecular bone and particularly in the vertebral bodies of the spine. Moreover, smokers harbour a higher concentration of substances harmful to bone: these include cadmium, lead and other toxic substances. It should be noted that, although there are many successful programs and strategies available today to help people stop smoking, no one can succeed without the one crucial requirement – the willpower to do so!

9.6
Step 6: Reduce Nutritional "Bone Robbers"!

These are substances in food that require calcium for their metabolism, neutralization and elimination. These substances are usually not recognized as damaging and therefore not avoided, which enables them to withdraw calcium from bone and thereby increase bone loss unobserved. *Bone robbers* include the following (see also Table 9.4):

High alcohol intake: This inhibits absorption of important building blocks for bone and damages the liver, an organ required for activation of vitamin D. Moreover, manifest hepatic cirrhosis also causes malabsorption by reducing the flow of bile. In addition, alcohol damages the bone cells directly. Many male alcoholics suffer from androgen deficiency, which in turn aggravates osteoporosis. Alcohol also has a negative effect on the immature skeleton. In contrast, small quantities (a drink a day) have been shown to have a beneficial effect on bone in older women.

Caffeine and other potentially harmful drinks: Caffeine acts as a diuretic causing an increased urinary excretion of calcium and magnesium. People with a low calcium intake are especially vulnerable to this loss. It would be prudent to avoid excessive intake >4 cups daily but patients who do not – for one reason or another – limit their consumption of coffee, are advised to drink a glass of milk for each cup of coffee to restore the calcium balance. Phosphate is the culprit in drinks made with cola, because the high content of phosphate binds calcium in the gut and thereby reduces its absorption. Many medicines, including aspirin and other pain relievers, diet aids and diuretics also have caffeine as an ingredient. On the other hand, tea – although also a caffeine-containing drink – is associated with a decrease in femoral neck fractures, possibly because tea contains flavonoids.

Sugar: Consumption of sugar has increased 1000-fold over the past 100 years. Approximately half of the intake of carbohydrates consists of sugar. Furthermore, the metabolism of sugar in the body utilizes vitamins and augments the renal excretion of valuable substances such as calcium, magnesium and other minerals. In addition, sugar also inhibits uptake of calcium in the intestines as well as stimulating the secretion of acids in the stomach – another "bone robber". In particular, the combination of coffee and sugar, as in very sweet black strong coffee or in "soft drinks" such as Coca Cola is a veritable "bone gobbler". Consequently, it is not surprising that healthy teeth and strong bones are characteristic of countries with a low overall consumption of sugar.

Salt: It has long been established that a high intake of salt is associated with an increased risk of high blood pressure and its associated disorders. In contrast to patients with normal blood pressure, hypertensives have a higher loss of calcium in the urine with its attendant risk of osteoporosis. In addition, some people seem to be more sensitive to the effects of salts than others. A sodium intake of less than 2400 mg/day is recommended. Every additional 500 mg of salt takes another 10 mg of calcium out of the bones, because sodium competes with calcium for reabsorption in the renal tubules. The latest studies have shown that limiting salt intake is directly associated with a decreased risk of osteoporosis.

Proteins: Acids, especially phosphoric and sulphuric acids, are produced during the metabolism and breakdown of proteins. These acids must first be neutralized – buffered – by combining with calcium before they are eliminated by the kidneys; otherwise the body would be "acidified". Meat protein is more acidic during digestion than protein from fish, dairy products, beans, nuts and seeds because these consist of different amino acids and different kinds of fatty acids. When protein intake is high while that of calcium is low, a "negative calcium balance" is created and the required calcium is mobilized from the bones. So, avoiding excessive protein intakes (>60 g/day) will improve calcium balance and overall health. Vegetarians, with their low consumption of animal proteins, always show a positive calcium balance and stable bones. On the other hand, Eskimos, with their high intake of animal protein and low consumption of calcium, suffer a 20% greater loss of bone than Europeans.

Phosphate: Combined with calcium it produces a strong crystalline substance which gives teeth and bones their hardness. Ideally, one part phosphate should combine with one part calcium. However, our diet contains far more phosphate than is required. This in turn triggers secretion of parathormone to neutralize the excess phosphate by mobilization of calcium and magnesium from the bones. Meat products, soft drinks and many prepared "ready-to-eat" meals and "fast foods" contain high levels of phosphate and their intake should be correspondingly restricted.

Lipids: Prior to absorption into the blood stream calcium is dissolved in the acidic gastric juices and combined with lipids. Only in this form can calcium be taken up by the gastric mucosa and pass into the circulation. But when too much fat is present, the opposite effect occurs – calcium and magnesium are lost and bone is also lost. The deleterious effect of fat on bone is illustrated by a comparison of the incidence of osteoporosis in the "low-lipid countries" of the Far East, with that of the USA, where it is significantly higher.

Over-acidification: In actual fact, our bodies are swamped by acids produced by the body itself or absorbed with food (proteins, sugars, fats) in large quantities. The acids have to be neutralized, and this is accomplished in the skeleton. The bones harbour a large quantity of alkaline salts such as calcium, potassium, sodium and magnesium, which are mobilized immediately to neutralize any acids in the blood. The connection between an acidic pH-value and osteoporosis is well-known and is taken into consideration in any program for the prevention of osteoporosis. These observations underline the importance of sufficient quantities of basic vegetables and fruits in order to supply the body with these alkaline substances, as well as with vitamins. It is clear, therefore, that vegetables and fruits are required for neutralization of acids and milk and its products for an adequate supply of calcium.

9.7
Step 7: Strive for an Ideal Body Weight!

All large osteoporosis studies have demonstrated the close connection between osteoporosis and low body weight. Underweight individuals consume insufficient calories and insufficient materials to maintain their bodies, in particular their skeletons. A low body weight and low muscle mass result in less stimulation of the bones, hence lower bone mass. Women with less body fat also tend to produce less oestrogen. However, obesity should not be encouraged because of its many harmful effects on overall health by way of the many possible co-morbidities, which in turn also effect the bones. The best course is to aim for a weight that is normal for height and body build.

Anorexia nervosa is an eating disorder triggered by an overwhelming fear of weight gain. It affects young women and disrupts the menstrual cycle, lowers oestrogen levels and so inhibits a normal peak bone mass. Up to 50 % of patients with anorexia nervosa have low bone density in their lower spine.

9.8
Step 8: Identify Drugs that Cause Osteoporosis and Take Appropriate Steps to Counteract Them When Possible and Necessary!

A comprehensive list of drugs associated with increased risk of osteoporosis in adults has been outlined by the National Osteoporosis Foundation. The most commonly used groups of drugs are given in Chap. 22.

Glucocorticoids: Excess of exogenous glucocorticoid is the most frequent cause of secondary osteoporosis. This group includes all substances derived from cortisone, such as prednisone and dexamethasone. Bone loss may be rapid, particularly in children, and in women over 50 years. The BMD should be measured in all patients before starting long-term therapy with glucocorticoids, and subsequently every 6 months thereafter during the whole course of treatment. Patients with a low bone mass or fractures should be considered for simultaneous therapy with antiresorptive agents. A study on the epidemiology of glucocorticoid adverse events noted that these may occur even under low dose therapy, depending on dose and especially duration, and possibly also presence of other risk factors. However, short-term local application of cortisone derivatives such as ointments or sprays are not damaging to bone. Not all patients experience the same degree of bone loss even with the same or similar medications and amounts of the drugs. Two major factors influence bone loss: the quantity of drug and the length of time during which the medication is taken. Therefore, the daily dose and period of administration should be kept to a minimum. When prednisone is unavoidable the patient should be advised to stop smoking, take calcium and vitamin D tablets and undertake (or to continue) regular sport or other physical activity.

Thyroid hormones: These have two applications – to prevent the development of struma and to treat hypothyroidism. Overdosage, which might occur with prolonged administration, should be avoided, as this may also lead to osteoporosis and fractures.

Anticoagulants: Heparin and warfarin given over long periods (years) may cause severe osteoporosis, as shown in some studies, but not confirmed in others. Therefore, as with glucocorticoids, the bone density is taken before starting therapy and at regular intervals thereafter. The patient is advised on preventative measures, while also considering co-morbidities.

Anticonvulsants: These include carbamazepine, phenytoin and barbiturates. They can damage bone over time and cause disturbances in mineralisation as well as bone loss ("osteo-poromalacia").

Many *other medications* also weaken the bones with prolonged use. This list includes: antidepressives, lithium, antibiotics, isoniazid, antacids containing aluminium, cytostatic drugs and certain diuretics.

Pain medications: The effects on bone vary from none to an increased risk of fracture. Any medication to be taken by a patient must first be checked for its potential to effect bone adversely, so that precautions may be taken in advance. Alternatively, a different medication may be substituted, but of course the same precautions apply.

9.9
Step 9: Recognize Diseases Which Damage Bones!

Primary chronic polyarthritis (PCP) is probably the most important representative of this group. Over the years PCP has consistently caused osteoporosis and fractures. Damage to bones is further aggravated by three additional factors: patients are treated with corticoids, they are limited in their movements and they are underweight. All three factors must be addressed by the physician in charge.

Chronic *pulmonary diseases*, especially bronchitis and emphysema caused by smoking, increase the risk of osteoporosis, which is further enhanced by the drugs often given as therapy. Chronic obstructive pulmonary disease (COPD) carries an increased risk of vertebral fractures.

Chronic cardiac insufficiency: This leads to increased resorption of bone because of limitations in mobility and secondary hyperparathyroidism. Consequently, when a heart transplant is considered, it is advisable to institute bisphosphonate therapy months in advance to avert the otherwise inevitable loss of bone.

Diabetes mellitus: This in itself constitutes a considerable risk for osteoporosis. The lack of insulin causes an increase in bone resorption as well as a decrease in the production of collagen. This affects mainly patients who are treated with oral insulin tablets.

Inflammatory bowel disorders and gastric/intestinal operations: these conditions almost inevitably lead to decreased absorption of calcium and vitamin D; therefore, particular attention must be paid to an adequate diet and sufficient vitamin intake, with supplements if required.

Renal insufficiency: The pathogenesis of renal bone disease is complex, multifactorial and as yet incompletely understood.

9.10 Step 10: Management of Patients Who Have Already Sustained a Fracture

Many reports have investigated the conditions and states of patients in the immediate and long-term post-fracture periods, and the overall conclusion was reached that the management of these patients could be much more effectively implemented with the aim of improving the quality of life, and most importantly of preventing further fractures. In fact, the Interactive Trial has recommended special nutritional and exercise strategies for early intervention in the post-fracture period, especially for older and vulnerable people: in particular by taking the individual risk profile of each patient into consideration. One retrospective study of patients after vertebroplasty demonstrated that significantly fewer fractures recurred if the patients had participated in a targeted exercise program. Wide application of such programs is highly recommended.

A recent follow-up study of 215 fracture patients has demonstrated the efficacy of such a program, and that the patients really took it seriously!

Physical Activity and Exercise Programs

10

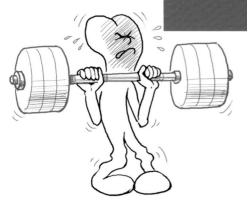

10.1
Strong Muscles Make and Maintain Strong Bones!

The human body is equipped with an impressive apparatus to overcome the forces of natural gravity on planet earth. This apparatus consists of the bones and joints of the skeleton, together with the tendons and muscles. Moreover, the physical stimuli of pressure, weight, and the "push and pull" of movements – controlled and uncontrolled, sudden and slow, continuous and interrupted – directly stimulate the bone cells to form new bone and thereby increase bone mass. Without adequate physical activity, 5–10% of the muscle mass may be lost per annum. This in turn leads to a decrease in bone mass. It should be noted that physical activity is just as, if not more, important for the prevention of osteoporosis as medication.

Immobilization, bed rest, spinal cord injury and a sedentary lifestyle inevitably induce rapid bone loss. The ultimate test of evaluating the effects of weight-bearing activity on bone occurred in space, where there is zero gravity. Before preventive measures were introduced, post-flight bone density of astronauts showed significant decrease in density after only 4–14 days in outer space!

In order to benefit the bones, exercise must be *weight-bearing*, together with special training to strengthen the muscles. Weight-bearing exercise is any type of exercise in which the bones must support the weight of the body against gravity. The most effective activities are those which challenge gravity such as climbing, walking, jogging, running, volleyball, basketball and especially going up stairs. Therefore, use the legs and not the lift. Whoever does not manage at least 30 min walking daily, should at least do some regular exercise at home. Giving up half an hour of TV every day is all that it takes! The importance of sustained exercise, especially with high impact loading, cannot be overemphasized for the prevention of osteoporosis as well as for its therapy, which has been extensively documented in various studies. No matter how you look at it, an effective exercise program takes approximately 3 h per week. Everybody should be able to manage that! As the age-old saying has it: "Where there's a will, there's a way!"

Muscle strength in older individuals responds dramatically to resistance exercise. Strength gains vary from 30% to more than 100% in various muscle groups. Training-induced strength gains are initially rapid but tend to plateau after 3 months, even with progressive increases in training loads. Thus, muscle strength can be improved and can also be maintained in older people without high-intensity training schedules.

The sense or the automatic ability to keep one's *balance* is gradually but systematically reduced from about 30 years onwards. However, the body is able to compensate, so that this deficit only becomes noticeable if and when other senses such as sight and hearing are also impaired. In osteoporotic patients, the consequences of the decreased ability to balance include falls

R. Bartl, B. Frisch, *Osteoporosis,* DOI 10.1007/978-3-540-79527-8_10,
© Springer-Verlag Berlin Heidelberg 2009

and possibly fractures. Clearly, appropriate measures must be taken to avoid this. Balance can be tested with the "*get up and go test*": Get up from a chair without using arms; walk several steps; turn around and walk back to the chair; sit without using arms. If this is accomplished successfully, balance is not a problem. Randomized clinical trials have shown that exercise can reduce the risk of falls by as much as 25%. Prospective observational studies suggest a U-shaped relationship of an increased risk of falls among people who are either very frail or sedentary, or extremely active. Trials have also shown that current or past physical activity is associated with a 20–60% reduction in hip fractures, but only a modest reduction in vertebral fractures.

10.2
The Muscle–Bone Unit and Sarcopenia

Recent studies (mainly in 2008) have presented evidence that intra-uterine and post-natal growth patterns and growth are associated with body composition later in life and this in turn with musculoskeletal disorders and their consequences. Most importantly, these include sarcopenia and osteoporosis. Moreover, a functional approach to densitometry has addressed the question of the mutual adaptation of muscle force with bone strength, and of how deviations of this adaptation may lead to disorders of bone, especially in paediatrics. Subsequently, taking into account Frost's "Mechanostat Hypothesis" as well as the modifications induced by hormonal signals, the quantified relationship between muscle force and bone strength has been suggested as a diagnostic parameter for distinguishing between primary and secondary disorders of bone. Other studies have reported on the association between birth weight and body mass index (BMI) with a tendency for large babies to become obese adults, while a low birth weight poses a risk for later development of the metabolic syndrome, itself associated with increased risk of osteoporosis. However, the results of many of these studies on the relationship of birth weight and its impact later in life on adult body composition still require confirmation.

There is one aspect of the muscle–bone unit which has global consequences and on which there is global agreement: *Sarcopenia*! Sarcopenia is the age-related

loss of skeletal muscle mass with concomitant decrease in muscle strength leading to a reduction in physical activity, which, with advancing age, is a major cause of osteoporosis and other disabilities (Fig. 10.1). Sarcopenia is internationally recognized as a major feature of human senescence. The mechanisms of this muscle loss are still under investigation, but various aspects and pathways have been described. These include biochemical aspects such as reduction in myosin heavy chain protein synthesis, changes in hormonal and neural activities, impaired post-traumatic regeneration, oxidative stress, mitochondrial abnormalities and dysfunctions and myositic apoptosis, as well as apoptotic loss of single nuclei in multinucleated cells. Decrease in telomere length with ageing may also occur in both muscle and bone cells. The good news is that long-term training within normal limits is not associated with abnormal telomere shortening in muscles, and in the elderly regular physical activity is also not associated with accelerated telomere loss in muscles and also not in leukocytes. In contrast, a sedentary lifestyle does have an effect on telomere length and may accelerate the ageing process! So that at least is one physiological risk factor that can be controlled!! Just get up and do it! Also important is endocrine-immune dysfunction involving both inflammatory and other cytokines, lifestyle factors, i.e. smoking, and, most significantly, nutritional deficiencies such as inadequate dietary protein and vitamins, in particular vitamin D. In addition to its function as a major regulator of calcium homeostasis, in the skeletal muscle actions of vitamin D are involved in protein synthesis, and in the kinetics of muscular con-

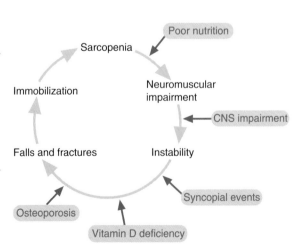

Fig. 10.1. Cycle of falls and fractures and their main contributors

tractions. Clinically, vitamin D deficiency is extremely common in the elderly in many countries, and is associated with neuromuscular functions and symptoms of osteoporosis. Recent studies have emphasized the positive effects of dietary supplementation, in particular amino acids and vitamins, especially vitamin D, on muscle mass and strength. In contrast, moderate calorie restriction and exercise have favourable effects on skeletal muscles, but studies have shown that an increase in muscle mass occurs only after resistance exercise. At the biochemical level, the beta-adrenergic signalling pathway is involved and it has been shown that beta agonists increase muscle mass while decreasing body fat. Further investigations of such pathways could identify therapeutic targets and indicate new approaches to counteract the decrease in skeletal muscle mass in many disorders, including involutional osteoporosis and especially the sarcopenia of ageing.

10.3
Exercise Programs – Preventive and Restorative

Before undertaking an exercise program at home, various aspects should be considered:
- Location: a place in the home which is suitable. This implies that there is enough free space, without furniture or appliances with sharp edges and no loose carpets or slippery surfaces.
- Clothing: use comfortable and non-restrictive clothing.
- Time: everyone has an individual biorhythm and daily schedule, so everyone should choose the most suitable time of day for him-/herself.
- Company: private or public, with a friend or a group, or with one of the many different commercial and other supervised facilities available today in many countries. However, these may involve cost.
- Grade of bone loss: when osteoporosis is already present, according to the bone density measurement or other imaging techniques, sports involving sudden or forceful movements and/or pressure on any skeletal area should be avoided. Such activities include volleyball, squash, jogging, cricket and others. Moreover, special care must be taken when physical activity involves bending the spine, in particular when the movement tends to be uneven, i.e. tilted more to

one side than to the other. Examples of daily activities during which this may occur include: filling and emptying washing machines and driers, dishwashers, lifting heavy cartons or boxes filled with bottles or other containers with drinks, carrying shopping or other heavy objects unilaterally on the arm or shoulder, bending unevenly when using the vacuum cleaner etc. In contrast, walking, dancing and golf are suitable as they induce bone formation, whereas cycling, swimming and rowing are more suitable and advantageous for the vascular system and for the muscles than for the bones, as these exercises do not carry the body's weight. Before beginning any training program, patients with severe osteoporosis must consult a doctor or an authorized trainer regarding which kind of exercise and training they should or should not carry out. With improvements in the state of the skeleton over time, such recommendations may obviously be modified.

10.4
Implementation of a Training Program

There are *five aspects* to consider:
- Warming-up period before doing the exercises, usually 5–10 min depending on physical condition, slow movements using the shoulders, hip and knee joints.
- Training for high-impact activities, e.g. volleyball, basketball or vertical jumping, risky for individuals with established osteoporosis!
- Training for strength (the stronger the muscles, the more powerful the stimulation of bone formation).
- Training for stretching (to avoid injuries and to improve flexibility).
- Training for balance (to prevent falls).

All of these can be carried out in *four positions*: Standing, sitting, supine on back or supine on all four limbs. The specific details of training programs can be found in various books and manuals and, of course, are given by any authorized trainer of any group or organization attended by the patient. As mentioned in the previous chapter, programs for patients after the first fracture should not be neglected, and especially adapted programs are required for the elderly.

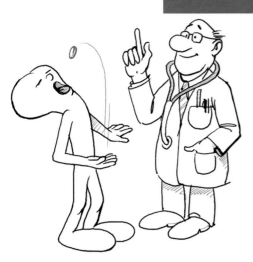

11.1
Evidence-Based Strategies for the Therapy of Osteoporosis

The major aim of therapy is the prevention of fractures. The properties of all *ideal therapeutic agents* include the following: the medication is well tolerated and safe with minimal side effects; it has oral and intravenous bioavailability; it has been proven to increase bone mass, improve bone quality and reduce fractures at all sites including the hip. It should be pointed out at the outset that there are considerable variations in both quality and credibility in results from randomized trials dealing with the efficacy of different treatment schedules. When results of these clinical trials are assessed and compared, questions and problems arise with respect to the following criteria:

- Duration of the study
- Number and age of the patients
- Definition of exclusion criteria
- Primary aim of the study
- Fracture incidence versus fracture rate
- Fractures prior to start of study
- Definition of "fracture"
- Definition of "control group"

- Status of vitamin D and calcium
- Risk profiles of the participants
- Method and accuracy of bone density measurements
- Differences in statistics used for analysis

It is now possible to evaluate results of studies and reports of experiences in an objective and balanced fashion ("*evidence-based medicine*") especially with reference to:

- Meta-analysis of randomized controlled studies
- Individual randomized controlled studies
- Studies based on observations
- Results of basic research
- Results and reports of clinical experience
- Results based on recommended guidelines, such as those issued by the National Institute for Health and Clinical Excellence (NICE) in the UK

With the continuing worldwide acceptance of evidence-based methodology, the classification of levels of evidence and the grading of recommendations are becoming better and more widely known and form the basis of an effective and rational treatment of osteoporosis:

Levels of evidence:
- Ia From meta-analysis of randomized controlled trials (RCTs)
- Ib From at least one large RCT
- IIa From at least one well-designed controlled study without randomization
- IIb From at least one other type of well-designed quasi-experimental study
- III From well designed non-experimental descriptive studies
- IV From expert committee reports or opinions

R. Bartl, B. Frisch, *Osteoporosis*, DOI 10.1007/978-3-540-79527-8_11,
© Springer-Verlag Berlin Heidelberg 2009

11

Grading of recommendations:
- A Levels Ia and Ib
- B Levels IIa, IIb and III
- C Level IV

When this rigorous approach of evidence-based medicine is adopted, the most conclusive evidence for

reducing fracture risk (*"A class" recommendation*) has been shown for the following antiresorptive and osteoanabolic drugs (Figs. 11.1 and 11.2; Table 11.1):
- Supplements with calcium and vitamin D
- Therapy with alendronate, risedronate, ibandronate and zoledronate
- Therapy with PTH and teriparatide

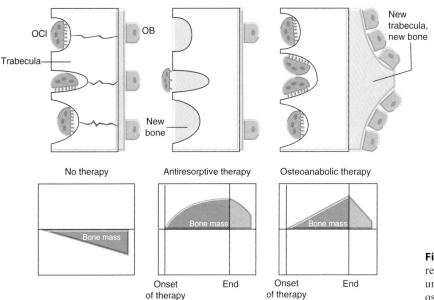

Fig. 11.1. Changes in bone remodelling and bone density under antiresorptive and osteoanabolic drugs

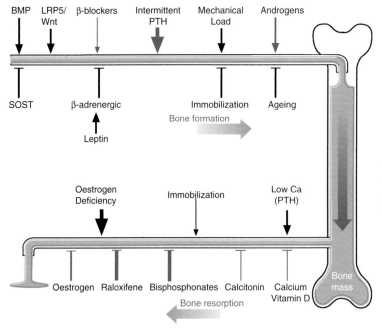

Fig. 11.2. Physiological factors, therapeutic agents and their influence on bone remodelling and bone mass. Physiological (black) and pharmacological (red) stimulators and inhibitors of bone formation and resorption are listed. The relative impact, where known, is represented by the thickness of the arrows. BMP, bone morphogenetic proteins; SOST, sclerostin; LRP5, low density lipoprotein (LDL)-receptor-related protein; PTH, parathyroid hormone; SERM, selective oestrogen-receptor modulator (modified from Harada and Rodan [2003])

Table 11.1. Evidence base for agents in the management of postmenopausal osteoporosis

Agent	Fracture site		
	Vertebral	Non-vertebral	Hip
Alendronate	A	A	A
Calcitonin	A	B	B
Calcitriol	A	A	nd
Calcium	A	B	B
Calcium+vitamin D	nd	A	A
Etidronate	A	B	B
Hip protectors	–	–	A
HRT	A	A	A
Ibandronate	A	A	nd
PTH	A	A	nd
Physical exercise	nd	B	B
Raloxifene	A	nd	nd
Risedronate	A	A	A
Strontium ranelate	A	A	A
Teriparatide	A	A	nd
Tibolone	nd	nd	nd
Vitamin D	nd	B	B
Zoledronate	A	A	A

nd, Not demonstrated; A, meta-analysis of RCTs or at least one RCT; B, well designed, controlled study or case-control, comparative or correlation studies

- Therapy with raloxifene (SERM)
- Therapy with strontium ranelate

These A-recommended drugs/substances should have first priority in osteoporosis therapy (Table 11.2). In contrast, no reliable or definite data are available as yet for calcitonin, etidronate, fluoride and calcitriol, so that no conclusions could be drawn as to fracture risk. Thus, it has now been conclusively shown that the N-containing bisphosphonates (e.g. alendronate,

Table 11.2. Large randomized controlled trials of antiresorptive therapies with fracture as an endpoint in postmenopausal women with osteoporosis

Agent	Study	First author Year	Patients (n)	Duration (years)	Primary endpoint	Completers	Age, mean	Prevalent Vert.Fx
Alendronate	FIT 1	Black 1996	2027 1022/1005 ALN/PLA	3	Vert.Fx –20%/4 mm	89% ALA 87% PLA	55–81, 71	0%
	FIT 2	Cummings 1998	4432 2214/2218 ALN/PLA	4	Clin.Fx –20%/4 mm	4272 96% 93% ALA 94% PLA	54–81, 68	0%
	FOSIT	Pols 1999	1908 950/958 ALN/PLA	1	BMD	?	–85, 63	?
	Liberman	Liberman 1995	994 526/355 ALN/PLA	8	Vert.Fx –20%/4 mm	89%	45–80,64	18%

Table 11.2. (continued)

Agent	Study	First author Year	Patients (n)	Duration (years)	Primary endpoint	Completers	Age, mean	Prevalent Vert.Fx
Risedronate	VERT-NA	Harris 1999	2458 813/815 RIS/PLA	3	Vert.Fx −15%	55% PLA 60% RIS	−85, 69	80%
	VERT-MN	Reginster 2000	1,226 407/407 RIS/PLA	3	Vert.Fx −15%	54% PLA 62% RIS	-85 71	98%
	HIP	McClung 2001	9331 5445 1812/1821 RIS/PLA	3	HipFx Secondary: NonVert.Fx, BMD	64% 57% RIS, 57% PLA	70–79	18% total, 31% group 1
			3886 1292/1313 RIS/PLA			41% RIS 42% PLA	>80	
Ibandronate	BONE	Chesnut 2004	2946	3	Vert.Fx (morphometric)	66% 66% IBN 65% PLA	69, 55–80	94%
	MOBILE	Miller 2004	1609	2	BMD		65, 55–80	48%
	DIVA	Recker 2004	1395	2 3	BMD Vert.Fx, HipFx	81%	66, 55–80	
Zoledronate	HORIZON	Black 2007	7765 3889/3876 ZOL/PLA	3	Vert.Fx, HipFx	81%	73, 65–89	37%
Raloxifene	MORE	Ettinger 1999	7705 5129/2576 RAL/PLA	3	Vert.Fx −20%/4 mm BMD Secondary: NonVert.Fx	89% 79% RAL 75% PLA	31–80, 67	
	MORE 1		3002/1522 RAL/PLA				65	11%

risedronate, ibandronate and zoledronate) achieve the greatest reduction in fracture risk: on average 50% reduction in vertebral and extravertebral fractures after 1-year of therapy (Table 11.3).

The concept of a placebo-controlled trial has been challenged on the basis that it is no longer ethical to place osteoporotic patients on placebo now that proven effective therapies are available.

Table 11.3. Drugs used and approved to treat osteoporosis

	Oral daily	Oral weekly	Oral monthly	Subcutaneous daily	Injection quarterly	Infusion annually
Alendronate	10 mg	70 mg				
Risedronate	5 mg	35 mg	150 mg			
Ibandronate			150 mg		3 mg	
Zoledronate						5 mg
Strontium ranelate	2 g					
Teriparatide				20 µg		
PTH				100 µg		

11.2
Comprehensive Approach to the Therapy of Osteoporosis

Successful therapy of osteoporosis (Fig. 11.3; Table 11.4) includes the following aspects:
- Treatment of pain
- Initiation of physical activity and exercises
- Prevention of falls
- Adaptation of lifestyle for skeletal health
- Bone-conscious nutrition
- Vitamin D and calcium supplements
- Hormone replacement therapy (HRT) for short periods only!

- Anti-resorptive therapy (bisphosphonates, raloxifene, calcitonin)
- Osteoanabolic therapy (strontium ranelate, parathormone)
- Other medications (statins, growth factors, tetracyclines, leptin)

Consultation with the patient on preference for the administration of the chosen medication is essential to ensure both short- and long-term compliance. This is crucial for patients with co-morbidities already taking other drugs, which in some cases might even have beneficial effects on the bones, such as statins. Patients with gastrointestinal problems might prefer i.v.

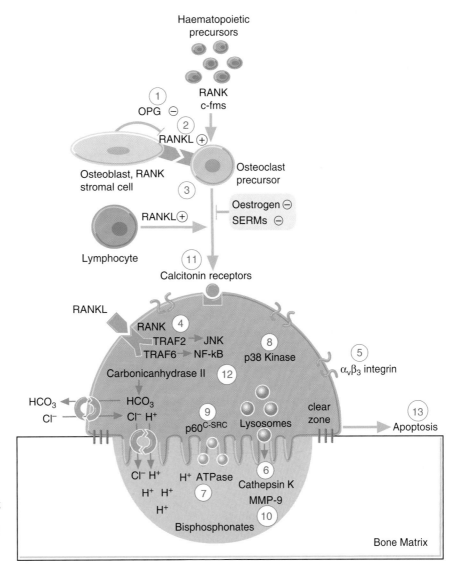

Fig. 11.3. Diagram of development and activation of the osteoclast: illustrating points of potential therapeutic targets indicated by numbers (modified from Rodan and Martin [2000])

11

Table 11.4. Anti-fracture efficacy of the first line drugs for postmenopausal osteoporosis when given with calcium and vitamin D, as derived from randomized controlled studies (updated from Kanis et al. 2008)

First line drugs	Effect on vertebral fracture risk		Effect on non-vertebral fracture risk	
	Osteoporosis	Established osteoporosis[a]	Osteoporosis	Established osteoporosis[a]
Alendronate	+	+	NA	+ (Including hip)
Risedronate	+	+	NA	+ (Including hip)
Ibandronate	NA	+	NA	+[b]
Zoledronate	+	+	+	+
HRT	+	+	+	+
Raloxifene	+	+	NA	NA
Teriparatide and PTH	NA	+	NA	+
Strontium ranelate	+	+	+ (Including hip)	+ (Including hip)

NA, no evidence available
[a] Women with prior vertebral fracture
[b] In subsets of patients only (post-hoc analysis)

administration, as already shown in some trials such as the Dosing Intravenous Administration (DIVA) study. Preference and adherence to monthly rather than daily or weekly tablets have been emphasized in reports from various European countries. Moreover, adherence difficulties may soon be a thing of the past, with the i.v. administration of quarterly, semi-annual, and annual doses of, for example zoledronate. The individual components of the therapeutic spectrum given above must be tailored to the special needs and requirements of each patient.

However, based on the results of the evidence-based medicine cited above, the following *treatment strategy* is employed in our out-patient clinic following patient examination, results of tests, medical history, family history and evaluation of personal risk profile:

- Patients are given vitamin D and calcium supplements
- HRT or its equivalent is discussed with each female patient, but is no longer advocated for treatment of osteoporosis alone
- Early administration of a modern (nitrogen-containing) bisphosphonate
- Alternatively, administration of raloxifene, strontium ranelate or parathyroid hormone (PTH) for a limited period and followed by a bisphosphonate

11.3 Indication for Treatment – Combining BMD with Clinical Factors

The WHO has defined osteoporosis as a T-score below -2.5, and osteopenia when T-scores vary between -1.0 and -2.5. This is a practical definition that allows researchers to classify degrees of low bone density within populations. However, from a clinical standpoint this definition lacks the ability to make decisions regarding fracture risk and treatment thresholds. The *NORA-study* of a cohort of about 150,000 postmenopausal women showed that 82% of those with fractures had T-scores greater than -2.5. Additionally, the *Study of Osteoporotic Fractures* showed that 54% of postmenopausal women with hip fractures did not have an osteoporotic T-score at the hip (as measured on dual-energy X-ray absorptiometry, DXA). Therefore, relying purely on T-scores to determine future fractures is inadequate and unreliable.

There have been several attempts to combine bone mineral density (BMD) values with clinical risk factors to allow clinicians to determine when to start specific treatment. The National Osteoporosis Foundation (NOF) has developed recommendations for treatment and these *guidelines* have been adopted by many health care organizations:

- T-score less than -2.0
- T-score less than -1.5 with at least one major risk factor (e.g. personal and family history of fractures, smoking, propensity to injurious falls, weight below 127 lbs/58 kg).

In German-speaking countries, factors such as BMD values (only DXA method accepted), age, sex, some risk factors and the presence of vertebral fractures are taken into consideration in order to determine indications for specific drug therapy (*DVO guidelines*). Therefore, based on currently available evidence of fracture prevention in randomized clinical trials, there are at least three groups of postmenopausal women who should receive the highest priority for osteoporosis treatment with pharmacologic agents:

- Patients with vertebral fractures
- Patients with a BMD defining osteoporosis according to the WHO (T-score of less than -2.5 at the hip or the spine)
- Patients with a T-score between -2.5 and -2.0 and other risk factors for fracture

The WHO is presently attempting to define a cost utility analysis that will combine BMD with clinical risk factors for fracture in order to determine a 10-year absolute risk of fracture. This study may eventually set the standard for pharmacologic therapy. Data regarding the fracture prevention value of initiating pharmacologic therapy for healthy postmenopausal women with T-scores between 0.0 and -2.0 are generally lacking. Therapeutic decisions for this risk group must be made on a case-by-case basis, and are usually made by the desire of the patient to prevent further postmenopausal bone loss or initial fractures. One of the most important determinants in therapeutic decisions is accurate assessment of the individual patient's fracture risk profile as emphasized in many recent investigations. In patients with secondary osteoporosis, for example due to a neoplasia, the potential extraskeletal benefits or disadvantages of the treatments required should also be considered, as already done for example in multiple myeloma.

Management of Pain in Osteoporosis

12

12.1
Start with the Patient, not the Disease!

Pain has been reported in up to 62% of female patients with osteoporosis. There are various causes for pain in osteoporosis, including concurrent degenerative disk disease, osteoarthritis and vertebral fractures. Osteoporotic back pain is usually acute, of sudden onset and caused by a fracture in the lower thoracic or lumbar vertebrae. On examination, there will be a painful spot in the area of the back where the vertebral fracture has occurred. The muscles next to the spine will be very tense and painful to touch. This pain can last for long periods ranging from a few weeks to months. In all patients an X-ray of the affected skeletal area should be taken to demonstrate or rule out a vertebral fracture and to document the extent of destruction of bone. A bone scan may demonstrate an acute inflammation around an area of fractured bone and may show the fractured vertebrae long before a regular X-ray, because of the increased uptake in that area. It has further been suggested that covert small fractures – microfractures – due to mechanical stress can also cause pain. When the intraosseous pressure exceeds a certain level, fluid in the bone enters the subperiosteal space and exerts pressure on the nerves and induces a painful periosteal reaction. Pain during healing of a fracture may well be related to local release of cytokines, prostanoids, histamine and bradykinin into the surrounding area.

12.2
Acute Phase

Before introducing measures for pain relief, the patient's pain should be evaluated for a drug-induced cause. Bisphosphonates are the agents of choice for most patients with osteoporosis, and although as many as 26% of patients taking these agents experience some sort of bone or back pain; discontinuation is usually not required. For immediate treatment of *acute pain*, peripherally active analgetics are generally administered first, as these reduce the pain faster and better than the centrally acting analgesics. These include acetylsalicylic acid, paracetamol, metamizol and especially non-steroidal anti-inflammatory drugs (NSAIDs), which act by local inhibition of prostaglandins. But these should only be taken for short periods of time, because of their possible harmful effects on the gastric mucosa, the kidney, the liver and the bone marrow (gastrointestinal ulcers, renal insufficiency, hepatotoxicity and aplastic anaemia). Especially in older patients the cardiovascular status may worsen secondarily due to overuse of these drugs. However, the latest in the series of anti-rheumatic drugs such as COX-2 inhibitors do not have these side effects. Bone pain can also be rapidly and effectively treated with bisphosphonates, which have largely replaced calcitonin for this purpose. When the pain is very strong, as in a recent fracture, any of the medications listed above can be combined with a weak opiate. In cases where patients require large doses or a combination containing *opioids* to control osteoporotic pain, a switch to an

R. Bartl, B. Frisch, *Osteoporosis*, DOI 10.1007/978-3-540-79527-8_12,
© Springer-Verlag Berlin Heidelberg 2009

12

opioid alone should be considered. Patients will still receive the analgesic effect, but without the increased risk of gastrointestinal bleeding and other adverse side effects. Caution should be used, though, as patients using opioid analgesics may be at higher risk for vertebral fractures secondary to falls related to the use of the opioids. Patients should regularly be assessed for risk of falls, and possibly for increased need of pain control, as well as for titration of maintenance medication. If the treatment outlined above is insufficient, a pain expert can be consulted and the treatment adjusted according to the advice given. It is advisable to avoid muscle relaxants as they increase the risk of falling because of their sedative action. Bed rest is recommended for the acute stage, but only until the acute pain has subsided. Subsequently, short periods of careful weight-bearing alternating with exercises are incorporated into the daily schedule. In the acute stage a wet dressing with cold water is applied to promote blood flow, while a warm-water dressing may be advantageous in the chronic phase.

Additional measures include physiotherapy, deep breathing exercises, yoga, acupuncture, electrotherapy and local anaesthetics. Many people have turned to complementary medicine for pain relief, either in the form of Chinese herbs, acupuncture or acupoint injection; the most effective sites recommended are those at the Jiaji points. In selected cases, *orthopaedic supports* may also contribute to alleviation of pain (Fig. 12.1a,b).

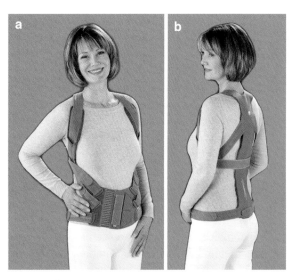

Fig. 12.1a,b. Orthopaedic support (Spinomed active) may also contribute to alleviation of pain

Acute pain caused by fracture usually resolves within 10 weeks. A different approach is required for patients with cancer-induced bone pain, as numerous factors must be taken into consideration: age and sex of the patient, type and stage of the cancer, location and degree of pain, as well as type, extent and duration of the therapy. It is expected that a greater understanding of the neuro-biological mechanisms underlying cancer-induced bone pain will shortly be translated into improved pain management.

12.3
Chronic Phase – Short Term

The pain gradually eases as the fracture heals, but can also merge into *chronic pain* due to the development of a skeletal deformity after the fracture, as well as unbalanced and disproportionate strain on the muscles and damage to the vertebral joints. Patients frequently complain of nocturnal pains (reminiscent of Sudeck-like pains) which respond to administration of NSAIDs. This chronic pain may be responsible for loss of sleep, irritability, fear and depression, which in turn highlight the pain even more. Moreover, sensitivity to pain varies greatly between patients and each must be evaluated and treated individually. Many patients with back and leg pains induced by osteoporosis have turned to complementary medicine and have been relieved by acupuncture and acupoint injection at the site of the Jiajii point group.

Various studies have compared the health-related quality of life as well as overall life satisfaction among elderly people who have suffered a fracture with controls who have not. The scores of the former were significantly lower than those of the latter, judged according to replies given to the questionnaires completed by both groups. The participation of the test group in social and leisure activities was significantly and independently lower than that of the control group without pain. To summarize: The first priority in all patients is to break the circle of pain and its consequences, and this is accomplished by physiotherapy and analgetics, calcitonin (either subcutaneously or nasally) or bisphosphonates (intravenously). Other treatments to decrease pain in vertebral fractures include percutaneous injection of artificial cement into the vertebral body (vertebro- and kyphoplasty). These invasive methods should be reserved for those patients unable to achieve adequate pain control after vertebral fracture by traditional pharmacologic and non-pharmacologic therapies. Further discussion of vertebroplasty and kyphoplasty is provided in Chap. 23.

12.4
Chronic Phase – Long Term

Once the pain has become bearable, the patient must be mobilized and the muscles strengthened. This is best accomplished by *physiotherapy*, special exercises and the ancillary measures noted above. Every patient should have an individualized program drawn up by the responsible physician in consultation with the physiotherapist. Swimming in particular, in warm or cold water, presents the ideal combination of relieving the vertebral column of weight while strengthening the muscles. As the pain lessens and the patient´s condition improves, more sport-oriented measures are introduced. Active training to strengthen bones and muscles also contributes to reduction of chronic pain. Exercises should be performed regularly and be adapted to the patient´s age and general condition. The program is developed and taught under specialist guidance to begin with and later should be continued by the patient in her/his home on a regular basis. A major aim is the stabilization and strengthening of the muscles of the back – especially those of the lower thoracic and lumbar spine. Care must be taken to avoid exercises which carry an increased risk of vertebral fractures, especially those which flex the lumbar spine, increasing thoracic kyphosis and forward flexion.

Low back pain is a major cause for seeking medical advice, and though it is frequently of musculoskeletal origin, additional or other causes must be ruled out before the assumption is made that it is due to osteoporosis and treated accordingly.

Chronic low back pain in the elderly may be accompanied by structural alterations in the brain, but their cause and relationship to any physical function or dysfunction have not yet been clarified. The site and possible cause of the pain must be investigated as in any other patient.

12.5
Electric Potentials in Bone

It has long been recognized that weight-bearing induces "stress lines" and thereby electric potentials in bone which is very important for healing and for new bone formation. This phenomenon is called "piezoelectricity" and it forms the basis for the theory that electrical charges constitute the impetus for bone resorption and formation. These electromagnetic fields in bone provide signals for neighbouring bone cells to "remodel" the bone according to the immediate need or requirement. The "trajection lines" seen in X-ray pictures represent these stress lines exactly. The compact bone is situated where the pressure points converge and the trabecular bone where they diverge. These characteristics have practical applications as they can be used to facilitate fracture healing as well as remodelling of newly-formed bone by means of a *"magnetic field therapy"*. The physician in charge must check to find out for which indications this therapy has been approved. Examples include:
- Delayed fracture healing
- Pseudoarthrosis
- Loosening of endoprosthesis

Calcium and Vitamin D

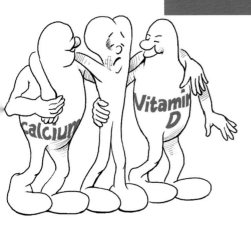

13.1
Calcium: A Lifelong Companion

Calcium is the most abundant mineral in the body and most of it (approximately 99%) is deposited in bone (Fig. 13.1). There is no doubt that calcium is a fundamental factor in the prevention and treatment of osteoporosis. However, there is less agreement regarding precise recommendations for appropriate calcium intake. The calcium recommendation for adults is about 1000 (800–1500) mg/day. The higher values are required by teenage girls, pregnant and lactating women, postmenopausal women who are not taking oestrogen and both men and women over age 50. Today, we ingest far less calcium than our ancestors did. In fact, studies reveal that three-quarters of Americans are deficient in calcium, with an average intake of only 500–600 mg/day in their diet. For adolescents and young adults, the National Institute of Health (NIH) consensus statement recommends 1200–1500 mg/day of elemental calcium.

Numerous studies have shown that a high calcium intake reduces postmenopausal bone loss and the risk of fractures, even in people who have already suffered fractures. Moreover, some evidence points to greater effectiveness of a high calcium intake perimenopaus-

ally before the decline in oestrogen secretion by the ovaries has stimulated unbalanced bone resorption. Supplements of calcium (1000–1500 mg/day) and vitamin D alone have been shown to decrease the risk of fracture by 40%! Calcium supplementation at levels of 1000 mg/day will suppress bone breakdown, probably by decreasing parathyroid hormone (PTH) secretion. Increased calcium intake during adolescence helps to build up the peak bone mass, and these mineral stores definitely decrease the risk of osteoporosis in later years. While calcium by itself cannot treat or heal established osteoporosis, it appears to enhance the effectiveness of other treatments which inhibit resorption and/or promote formation of bone. In addition to calcium, sufficient protein, at least 1 g/kg body weight, is necessary to maintain the function of the musculoskeletal system. An adequate diet, together with the required supplements, can shorten the duration of the stay in hospital of elderly patients with hip fractures.

The best way to get sufficient calcium is to eat calcium-rich foods. Moreover, getting enough calcium with meals entails consumption of many other nutrients at the same time. Bottled mineral waters with high calcium content, low-fat dairy products, green leafy vegetables and calcium-fortified juices will help to provide plenty of calcium. However, experience has shown that most patients do not get the required amount of calcium by nutrition alone. In this situation, *calcium supplements* are recommended and are available in tablet, powder as well as in several other forms, each with its own advantages and disadvantages (Table 13.1):

- Naturally derived calcium (dolomite, bone meal, oyster shells): this type of supplement is inexpensive and easy to swallow, but is harder to absorb and

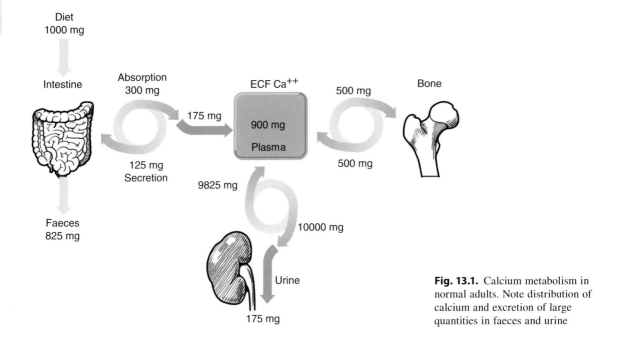

Fig. 13.1. Calcium metabolism in normal adults. Note distribution of calcium and excretion of large quantities in faeces and urine

may contain significant amounts of lead and other toxic minerals.

- Refined calcium carbonate is the least expensive form of calcium and has the highest percentage of elemental calcium, but is poorly absorbed. It often causes constipation and because it is an antacid, in the long run it may lead to "rebound hyperacidity" and gastric irritation. It requires acid in order to dissolve. Taking calcium carbonate supplements together with vitamin C or with meals helps to some extent, because that is when the acid levels in the stomach are at their highest.
- Chelated calcium is calcium bound to an organic acid, including citrate, citrate malate, lactate, gluconate and others. Although chelated calcium is bulkier than calcium carbonate, it dissolves easily and therefore may be easier to absorb. In older patients, calcium citrate is preferred.

Very few patients cannot take calcium, or only under medical supervision. Patients with hypercalcaemia, nephrolithiasis and renal insufficiency belong to this group. The following points may help in the choice of calcium supplements:

- Calcium is primarily absorbed in the small intestine, especially in the duodenum and proximal jejunum. Absorption of calcium is complete within 4 h. During periods of rapid skeletal growth, children absorb about 75% of ingested calcium, this value decreases to 30% in adults.
- Avoid taking more than 500 mg of calcium in one dose. Take one dose before bedtime to prevent bone loss at night. If more is needed, take several doses throughout the day.
- Calcium supplements should be taken with meals to boost their absorption, which is increased by lactose and proteins.

Table 13.1. Amounts of elemental calcium in calcium salts used as supplements

Calcium salt	Calcium mg/1000 mg calcium salt	% Calcium
Calcium carbonate	400	40.0
Calcium phosphate tribasic	388	38.8
Calcium lactate	184	18.4
Calcium gluconate	93	9.3
Calcium citrate	241	24.1

- Certain substances can hinder absorption of calcium: foods rich in fibres and fat, zinc, iron, spinach, coffee, alcohol and antacids. Therefore, calcium should not be taken together with these.
- Patients should be advised to aim for a calcium: phosphorus ratio of 2:1. The easiest way to achieve this is to avoid excesses of cola drinks and foods with phosphorus additives – check the labels before buying the products!
- Calcium may interfere with certain drugs, including: thyroid medications, tetracycline, anticonvulsants and corticosteroids. Therefore, these should always be taken separately.
- There is no need to worry about development of kidney stones if the correct dosage in the suitable form of calcium is taken together with sufficient fluid.
- The amount of calcium in blood and urine should be checked regularly when supplements are regularly taken.
- Calcium supplements can cause gas, abdominal distension and constipation in some individuals. In this situation, it is reasonable to switch to a different preparation.

Despite the linkage between calcium intake and bone mass, the incidence of osteoporosis is low in many areas, particularly in developing countries, where calcium intake is also low. There may be many possible explanations for this apparent paradox:

- Inadequate reports
- Lower life expectancies
- Non-dietary factors (genetic differences, exercise patterns, exposure to sunlight)
- Dietary factors (consumption of soy and other natural products)

13.2
The Concept of Vitamin D in the 21st Century

The structure of vitamin D was identified in 1900. In the course of the subsequent decades right up to the end of the last century, numerous studies elucidated its metabolism and its effects on calcium-phosphate homeostasis and its correlation to skeletal mineral metabolism. Indeed, some authors have claimed that the skeleton is an "intracrine organ" for vitamin D metabolism, based on its direct effects on the bone cells and on the fact that the bone cells themselves can convert 25D into 1,25D by means of the 25-hydroxyvitamin D 1alpha-hydroxylase (CYP27B1), thereby participating in the autocrine and paracrine loops of vitamin D metabolism.

Moreover, with the start of the new century, an impressive accumulation of work has now established a role for *vitamin D in multiple (if not all) organ systems* and in their physiological (and pathological) molecular processes. This is accomplished by way of the cellular vitamin D receptors which are present in many organs and tissues. By attachment to its receptor(s), vitamin D initiates and/or participates in numerous processes such as proliferation and differentiation, inflammation in the immune system, as well as various functions in the endocrine systems, including the angiotensin system, in glucose and insulin metabolism and in the metabolism of lipids, to mention some of its more prominent activities.

With regard to the *reproductive systems*, vitamin D is a secosteroid hormone and affects pregnancy, the foetus and lactation. The association between ultraviolet B irradiance (UVB), vitamin D status and incidence rates of type 1 diabetes in children up to 14 years old was studied in 51 regions all over the world by the Diabetes Mondial Project Group. The results demonstrated that the incidence rates approached zero in regions with high UVB, confirming the action of vitamin D in risk reduction for diabetes type 1 in children – a graphic illustration of the skin's ability to produce vitamin D under the influence of sunshine! These numerous biological activities have suggested almost as many potential therapeutic interventions for vitamin D.

The far-reaching effects of vitamin D in *oncology* have only recently been recognized, as represented by some reports in the 1980's and 1990's, but numerous publications in the first decade of the 21st century. At the cellular level, these reports describe specific actions of vitamin D including pro-apoptotic, anti-metastatic, anti-angiogenic, anti-inflammatory, pro-differentiating and immunomodulating effects. These anti-cancer properties have been attributed to calcitriol, the "hormonal" form of vitamin D. Equally significant – probably even more so – is the preventive effect of an adequate amount of vitamin D in the daily food intake on the incidence of various cancers at the individual and population levels! In addition, this is definitely not the present situation, because vitamin D deficiency is now recognized as a worldwide pandemic! The preventive affect of vitamin D has now been demonstrated by evidence-based investigations for a number of malignancies including colon, pancreatic, renal and breast cancers. But so far, studies of vitamin D and risk of prostate cancer have not shown a protective effect; on the contrary. Apparently higher circulating 25(OH)D concentrations have been associated with an increased risk of a more aggressive type of prostate cancer. Recent results of the pooled data taken from 45 observational studies of 26,769 men on the effects of dairy products, vitamin D and calcium intake found no support for any association with risk of prostate cancer. However, the situation is more complex, because calcitriol and its analogues exert several anti-inflammatory actions in normal prostate cells, and it is thought that these reactions could contribute to a putative preventive or therapeutic effect also in prostate cancer cells. Investigations of the effects of calcitriol and its analogues are now underway on prostate cancer cells in animals. Moreover, there is also a genetic component, as polymorphisms of the vitamin D receptor (VDR) gene have been shown to affect the risk of, for example renal cell carcinoma, while other polymorphisms in VDR genes also appear to reduce the risk for recurrence of colorectal carcinoma.

Genetics has recently revealed the existence of another significant factor linked to *ageing*, and also involved in mineral and vitamin D metabolism, namely alpha-Klotho, an age-suppressing gene which participates in the regulation of 1,25(OH)(2)D(3) production and thereby in calcium homeostasis by maintaining the extracellular level of calcium in blood and body fluids. Studies have now demonstrated that klotho-deficient mice exhibit multiple pathologic changes resembling human ageing. These findings have significant implications for musculoskeletal metabolism including involutional osteoporosis in humans. Animal studies have already demonstrated the involvement of klotho in dentinogenesis and its mineralization, which could also be significant in pathologic conditions of the jaw bones and teeth. One study in human elderly people has described down regulation of CD4(+) T lymphocytes especially in patients in association with rheumatoid arthritis. Further investigations of the functions of klotho are expected also to indicate possible future therapeutic applications.

According to the international literature, vitamin D is now considered an endocrine system. Vitamin D itself is the pro-hormone, which is converted into the active hormonal form: 1.25(OH)(2)D(3), or 1,25 (OH)(2) D(3) in various tissues, for example the skin, which is now considered the largest endocrine organ of the human body!

13.3
Vitamin D: Don't Rely on Sunshine, Take Supplements

Vitamin D, as the most important regulator of calcium homeostasis (Fig. 13.2), has the following actions which affect the skeleton:
- Promotes absorption of calcium from the gut into the blood stream
- Decreases the excretion of calcium in the kidney
- Promotes the recruitment, maturation and action of bone cells and protects osteoblasts from apoptosis
- Promotes the incorporation of calcium into bone (mineralization)
- Protects microstructure of trabecular bone

Additional beneficial *actions of vitamin D* include:
- Increase of muscle mass and strength by support and maintenance of type 11 fibres.
- Improvement of coordination and balance.
- Lower risk of falling.
- Lower risk for hypertension and heart failure.
- Lower risk of type 1 diabetes mellitus.
- Lower risk of breast, lung, colon, breast and possibly other cancers by its anti-proliferative effect mediated by the VDR. In a recent comprehensive study, the chemo-preventive effect of calcitriol on the development of lung cancer was indicated.
- Anti-inflammatory action (immunomodulatory effects in immunological and autoimmune conditions, e.g. in gastrointestinal inflammations)
- Antithrombotic effect
- Participation in the treatment of psoriasis, tuberculosis and Alzheimer's disease
- Anti-ageing effect

Vitamin D is measured in international units (IU). The recommended daily intake of vitamin D is 200–400 IU, but this is a maintenance dose; therapeutic ap-

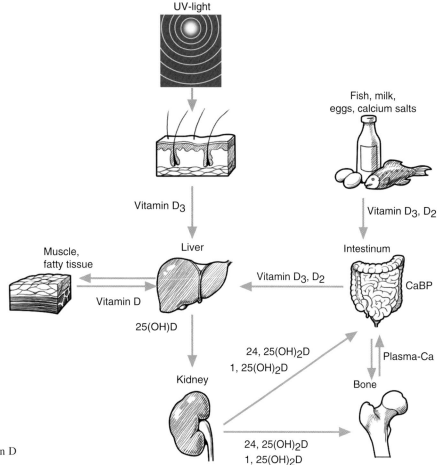

Fig. 13.2. Pathways of vitamin D metabolism

plications require higher amounts, e.g. 400–1000 IU (10–25 µg) are considered to be effective. These values may vary depending on age, ethnic group, nutritional status and skeletal size. Most people with vitamin D deficiency readily agree to take supplements and not to rely on dietary intake. The best assay to determine vitamin D status is to check the level of 25(OH)D in the blood. The normal range for 25(OH)D in most laboratories is approximately 8–57 ng/ml. However, patients with levels of 25(OH)D between 8 and 25 ng/ml are most probably vitamin D-deficient. Moreover, levels of vitamin D of <20–25 ng/ml have been shown to be associated with secondary hyperparathyroidism, which may result in bone loss over time. Serum 25(OH)D levels below or equal to 12 ng/ml were associated with an increased fracture risk in persons aged 65–75 years, as shown in a recent study. Although there are a variety of other metabolites of vitamin D

in the circulation, the measurement of these has not proved to be of any significance.

13.4
Rickets

Rickets is a childhood disease resulting from vitamin D deficiency characterized by inadequate mineralization of osteoid. In adults, the resulting disease is called *osteomalacia* or *osteoporomalacia* when there is component of osteoporosis. A relative vitamin D deficiency often occurs in older age groups and in people with disorders of the gastrointestinal tract. Moreover, inadequate vitamin D levels are more common than has been previously appreciated. Based on many large studies, the prevalence of vitamin D insufficiency proved to be >25%, and it has been as

13

high as 70% in studies done in northern latitudes in the winter. If vitamin D deficiency is suspected, the level of 25(OH)D in the serum must be checked. The following factors contribute to a *calcium/vitamin D deficiency in older people*:
- Inadequate consumption of calcium-rich foods
- Reduced absorption capacity of the intestinal mucosa
- Reduced exposure to sunlight and therefore
- Reduced synthesis of vitamin D in the skin
- Reduced metabolism of vitamin D to its active form

As a consequence of these factors, most elderly patients have some degree of vitamin D deficiency and secondary hyperparathyroidism with increased bone resorption (Fig. 13.3). Consequently, correction of the deficiency by vitamin D supplements causes a decrease in the serum PTH concentration, a decrease in bone turnover and an increase in bone mineral density. Vitamin D and calcium supplements could reduce the incidence of hip and other peripheral fractures in an elderly nursing home population. Therefore, prescription of 1000 mg calcium and 1000 IU vitamin D daily for the prevention of involutional, age-related osteoporosis is indicated and highly recommended. Alternatively, 50,000 IU i.m. can be administered every 6 months if there are difficulties in compliance, or in order to avoid them. Calcium and vitamin D should always be considered as adjuncts together

with other specific treatments for osteoporosis and osteomalacia.

Vitamin D is especially important in *childhood* during growth. Growing children need vitamin D for:
- Increased absorption of calcium from food
- Recruitment, maturation and activation of bone forming cells
- Mineralization and hardening of newly formed bone (osteoid)

An adequate supply of vitamin D (recommended dose of 1000 IU daily) is therefore extremely important for normal development of the skeleton.

Vitamin D belongs to the group of fat-soluble vitamins such as vitamins A, E and K and therefore can be stored in the body for long periods. Nevertheless, many obese persons are vitamin D-deficient because the vitamin is kept in the large body-fat pool and therefore is not available for metabolic activity. Patients suffering from conditions which reduce absorption of fat usually also have deficiencies in the fat-soluble vitamins. Such patients are best treated by one of the many multivitamin preparations available. The conclusion which must be drawn from this brief review of calcium and vitamin D is that everybody in the framework of osteoporosis prevention and therapy must receive 1000 mg calcium and 1000 IU vitamin D either in food or in supplements every day throughout the year. In the elderly with poor nutritional status there may be some additional benefit from protein and multivitamin supplementation, taking into consideration that vitamin D3 is more potent than vitamin D2.

Recently, *upper limits* for both calcium and vitamin D have been recommended for children of 1 year and older: calcium = 2500 mg/day and vitamin D = 2000 IU (50µg)/day. When consumed in very high quantities, both calcium and vitamin D can cause health risks. High calcium intake may decrease absorption of other minerals such as iron and zinc. The risk of kidney stones, however, is a complex issue because there are many possible causes of renal stones. In general, dietary calcium does not increase the risk of calcium oxalate stones by binding to oxalate in the intestine. The potential risk of excessive vitamin D intake (in some reported cases more than 20,000 IU/day) is unpredictable and may include damage to the central nervous system, which in turn can result in depression, nausea and anorexia. With increasing availability

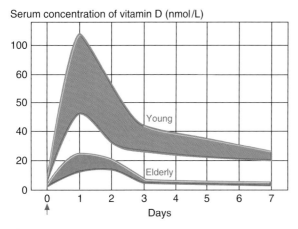

Serum concentration of vitamin D (nmol/L)

Fig. 13.3. Graph illustrating the decreasing ability of the skin to produce vitamin D in response to exposure to sunlight (modified from Holick et al. [1989] Lancet 4:1104–1105)

of supplements and fortified foods, it will be important to monitor intakes of these substances. The dose of a calcium supplement should be adjusted on the basis of dietary intake, age, sex, physical condition, lifestyle, existing disorders and co-morbidities if present.

Vitamin D metabolism is inhibited in patients with chronic renal and hepatic disorders, so that they require the activated form of vitamin D to stabilize and perhaps even to increase bone mass. *Activated vitamin D metabolites* are physiological and therefore non-toxic substances, but they are metabolically highly active so that levels of calcium in blood and urine must be checked regularly to exclude hypo- or hypercalcaemia and/or the hypercalciuria conducive to stone formation. No more than 500 mg calcium per day should be given to patients with chronic renal or hepatic disorders. Recommended dosages are:

Alfacalcidol	0.5–1.0 µg/day orally
Calcitriol	0.5 µg/day orally

Several studies have shown decreases in vertebral fractures, while others have not. A few reports have suggested that alfacalcidol and calcitriol have a direct action on muscle strength and decrease the rate of falling in elderly patients. The major problem with the use of active vitamin D derivates is the narrow therapeutic window with the risk of hypercalcaemia and hypercalcuria, impairment of renal function and nephrocalcinosis. However, recommendations are fairly frequently published in the literature by recognized authorities, taking into consideration sex, age, race, ethnicity, geographic location, climate, economic and social factors, the individual medical history and family history, medical examination and results of relevant tests.

13.5
Other Vitamins Involved in Skeletal Health

Vitamin K is also important in normal bone formation. A higher vitamin K intake helps prevent hip fractures. Vitamin K appears to be essential for conversion of osteocalcin to its active form in bone. There are three major forms of vitamin K:

- K1 (phylloquinone) is the natural form found in plants, especially in leafy dark-green vegetables.
- K2 (menaquinone) is produced by bacteria in the gut.
- K3 (menadione) is a synthetic form.

The recommended dose for vitamin K is 100–300 IU daily. Vitamin K is particularly important for the management of bone loss in patients with hepatic cirrhosis.

Vitamin A in excess may be detrimental to bone; in some studies intakes of more than 1500 µg RE/day were related to a two-fold increase in the risk of hip fractures.

Further nutritional supplements for healthy bones are *magnesium* and four essential *trace elements*: boron, silicon, zinc and copper. Magnesium plays several roles in the metabolism of vitamin D and in the regulation of PTH. Finally, osseous alkaline phosphatase is activated by magnesium. Some studies have found that higher magnesium intakes are associated with higher bone mineral density in the elderly. However, magnesium supplementation is only recommended in magnesium-depleted individuals. The recommended daily dose of magnesium is 200–500 mg.

Hormones for Replacement Therapy

14

14.1
Hormone Replacement Therapy for Women – Now Recommended for Symptoms Only!

Decrease in oestrogen production starts well before the menopause and initiates a continuous loss of bone. After the menopause, and in the absence of therapy, 1–4% of the bone mass may be lost annually. In general, the indications for hormone replacement therapy (HRT) used to be:

- Relief of postmenopausal symptoms and signs attributable to oestrogen deficiency
- Reduction of risk of diseases associated with oestrogen deficiency (osteoporosis, cardiovascular and cerebrovascular disorders).
- HRT was thought to delay cognitive decline, but this has not been substantiated.

Long-term use (5–10 years) of oestrogen results in a reduction of fractures of the hip, vertebrae and arm by about 50%. The greatest effect is seen in the vertebral column: within 2 years of HRT increases of up to 10% in bone density of the lumbar vertebrae, and up to 4% in the femoral neck have been reported. The effect of HRT is more pronounced in skeletal sites with mainly trabecular bone. On cessation of HRT, bone loss resumes at the postmenopausal rate.

A significant reduction in the incidence of fractures had occurred in the years during which HRT was widely taken, confirmed by many studies, for example from Norway. In contrast, other studies, one from Australia, showed a decrease in the incidence of breast cancer after the decrease in use of HRT. Other analyzes of mainly European women showed that many who had been on HRT switched to bisphosphonates and/or raloxifene, as described in a French study. Raloxifene is the only selective oestrogen receptor modulator (SERM) that has been officially approved and covered by insurances in some countries, such as Japan, for the prevention and management of osteoporosis.

Although oestrogen is considered to be the gold standard for osteoporosis prevention, not all patients experience an increase in bone mass. Because of this, the National Osteoporosis Foundation recommends bone mineral density (BMD) testing for all women on long-term HRT to assure that patients have responded to this treatment. In patients who have not responded adequately to oestrogen therapy (also referred to as ERT when only oestrogen is used) or in those found to have a low bone mass, a combination of HRT and alendronate has additive benefits on bone and could be considered, together with anabolic therapy with parathyroid hormone (PTH). Every woman who reaches the menopause is therefore confronted with the far-reaching decision as to whether or not to begin HRT. It is advisable to reach a decision concerning HRT and ERT only after consultation with the patient and a gynaecologist. A BMD measurement and evaluation of the patient's risk profile, including family history, also contribute to the decision. But today, the indications are far more limited and the operative principles are:

- Who should get HRT? – As few women as possible.
- How much HRT? – As little as possible.
- For how long? – As short as possible.

The *mechanisms of action* of oestrogen on bone and tissues related to maintenance of bone are complex and include (Figs. 14.1 and 14.2):

R. Bartl, B. Frisch, *Osteoporosis*, DOI 10.1007/978-3-540-79527-8_14,
© Springer-Verlag Berlin Heidelberg 2009

14

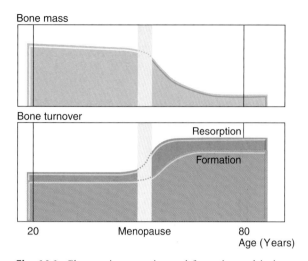

Fig. 14.1. Changes in resorption and formation and in bone mass before and at the menopause, without therapy

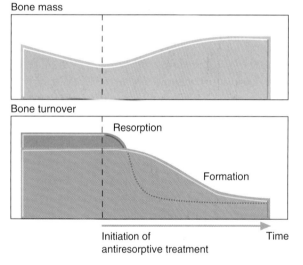

Fig. 14.2. Preservation and/or increase in bone mass, decrease in bone turnover at and after the menopause under the influence of bisphosphonate therapy

- Induction of FasL in osteoblasts, leading to apoptosis in preosteoclasts
- Inhibition of osteoclast activity
- Stimulation of collagen synthesis by osteoblasts
- Promotion of gastrointestinal absorption of calcium
- Stimulation of calcitonin secretion
- Modulation of PTH secretion
- Improvement of central nervous functions and therefore decrease in tendency to fall
- Increased blood flow through the bones

The data from the oestrogen/progesterone arm of the *Women's Health Initiative (WHI) Study (2003)* has influenced perceptions on the effects of HRT and its role in patient management. The study confirmed that HRT reduces the risk of vertebral, non-vertebral and hip fractures. This was a major advance in the evidence base concerning the effects of HRT on bone, but at the same time, cardiovascular and breast cancer data from the trial have had a negative effect on perceptions and, as a consequence, the use of HRT and ERT is now strictly limited. This is all the more so, as alternatives are readily available and do not have the potentially dangerous side effects of HRT and ERT. As a result, women who do use HRT, limit their use to a short time after the menopause. Women at high risk of osteoporosis who wish to minimize postmenopausal bone loss now have the option of transferring to raloxifene or a nitrogen-containing bisphosphonate, or the combination of the two, as well as the latest anabolic therapy, if osteoporosis is already established.

14.2
Which Oestrogens and Progestins, and How to Take Them?

The main groups of oestrogen preparations given orally or transdermally are:
- Synthetic oestrogen analogues with a steroid skeleton
- Non-human oestrogen, produced from an equine source (conjugated equine oestrogens)
- Native human oestrogens or compounds that are transformed to native oestrogens in the body

Effective daily doses of commonly used oestrogens are:
- Oestradiol Orally 2 mg
- Patch 50 µg
- Gel 1 mg
- Conjugated equine oestrogens 0 625 mg
- Oestradiol valerate 2 mg

For women with an intact uterus, oestrogen should be combined with *progestin* to prevent the risk of endometrial hyperplasia and cancer. Cyclic treatment is recommended for women immediately after the menopause, while continuous daily intake is suitable for older postmenopausal women when regular uterine bleeding is undesirable. Most clinical experience has been gained with the use of medroxyprogesterone acetate, norethisterone acetate and levonorgestrel. However, as pointed out previously, women should be informed about the alternatives to HRT but, if used, then as little as possible, for as short a time as possible! All the above refers to the use of oral medications. However, many studies, but no clinical trials, have now demonstrated the effects of non-oral hormone therapy, in much lower doses, on bone and on the maintenance of BMD.

Tibolone is a synthetic analogue of gonadal steroids with combined oestrogenic, progestogenic and androgenic properties. The endometrium is unaffected and combination with progestin is not necessary. At a dose of 2.5 mg daily it reduces bone turnover by 30–50% and so increases bone mass by 2–5% during the first 2 years. This effect on bone is similar to that of conventional HRT. The effect on fracture risk remains to be determined.

14.3
Which Women to Treat?

Early treatment is warranted for the following indications:
- Premature and surgically induced menopause, especially under the age of 40
- Women with osteopenia: T-score <−1 SD
- Loss of bone density in excess of 1% per year (DXA)
- Women at high risk due to lifestyle or other factors

14.4
How Long to Treat?

Every patient must decide for herself how long to continue to take HRT. For effective prevention and management of osteoporosis a period of 5–15 years was previously recommended, possibly even for life. The longer the therapy, the longer the bone is protected. HRT can be started even at 75 years of age, but must be continued and taken regularly to pre-

serve the beneficial effects on the skeleton. As soon as HRT is discontinued, bone resorption begins again, so that the bone density returns to its starting value 3–4 years after cessation of therapy. Research on the discontinuation of HRT has demonstrated that the rate of loss of bone mass is similar to the rate of loss at the menopause.

General compliance with HRT is low and it is often rejected by women:
- Only 15% of women who would benefit from HRT actually take it.
- Only 70–50% of the various oestrogen preparations prescribed are actually taken.
- Only 20% of women who embarked on therapy with oestrogen take it for more than 5 years.

Since HRT is no longer recommended except in low doses for short periods and only for oestrogen deprivation symptoms, such as hot flushes, but not for the prevention of osteoporosis, the issue of compliance is no longer relevant. For many women, lifestyle changes, increased physical activity, proper nutrition and supplements would prevent osteoporosis and obviate the need for hormones. Should osteopenia or osteoporosis be diagnosed by routine bone density measurements, treatment with bisphosphonates or other anti-resorptive and anabolic agents is now readily available.

14.5
How to Monitor HRT?

Oestrogen replacement therapy, with or without progestin, needs to be monitored annually for efficacy and safety:
- *Efficacy*: dual-energy X-ray absorptiometry (DXA), alkaline phosphatase and CrossLaps in the serum, selectively oestradiol and sex hormone-binding globulin (SHBG)
- *Safety*: Annual breast examination and mammogram, vaginal ultrasound

Some patients may not respond to oral oestrogens because of gastrointestinal side effects, malabsorption or enterohepatic binding of oestrogen. Alternative routes of administration include oestrogen patches or gel.

14.6
What are the Risks and Adverse Events of HRT?

Over the past few years, many studies have been designed, carried out and published on the risk and benefits of HRT, especially long-term. HRT had previously been taken for many years by millions of women after cessation of the menses. Results of controlled trials did not show a protective effect of HRT on reducing risk of coronary artery disease, but there was a decreased risk of colorectal cancer and of osteoporotic fractures. Most importantly, however, there was an increased risk of heart disease, stroke, invasive breast cancer and venous thromboembolism. The findings of these extensive controlled trials have seriously undermined the indications for long-term HRT, which should no longer be prescribed. "Better safe than sorry", as the proverb has it!

In spite of some 50 observational studies, there is still no complete consensus on breast cancer risk with HRT. Most experts agree that oestrogen may be a promoter rather than a cause of breast cancer. The risk of breast cancer for ERT-treated women appears to be time- and dose-dependent and increases by 25–70% after 10–15 years of ERT. In the *HERS study*, the use of oestrogen in women with serious cardiovascular disease did not result in protection against myocardial infarction. A further large prospective study *(Woman's Health Initiative)*, designed to answer many questions related to oestrogen replacement, included more than 27,000 older, generally healthy postmenopausal women. The oestrogen-plus-progesterone segment was stopped when results showed that hormone therapy caused small increases in the risk of coronary events, stroke, pulmonary embolism and breast cancer. There were also some small decreases in the risks of hip fracture and colon cancer, but the overall harm outweighed these benefits. There was also clear evidence that hormone therapy does not result in better quality of life among older women without menopausal symptoms, and does not improve cognition, depression or sexual function. At present, women with postmenopausal vasomotor symptoms must weigh the risks associated with HRT treatment against the benefits of symptom relief. They require treatment for a much shorter duration than 5 years, and therefore the risk will be smaller. Given the availability of other effective drugs, the use of hormone therapy for the prevention or treatment of osteoporosis

is not appropriate for most women. Obviously the indications for HRT have changed, as have the variety of choices available and alternative therapies. HRT is only recommended for climacteric symptoms, at a dose as small as possible and for a limited period of time (less than 4 years). As regards osteoporosis, comparative trials have now shown that the bisphosphonates produce a similar reduction in fracture risk, without the possible adverse events of HRT. It must be unequivocally stated that HRT is no longer recommended as a first-line therapy for the prevention and therapy of osteoporosis.

14.7
What are the Main Contraindications?

- Vaginal bleeding of unknown origin
- Thrombotic tendency and pulmonary emboli in the patient's history
- Family history of breast cancer
- Hypertension
- Acute or chronic hepatic disorders
- Hypertriglyceridaemia
- Malignant melanoma

14.8
Natural Oestrogens – How Effective are They?

There is much interest among postmenopausal women in "natural" alternatives to oestrogen. *Phytooestrogens*, also known as plant oestrogens, are non-steroidal molecules (isoflavones, lignans, coumestans, stilbenes and resorcylic lactones) and occur naturally in plants and vegetables, for example in soy products, some types of peas and beans as well as in tea, milk and beer. The plants contain three main classes of phytooestrogens: isoflavones, lignans and coumestans, which resemble oestrogen chemically and are converted in the body into very weak forms of oestrogen. These molecules do not share the common chemical structure with oestrogens, but they have two structural features that resemble oestrogens (Fig. 14.3):

- An aromatic A ring with a hydroxyl group, and
- A second hydroxyl group in the same plane of the A ring

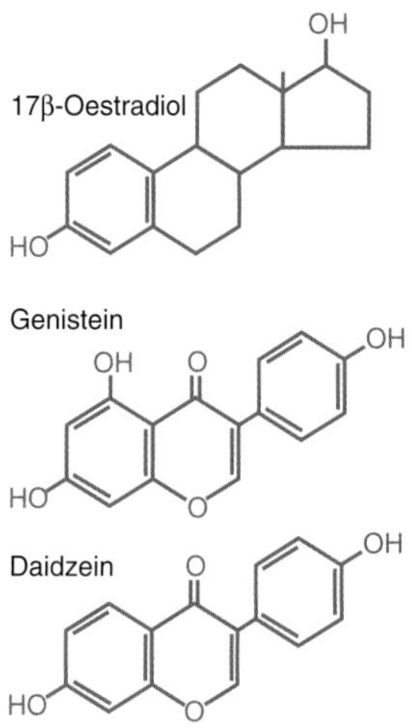

Fig. 14.3. Structures of the 17β-oestradiol and the two main natural oestrogens Genistein and Daidzein present in soy

17β-Oestradiol

Genistein

Daidzein

These similarities allow the molecules to bind to the oestrogen receptors (ER) and thereby lead to biological activity (nuclear DNA-stimulated protein synthesis).

Although these plant oestrogens are a thousand times weaker than animal oestrogens, they do exercise

a positive effect on the vegetative manifestations of the menopause and also have positive effects on bone-building. Some observational studies have related the lower incidence of osteoporosis in women in Eastern countries with a diet rich in phytooestrogens. *Isoflavones* are found principally in legumes and soybean products. In terms of dietary sources, most soy products contain about 2 mg/g of isoflavones, and the upper limit of iso-flavone intake should be approximately 50 mg/day from diet and supplements (Fig. 14.4). *Lignans* are found in fruits, vegetables and beer, and *coumestans* in bean sprouts and fodder crops. Two small studies have demonstrated that they significantly reduced fracture risk. An additional advantage is that, presumably, they have no tumour-promoting activity. The recommended dose of ipriflavone is 600 mg daily, taken in two or three separate doses. Though these results are promising, larger studies are necessary to demonstrate the value of phytooestrogens in osteoporosis, in particular in Western countries. Phytooestrogens have the potential of significant biological effects, although the spectrum of these

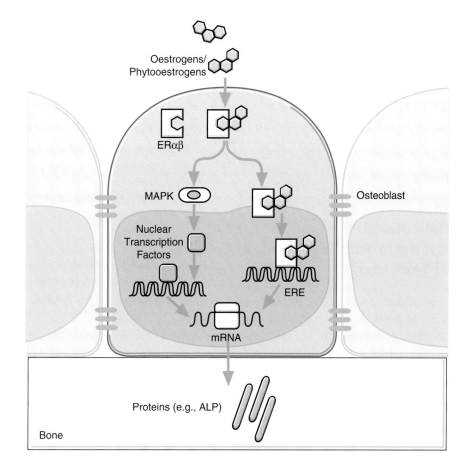

Fig. 14.4. Similar action of oestrogens and phyto-oestrogens in stimulating osteoblasts to produce the proteins which constitute the bone matrix. *ER*, oestrogen receptor; *MAPK*, mitogen-activated protein kinase (modified from Migliaccio et al. [2003])

effects may be quite different from that of oestrogen or SERMs. However, cell and animal studies have shown that this effect is mediated, at least in part, via the classical oestrogen receptor mechanism, presumably via the osteoblasts. Stimulation of both cell proliferation and alkaline phosphatase, a marker of osteoblastic cell differentiation, suggests that *genistein* may enhance bone formation activities. Genistein also inhibits the synthesis and secretion of interleukin-6, which further indicates that this substance may decrease osteoclast differentiation and function through an osteoblast-mediated effect, as already suggested for E_2.

Recommendations for the medical community and the general public concerning the use of soy and other isoflavone supplements to help postmenopausal women with low BMD must await further randomized clinical trials, to satisfy objectively the needs for evidence-based medicine. One must also keep in mind that herbal products are not regulated by the FDA, which means that the purity, safety and effectiveness of the herb is not necessarily assured and the amount of active drug per milligram dose may vary with different manufacturers. There may also be the possibility of contamination with other compounds when collected, distilled and manufactured in capsules. Furthermore, the metabolism of the active drugs and consequently their action appear to be highly influenced by other factors of diet, intestinal function, intestinal bacteria and individual variations. However, standardized plant extracts as substitutes for HRT are now available and results of trials are awaited.

14.9
Dehydroepiandrosterone (DHEA) – Is it Useful for the Prevention of Bone Loss?

This substance has gained a great deal of attention from the media and the public and many people now take DHEA to prevent or reverse various age-related changes. DHEA is one of the major circulating adrenal androgens. Serum DHEA levels peak by the second decade of life and then steadily decline by about 10% per decade. The regulatory role of DHEA in bone metabolism has been evaluated in several studies, indicating that adrenal androgens may prevent bone loss induced by oestrogen deficiency. When using pharmacologic doses of DHEA, variable effects on blood lipids and body composition have been reported, but none of these studies investigated the effects on bones. Consequently, DHEA supplements should be deferred until the results of ongoing studies with this hormone are published.

14.10
Testosterone – Good for Bones and Well-Being in Men!

Secondary osteoporosis should always be suspected if a decrease in bone density occurs in a young male. Possibilities are hypogonadism or Klinefelter syndrome, for which the therapy of choice is early institution of *testosterone replacement therapy*. Hypogonadism in the male is associated with low values of calcitriol and decreased intestinal absorption of calcium. Under therapy with testosterone, gains in BMD correlated better with serum oestrogen levels than with testosterone, indicating that conversion of testosterone to oestrogen may be an important factor. Treatment with testosterone may also increase muscle mass and improve well-being. The use of testosterone therapy should be limited to men with low levels of free testosterone who have no contraindications such as benign prostatic hypertrophy or prostate cancer. Safety of treatment should be monitored by blood tests, and by levels of glucose and prostate-specific antigen (PSA) in the serum. Recommendations for testosterone replacement in patients with low serum levels include: intramuscular injections 100–250 mg every 3–4 weeks or testosterone gel 5 mg daily.

14.11
Anabolic Steroids – Strong Muscles for Healthy Bones!

The efficacy of these drugs in osteoporosis has long been recognized and is due to their effect on the muscles, although a direct action on bone-forming cells has also been described. These drugs are indicated in the elderly when there is reduction in muscle mass (sarcopenia), muscular weakness or even cachexia. Anabolic steroid therapy in the elderly has a significant anabolic effect on bone in addition to its anti-catabolic effect. Treatment should be restricted to 3 years, and the well known side effects (virilization in women) and hepatic damage must be taken into consideration. Moreover, men may experience a reduction in sexual function. In addition, cancer of the prostate must be ruled out before therapy is started, because it could be stimulated by anabolics. *Nandrolone* decanoate is the preparation most frequently prescribed: 50 mg i.m. every 4 weeks. This drug can be used as an adjuvant treatment in elderly women, as well as in male patients with osteoporosis.

In the years that have now passed since the publication of the WHI trial results in 2002, many different types, combinations, formulations and ways of administering HRT have been described, as well as who should receive them, why they should receive them and exactly for what they should receive them, and precisely for how long they should receive them! All have one goal – effective hormone therapy targeted for specific conditions without the adverse side effects disclosed by the WHI trials. Also, over the years various authorities have regularly published position papers on HRT, as up to date results of more trials and investigations were made public. A few are listed below, all published in 2008. One of the latest, which is very comprehensive and also includes a discussion of the risk–benefit concepts, is the Position Statement of the North American Menopause Society, dated July 2008. The results and conclusions reached do support the use of HRT to treat or reduce the risk of specific disorders such as osteoporosis and fractures, but only in selected populations of postmenopausal women. Conditions and reservations concerning the recipients, as well as the therapies, are also outlined in the report. In another study, 600 US and European gynaecologists, who participated in an enquiry on HRT, confirmed that they still utilize HRT as therapy for postmenopausal women, but only for specific aims, at much lower doses and for limited periods of time. A novel combination consisting of minimal quantities of hormones – oestradiol 0.5 mg and norethisterone acetate (NETA) 0.1 mg – has been approved by the FDA, the European Medicines Agency, The International Menopause Society and the North American Menopause Society. As a first-line oral therapy for post-

menopausal women, its effectiveness, tolerability and safety have already been demonstrated in a 6-month trial. Results of longer trials are awaited.

The *hormone-dependent or -related problems in the ageing population*, especially in women, are also addressed. According to some authors, these include osteoporosis, Alzheimer's disease, urinary incontinence and generalized as well as coronary atherosclerosis. In fact, many studies have concluded that cardiovascular or coronary heart disease constitutes a major group in the category of hormone-related problems in the aged. Extensive animal studies have demonstrated the significant role of HRT on vascular endothelium and vascular smooth muscle, but have emphasized that in women the type, dosage, administration and timing must be adapted to the individual patient's age and cardiovascular condition in order to enhance the benefits of HRT also in elderly women. Recent investigations and reviews have emphasized that the risk for coronary heart disease is highest in 70- to 79-year-old women, often together with risk of fractures due to osteoporosis. Therapy for these patients is specific: for the cardiologic conditions, for osteoporosis and for any other specific condition, as well as serious attention to lifestyle factors such as nutrition and exercise. Other incidental conditions such as infections and their consequences, e.g. hepatitis C followed by hepatic steatosis or fibrosis, are also candidates for consideration of HRT. Hormone therapy is also an option for adolescents under special circumstances.

There is a beneficial effect of HRT and of exercise training (ET) on insulin action, and this has also been observed in overweight adults with sedentary habits. Moreover, the ET effects on insulin are different for men and women on or off HRT, which is taken into account in the preparation of treatment strategies for these patients. The combination of low dose HRT and exercise training also has beneficial effects on BMD and muscle mass in postmenopausal women.

In summary, as time has passed, and the results of the WHI investigations are seen in greater perspective, HRT and ERT are prescribed, but more specifically, in minimal effective dosages and for the shortest possible period of time.

Bisphosphonates

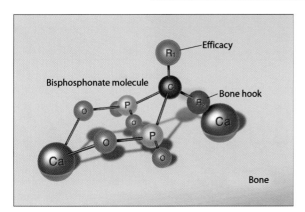

A new era in the treatment of disorders of bone began about 30 years ago with the introduction of bisphosphonates into clinical practice. Bisphosphonates are deposited on the surface of the bones, inhibit osteoclasts and thus resorption of bone. Consequently, these drugs have long been given to patients with Morbus Paget, hypercalcaemia, multiple myeloma and osseous metastases. Bisphosphonates not only inhibit resorption of bone, they also inhibit growth of metastases in the bone and bone marrow.

Bisphosphonates inhibit resorption in osteoporosis and – in particular the latest aminobisphosphonates – have no adverse effects on bone formation and therefore lead to a long-lasting (periods of years) positive bone balance. Bisphosphonates have been successfully used for the prevention and therapy in all forms of osteoporosis. Compact and spongy bone show equal increases in bone density (Fig. 15.1). Moreover, the long-term incorporation of bisphosphonates into the bones has no detectable deleterious influence on bone quality and strength. The concept of "frozen bone" under bisphosphonate therapy is simply not true. A basic level of remodelling is consistently maintained even under long-term bisphosphonate therapy. Disturbances of mineralization have not been observed with the new bisphosphonates currently in use.

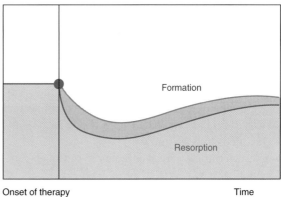

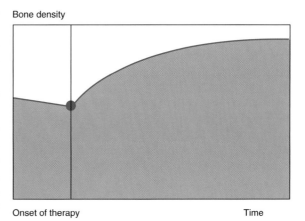

Fig. 15.1. Bone remodelling and bone density under antiresorptive therapy with bisphosphonates

The nitrogen-containing bisphosphonates are today the most effective medications available for the

R. Bartl, B. Frisch, *Osteoporosis,* DOI 10.1007/978-3-540-79527-8_15,
© Springer-Verlag Berlin Heidelberg 2009

15

treatment of all forms of osteoporosis in both men and women, young and old, congenital and acquired osteoporosis, primary and secondary, high and low turnover, and in pre-, peri- and post-menopausal and involutional osteoporoses. Bisphosphonates have also been given to children – even very young ones – but this should only be done in authorized paediatric centres under strictly controlled indications and conditions.

15.1
A Brief Survey of Bisphosphonates

These are synthetic compounds, analogues of pyrophosphate in which the oxygen atom of the central P–O–P bond has been replaced by carbon, resulting in a P–C–P group. This exchange has made the bisphosphonates resistant to enzymatic hydrolysis. In addition, different bisphosphonates can be synthesized by substitution of both hydrogen atoms on the carbon atom, and these bisphosphonates differ in their biological properties, activities, pharmacodynamics and toxicity. There are two side chains (Fig. 15.2):

- One binds to bone mineral
- One determines class and potency (nitrogen molecule)

The dynamics of these new bisphosphonates manifest themselves in their potency – they are 20,000 times more potent than etidronate, the first generation bisphosphonate (Table 15.1). Bisphosphonates have a high affinity for certain structures on the surface of bone. Most of the bisphosphonate absorbed in the gastrointestinal tract is deposited on bone within

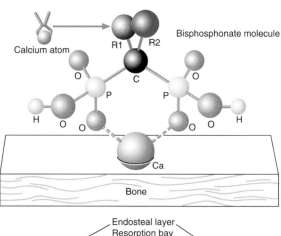

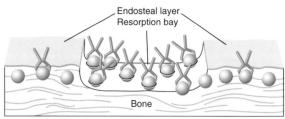

Fig. 15.2. Molecular structure of bisphosphonates. Note structural resemblance to tongs. Deposition of bisphosphonates on osseous surface: subsequently bisphosphonates are phagocytosed by osteoclasts or incorporated into the bone

hours, especially in resorption bays (Howship's lacunae) or in the acid environment under the osteoclasts. This causes a very effective inhibition of osteoclasts and resorption, as well as re-activation of the suppressed osteoblasts and thereby leads to an overall positive "bone balance" and increase in bone mass. The bisphosphonates deposited on the surface are later (weeks or months) built into the bone and may remain there for many years, until eventually they may reach the surface again in a remodelling cycle. However, due to their extremely low concentrations, these bisphos-

Table 15.1. List of available bisphosphonates according to side chains and relative potency

Substance	Trade name	R1	R2	Relative potency
Etidronate	Didronel®	–OH	–CH$_3$	1×
Clodronate	Ostac®	–CL	–CL	10×
Pamidronate	Aredia®	–OH	–CH$_2$–CH$_2$–NH$_2$	100×
Alendronate	Fosamax®	–OH	–CH$_2$–CH$_2$–CH$_2$–NH$_2$	1000×
Risedronate	Actonel®	–OH	–CH$_2$–$\langle$=N$\rangle$	5000×
Ibandronate	Bondronat® Bon(v)iva®	–OH	–CH$_2$–CH$_2$–NH$_2$–CH$_3$ C$_5$H$_{11}$	10000×
Zoledronate	Zometa® Aclasta®	–OH	–CH$_2$–N$\langle$=N$\rangle$	20000×

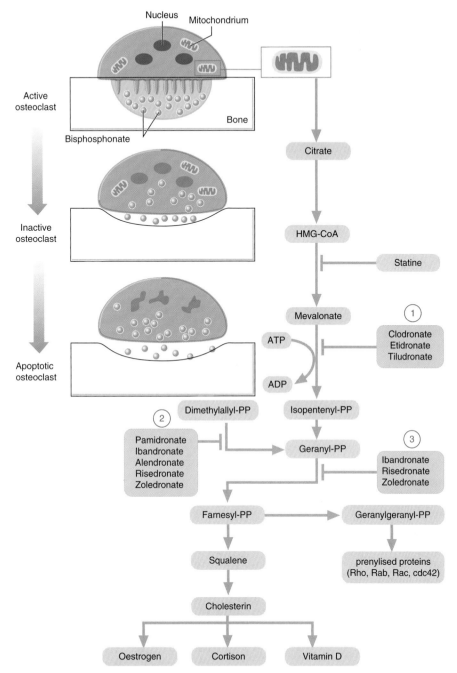

Fig. 15.3. Cellular and biochemical mechanisms of action of the nitrogen-containing bisphosphonates: *Left*, layer of bisphosphonate (*blue dots*) on bone beneath osteoclasts in resorption lacunae. The bisphosphonates are taken up by the osteoclasts, which leads to their inactivation and retraction of the ruffled membrane. Higher doses lead to increased apoptosis of the osteoclasts. *Right*, biosynthetic pathway for sterols and isoprenoids, which takes place in the cytoplasm of the osteoclasts. Steps of inhibition by statins and bisphosphonates. *HMG CoA*, 3-hdroxy-3-methylglutaryl-Co-A; *PP*, pyrophosphate. 1, 2 and 3 show the different generations of bisphosphonates, each with its own specific targets. Effects of the 2nd and 3rd generation lead to an accumulation of isopentenyl-PP, which in turn stimulates the acute phase reaction. However, this may be reduced by simultaneous administration of clodronate

phonates remain inactive, even when "recycled", that means when the bone on which they are deposited undergoes remodelling again.

The *mechanism of action* is not yet completely understood, but some aspects have been elucidated (Fig. 15.3):

- Incorporation of bisphosphonates into hydroxyapatite crystals and the bone matrix leads to decreased solubility of the bone substance and disturbances of mineralization – physical–chemical effect.
- Reduction in recruitment and fusion of osteoclast precursors – direct influence on the monocyte–macrophage system.
- Inhibition of osteoclast activity by means of inhibition of the proton-ATPases – a direct toxic effect.
- Inhibition of enzymes of mevalonic acid metabolism – by the aminobisphosphonates.
- Shortening of osteoclastic survival by induction of apoptosis, probably associated with a lengthening of osteoblastic survival (alterations in the periods of the phases of remodelling cycles).
- Indirect inhibition of osteoclastic resorption by way of factors produced by osteoblasts – interference with "coupling" in the osteoblast–osteoclast cycle.
- Increased synthesis of collagen type I by osteoblasts.
- Inhibition of production of prostaglandin E2, proteolytic enzymes, interleukin 1 and 6 and many other cytokines.
- Inhibition of adherence of osteoclasts and tumour cells to the surface of bone.
- Effect on afferent nerve fibres in bone with inhibition of release of neuropeptides and neuromodulators at the nerve ends.
- Bisphosphonates have an anti-apoptotic effect on osteoblasts and osteocytes, for which connexin 43 is required.
- Individual bisphosphonates may also exhibit particular individual activities.

From a laboratory point of view, inhibition of osteoclastic resorption results in decreased excretion of the breakdown products of collagen in the urine and a reduction in the level of calcium in the blood in patients with hypercalcaemia. In the long term, inhibition of resorption results in a positive calcium balance with a continuous increase in bone mass, especially in trabecular bone because of its large surface area. Moreover, the increase in bone mass is accompanied

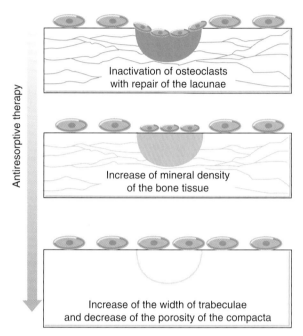

Deep resorption cavities with active osteoclasts

Inactivation of osteoclasts with repair of the lacunae

Increase of mineral density of the bone tissue

Increase of the width of trabeculae and decrease of the porosity of the compacta

Antiresorptive therapy

Fig. 15.4. The sequence of effects of bisphosphonate therapy

by an increase in mechanical resistance of the bone. Bisphosphonates and other antiresorptive agents improve *bone strength* by various effects (Fig. 15.4):

- They reduce the size of the remodelling space and repair the resorption cavities caused by increased osteoclastic activity.
- They maintain the trabecular architecture, especially the horizontal trabeculae.
- They decrease cortical porosity.
- They increase mineralization density by a prolongation of the bone formation period.
- They maintain osteocytic viability. Indeed, recent studies indicate that osteocytes act as mechanosensors and thereby participate in the regulation of bone remodelling. There is also evidence that oestrogen, bisphosphonates and raloxifene all prevent osteocytic apoptosis.
- They significantly alter maturation and properties of bone collagen, suggesting a contribution of the organic matrix to the anti-fracture efficacy of these drugs. Bisphosphonates exert more profound chang-

es in the organic matrix than raloxifene, probably due to their more potent suppression of turnover (>50% suppression).

The osteomalacia (disturbance of mineralization) observed after long-term use of the first generation of bisphosphonates has not occurred with the latest aminobisphosphonates (i.e. those with an amino group in one of the side chains) even after 8 years of therapy. Increases in mineralization, collagen maturity and non-enzymatic cross links have been observed after 3 years of therapy. Changes in lamellar structure of the trabeculae were also not observed. It has recently been reported that in dogs given a six-fold greater than the normal therapeutic dose of alendronate or risedronate, both drugs substantially decreased bone turnover, but there was an increase in histological microcracks. Moreover, there was a greater increase in bone strength in the alendronate and risedronate groups than in controls. To summarize, in humans, none of the currently used aminobisphosphonates were found to have any deleterious effects on bone quality, estimated by preclinical mechanical testing and clinical fracture risk. Studies are available on the determination of the active ingredients in bisphosphonates as well as reviews of the analytical methods applied.

However, one cautionary note: a recent investigation on the in vitro effects of pamidronate and alendronate on osteoblasts showed that these aminobisphosphonates inhibited osteoblast growth and caused osteoblast apoptosis. These inhibitory effects were observed at the same concentrations of bisphosphonates that caused osteoclast inhibition. To what extent these in vitro studies reflect the in vivo situation remains to be determined.

The most recent investigations have shown an antiproliferative effect of bisphosphonates on growth of tumour cells. The inhibition of osteoclasts results in a reduction in the production of IL-6 and in the release of growth factors from the bone matrix. Evidence is also accumulating that bisphosphonates have a negative influence on osseous and probably also on visceral metastases, possibly by way of interactions with adhesion molecules on the tumour cells and/or by forming a film on the surface of the bone, which inhibits attachment of the tumour cells to the osseous surface.

Data from studies on hyperlipidemic patients with osteoporosis and on therapy with bisphosphonates showed that these also have a beneficial effect on lipid metabolism.

15.2 Pharmacokinetics

As mentioned above, the P–C–P bond is completely resistant to enzymatic hydrolysis. Consequently, the currently used bisphosphonates are absorbed unchanged, are deposited on bone and eventually excreted. They are not metabolized in the body and interactions with other medications do not occur. Intestinal absorption is minimal – somewhere between 1 and 10% – and with the latest bisphosphonates probably less than 1%. Absorption may be further reduced if bisphosphonates are taken with food or drink especially with bivalent salts such as calcium and magnesium. Consequently, it is essential to ingest the bisphosphonates on an empty stomach and only with water. The manufacturers recommend taking alendronate and risedronate with a full glass of tap water on an empty stomach half an hour before breakfast. The patient must remain in the upright position to ensure absorption and to avoid adverse reactions. The tablet should not be regurgitated together with gastric juices and remain in the oesophagus, because that could damage the mucus membrane. If a patient has difficulties in swallowing or there is a pre-existing reflux esophagitis, an alternative method of administration, or a different therapy, should be chosen. Between 20 and 50% of the absorbed

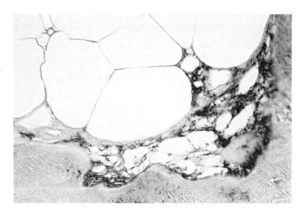

Fig. 15.5. Deposition of bisphosphonate (*red*) on bone in a resorption lacuna and in the cytoplasm of an osteoclast visualized by means of an antibody to ibandronate, as seen in sections of a plastic embedded undecalcified iliac crest biopsy

15

bisphosphonate adheres to the surface of the bone (Fig. 15.5), while the rest is excreted in the urine or faeces over the course of the day.

In contrast to its short stay in the peripheral blood (half-life of 1–15 h) the *half-life of bisphosphonates in the skeleton* is much longer – a matter of years, as is the case for other substances, such as tetracycline, which have a high affinity for bones. Individual bisphosphonates may have different interactions with bone that result in differences in their pharmacologic behaviour. For example risedronate has a lower kinetic binding affinity for the mineral substrates on the bone surface than alendronate does. These differences may contribute to the apparently shorter half-life of risedronate and to its faster clinical on and off responses compared to alendronate. Preliminary results suggest that ibandronate and zoledronate have higher kinetic binding affinities than alendronate and risedronate.

15.3
Toxicity and Contraindications

Bisphosphonates are very well tolerated when taken as prescribed. Side effects and adverse reactions are few and rarely severe:

- *Gastrointestinal complaints*: these have been reported in 2–10% of patients and include nausea, vomiting, stomach aches, and diarrhoea. However, in large placebo-controlled studies, these were reported equally by both test and control groups. Inflammation and ulceration of the oesophagus, occasionally reported, can easily be avoided by strict adherence to the directions for taking the medication. Lesions of the mucus membrane occur in two stages. Firstly, regurgitation of gastric acid damages the oesophageal epithelium; secondly, amino-bisphosphonates diffuse into the adjoining epithelial cells and inhibit synthesis of cholesterin (inhibition of the mevalonic acid pathway), which in turn prevents cholesterin-dependent repair of the damaged mucosal cells. Bed-ridden patients or patients with reflux esophagitis should not be given oral amino-bisphosphonates, or at best only under the strictest medical supervision.
- *Acute phase reaction*: This can occur within 24 h of the first intravenous infusion of an aminobisphos-

phonate. The reaction consists of a rise in temperature, joint and bone pains, myalgias, increase of IL-6 and C reactive proteins in the blood, as well as changes in lymphocyte counts.
- Very rarely, an infusion or oral treatment must be stopped because of the outbreak of a *skin allergy* or photosensitivity.
- *Ocular reactions* have been observed, but very rarely (1/1000 patients). Uveitis scleritis and episcleritis have been observed after pamidronate. With cessation of the infusion and administration of glucocorticoids the ocular inflammation improved rapidly.
- About 3% of patients who receive infusions of bisphosphonates experience *moderate hypocalcaemia and hypomagnesemia*, which however do not require any medical treatment. Aminobisphosphonates should not be given together with aminoglycosides since both medications reduce the calcium level in the blood which may last for considerable periods of time. We have not observed any clinically significant hypocalcaemia as a consequence of infusion of bisphosphonates.
- *Renal function* should be checked before intravenous infusion of bisphosphonates. At high dosages kidney pain may occur as well as mild, clinically non-significant albuminuria.
- No data on humans suggest that the administration of modern bisphosphonates, at least in doses used for osteoporosis, interfere clinically with *fracture repair*. The amount of callus formed was either unchanged or was increased, but never decreased. The slowing of callus turnover was accompanied paradoxically by a higher mechanical strength.
- *Acute and chronic toxicity studies* using oral alendronate in female animals showed no evidence of mutagenicity, including those most relevant to human carcinogenic potential. Carcinogenicity studies in rats and mice at maximum tolerated doses showed no increase in tumour incidence associated with alendronate treatment. There was also no effect on fertility or reproductive performance in male or female rats.
- *Low energy fractures of the femoral shaft* have recently been observed in some patients on long-term therapy (> than 6 years) with alendronate. The fractures had a simple transverse pattern and were presumed to result from propagation of a stress fracture presumed to be due to impaired repair of microdamage. One other previous study had iden-

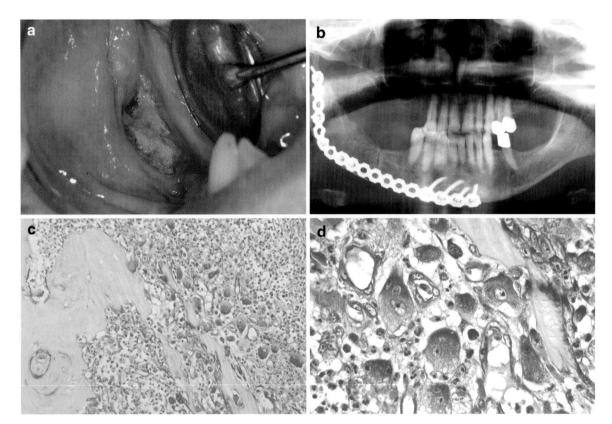

Fig 15.6a-d. (a) Osteoporosis of the jaw in a patient with breast cancer, 1 year after therapy with a bisphosphonate given monthly i.v. **(b)** Surgical stabilization of the necrotic area of the jaw. **(c)** Histology of the necrotic jaw in the same patient show-ing chronic osteomyelitis with necrotic bone and osteoclastic re-sorption, Giemsa staining. **(d)** At higher magnification, increase of large, multinucleated macrophages, lymphocytes and granu-locytes in the surrounding bone marrow, Giemsa staining

tified low energy femoral shaft fractures in some patients after an average of 4.8 years of therapy with alendronate. There has been speculation that these atypical fractures of the femur were due to atypical skeletal fragility as a result of severely suppressed bone turnover, due to inherent conditions as well as to prolonged antiresorptive therapy.

15.4
Osteomyelitis/Osteonecrosis of the Jaw (ONJ)

Numerous articles on the association of therapy with bisphosphonates and the occurrence of osteonecrosis of the jaw (ONJ) have appeared in the international medical press since the publication of the first report of a single patient in 2003 (Fig. 15.6a–d). Many of these reports were published in the last few years, especially in 2008. Included are studies of related and possibly causative factors as well as retrospective investigations of large numbers of patients. The sug-gested associated factors include:

- Suppression of the activity of local macrophages by bisphosphonates.
- Microfractures in heavily burdened jaw bones.
- Anomalies of the vascular system in the jaws. Stud-ies have shown that the jaw bones have a greater blood supply than other bones, as well as a high bone turnover rate and therefore there is a high concentration of bisphosphonates in the jaws.
- Infectious inflammatory processes during immuno-suppression.
- Anti-angiogenic effects of bisphosphonates leading to local necrosis.
- Inhibitory effect on local physiological processes in bone.

15

- Administration of bisphosphonates oral or, mostly, intravenous.
- Enhancement of inflammatory/necrotizing processes caused by prior or current chemotherapy and/or corticosteroids already present before administration of bisphosphonates leading to an increased concentration of bisphosphonates.

Many articles and position papers have been published on how to deal with the problem of ONJ. These include specific up-to-date practice guidelines. An excellent example is the Canadian Consensus Practice Guidelines for Bisphosphonate-Associated Osteonecrosis of the Jaw, June 2008. It should be stressed that the guidelines in this Consensus were compiled with the collaboration of recognized, established authorities from all over the world. The guidelines include recommendations given by international experts and results obtained from evidence-based investigations on the prevention of ONJ, its diagnosis and therapy, as well as the management of gums, jaws and in particular patients themselves. However, relatively little attention has been given to the possible association of periodontal conditions with systemic disorders that may also be present, perhaps even for longer periods of time and whether their management took the state of the jaws into consideration. These systemic disorders include diabetes, renal, respiratory and cardiovascular diseases. In elderly patients, such co-morbidities may have been present for a significant length of time and their presence, as well as their therapy, given could very well have impacted the state of the gums and jaw bones.

As mentioned previously, the vast majority of the cases of ONJ reported so far represent only a minuscule percentage of the more than 20 million patients already treated with bisphosphonates for many years. Many studies have confirmed that nearly all patients who developed ONJ had malignancies. In one recent report in which the medical records of 1086 patients were evaluated, the following percentages were calculated: 3.8% per 100 with myeloma, 2.5% per 100 with breast cancer, and 2.9% per 100 with prostate cancer had developed ONJ during the 5-year study. All these patients received bisphosphonates i.v., which led to the hypothesis that there could be complex interactions between the bisphosphonates and the chemotherapies the patients were receiving at the same time, and this possibly warrants further investigation.

In contrast, another study concentrated only on patients who were prescribed oral, not i.v., bisphosphonates, and only for indications other than malignancies and who had developed ONJ. These patients were studied in order to identify potential contributing factors. The cases included 85 patients with osteoporosis, 10 patients with Paget's disease and individual patients with other conditions. Most of the patients (9% of 63 patients) who supplied dental information had undergone a dental procedure before the onset of the ONJ and in addition 81% of these patients had co-morbidities and were taking at least one other drug which affects bone turnover. The authors concluded that the circumstances of each patient must be taken into consideration, and that a multiplicity of factors may be associated with the development of ONJ (Fig. 15.7). Another study pointed out that ONJ is rare

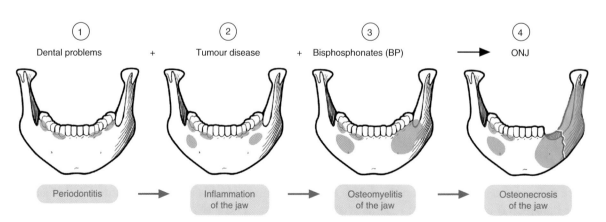

Fig. 15.7. Cascade of events and reactions in the development of osteoporosis of the jaw in patients with neoplasias

in metabolic bone disease and in Paget's disease, i.e. 1 per 100,000 person years. Interestingly, according to another study, smoking and obesity are strong risk factors for ONJ, which suggests that patients should be asked and, if necessary, advised about lifestyle factors before initiation of bisphosphonate therapy.

To summarize: ONJ has been reported in cancer patients receiving high doses of intravenous bisphosphonates, especially pamidronate or zoledronate. However, this situation may change as a novel bisphosphonate, TRK-530, which has recently been developed, has both anti-inflammatory as well as antiresorptive effects, and animal studies have already demonstrated its efficacy in preventing alveolar bone loss in animals with experimental periodontitis, by both topical and systemic administration. The incidence of ONJ in osteoporotic patients treated with oral and/or intravenous bisphosphonates is extremely low (in the order of 1/100,000 cases), and its causal relationship with bisphosphonate therapy has not been established. No causative relationship has been unequivocally demonstrated between ONJ and bisphosphonate therapy. ONJ occurred after tooth extraction. Furthermore, the underlying risk of developing ONJ may be increased in osteoporotic patients by co-morbid diseases. Finally, two studies have confirmed the hypothesis that genetic susceptibility may also participate in the host's reaction to bacteria: complex interactions between pathogenic bacteria and factors in the host's inflammatory reaction such as polymorphisms of IL-6 were shown to participate in the aggressivity of periodontitis, and this could represent one important genetic determinant in the individual patient's propensity to develop ONJ. On a more optimistic note, the FDA has recently approved the use of recombinant human platelet derived growth factor (rhPDGF) for the repair of periodontal defects. PDGF is a crucial factor in the biological repair of many skeletal conditions, and it is anticipated that it will prove effective in the prevention and/or therapy of ONJ.

15.5
Contraindications

Bisphosphonates should be avoided during pregnancy and breast-feeding, although adverse reactions in these conditions have not been reported. On the contrary, they have been used successfully in some patients both during pregnancy and lactation without any detrimental effect on mother or baby, as recently reported.

15.6
Oral Bisphosphonates Currently Used in Osteoporosis

Bisphosphonates are now regarded as the treatment of choice for postmenopausal osteoporosis, due to proven efficacy and a good safety profile. The National Institute for Health and Clinical Excellence (NICE) in the UK has recently recommended bisphosphonates as the first-line therapy in patients with established osteoporosis. The following oral bisphosphonates have been approved to date:

- Alendronate (Fosamax®) 10 mg daily or 70 mg once weekly (Fosamax once weekly 70 mg®)
- Risedronate (Actonel®) 5 mg daily or 35 mg once weekly (Actonel® once weekly 35 mg or 150 mg once monthly)
- Etidronate (e.g. Didronel®) 400 mg daily for 14 days every 3 months
- Ibandronate (Boniva® 150 mg monthly).

15.7
Alendronate

This aminobisphosphonate has been tested in clinical trials involving more than 17,000 patients and has been prescribed for millions of patients in 80 different countries worldwide. It has been approved for treatment of postmenopausal osteoporosis as well as cortisone-induced and involutional bone loss in both men and women.

Alendronate 10 mg orally for 1–3 years resulted in an increase of bone density of 5–9% compared to the control group who received only calcium and vitamin D. After the first year of alendronate therapy, the vertebral fracture rate was reduced by 59% and the hip fracture rate by 63% after 18 months. Significant increases in bone density were seen after 3 months of therapy and the success rate was 95% after 1 year. Moreover, as shown by the FIT study (Fracture Intervention Trial), many patients reported decreases in pain and morbidity. Alendronate achieved significant decreases in fracture rates of vertebrae, hip and fore-arm in post-menopausal women. Similar results were reported in men and in patients with cortisone-induced osteoporosis. The results have been confirmed by several large international trials.

Alendronate 5 mg orally daily has also been approved for the prevention of osteoporosis. Because of the low side effects, 5 mg alendronate daily is especially useful in women who do not take hormone replacement therapy (HRT).

A recent study has shown that combining HRT with alendronate therapy results in a significantly greater increase in bone mineral density (BMD) compared to either oestrogen or alendronate alone.

A significant advance in therapy has been the development of the alendronate once-weekly dose of 70 mg. Numerous animal and clinical studies have shown that alendronate given once weekly as a single tablet produces less irritation of the oesophageal mucosa. Pharmacological studies have also shown that 0.5–1% is absorbed of which 50% is deposited on the resorptive surfaces of bone, where it inhibits the osteoclasts. The same local concentration of alendronate is achieved by daily as by weekly intake. Similarly, the rate of increase in bone density was also equal after daily or weekly administration. Moreover, bone remodelling, i.e. resorption and formation, was also identical. A very important aspect of the once-weekly dosage is that patient acceptance, compliance and tolerance are greatly increased. In the *first head-to-head trial*, the efficacy of alendronate and risedronate was compared (FACT trial). In this study, alendronate 70 mg once weekly produced significantly greater BMD increases at the spine and hip after 12 months therapy than did risedronate 5 mg daily. These differences may be due to the antiresorptive efficacy of alendronate 70 mg once weekly as opposed to reduced absorption and bioavailability of risedronate resulting from postprandial ingestion.

15.8
Risedronate

Risedronate has a nitrogen molecule in a pyridinyl ring in the R2-position and belongs to the third generation of bisphosphonates. This bisphosphonate has also been tested in large clinical trials (VERT trials) involving 15,000 patients. At a daily oral dose of 5 mg

it increased spinal BMD by 4–5% and hip BMD by 2–4% over 3 years. It reduced bone turnover markers by 40–60%. Risedronate (5 mg/day) was shown to reduce vertebral and non-vertebral fractures by 40–50% and 30–36%, respectively, in two 3-year trials that included approximately 3600 women with prevalent vertebral fractures. The reduction was evident as early as 1 year after initiation of therapy. Osteoporotic non-vertebral fractures were reduced by 39% in one of these studies. In the HIP study, risedronate showed a 30% overall reduction in hip fracture. In the subset of women with very low BMD (hip T-score below –3 or –4), there was a 40% reduction. Risedronate is well tolerated even by patients with gastrointestinal problems. It is effective in cortisone-induced osteoporosis and has been approved by the FDA for treatment of post-menopausal osteoporosis, corticosteroid-induced osteoporosis and osteoporosis in men. Risedronate 35 and 50 mg once a week provided the same efficacy and safety as the daily 5-mg regimen. Therefore, the lower dose, *35 mg risedronate once a week*, is considered to be the optimal dosage for pa-

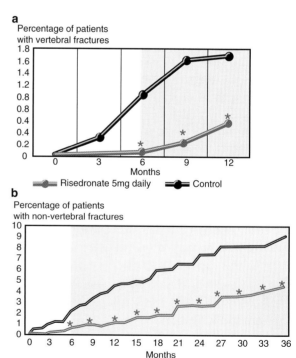

Fig. 15.8a, b. Early reduction of vertebral fractures (**a**) and non-vertebral fractures (**b**) under risedronate. Significant values already after 6 months of therapy

tients with post-menopausal osteoporosis. In a recent study, risedronate *150 mg once a month* was similar in efficacy and safety to daily dosing and may provide an alternative for patients who prefer once-a-month oral ingestion.

Analyses of data from several large trials in osteoporotic post-menopausal women indicate that treatment with risedronate reduces the incidence of vertebral and non-vertebral fractures within 6 months of the start of treatment, and the benefit continues for at least 3 years. The mechanisms for this early significant effect within 6 months are not known, but appear to be related to an early bioavailability as well as to a preservation of micro-architecture, thus avoiding progression of trabecular thinning and loss of connectivity. This *early onset of action* is clinically important for patients with high risk for osteoporotic fractures (Fig. 15.8a and b).

Meanwhile, the results of a 7-year placebo-controlled clinical experience have demonstrated that the *long-term efficacy* and the beneficial effects of risedronate treatment are sustained over this 7-year long period.

15.9
Etidronate

This first generation bisphosphonate is the only one which is administered intermittently. It is given daily 400 mg for 2 weeks every 3 months. It has been shown to reduce vertebral fractures, but with no significant effect on non-vertebral fractures. Etidronate is being replaced by the newer aminobisphosphonates as described above and is not recommended as a first-line therapy for osteoporosis.

15.10
Ibandronate

Ibandronate is a potent nitrogen-containing bisphosphonate that possesses a tertiary nitrogen group on its R_2 side chain and a hydroxyl group on its R_1 side chain, which together confer on ibandronate one of the highest antiresorptive potencies of all bisphosphonates. Due to this greater potency, ibandronate can be given in lower dosages and at longer intervals than the other bisphosphonates already approved for osteopo-

rosis. Ibandronate was the first *to become available as a once monthly tablet*, as well as having the option of i.v. administration. It can be taken orally once a month, for which it has already been authorized; and it is currently being tested both orally and intravenously for the therapy of post-menopausal osteoporosis, as an infusion or as a bolus given i.v. every 3 months. In a previous placebo-controlled trial, the optimal daily dose was shown to be 2.5 mg, which resulted in increases in bone density of up to 10% after 2 years. In the BONE Study, the efficacy of ibandronate was established with respect to reduction of fractures, increase in bone density and decrease in risk parameters. The outcome of the BONE Study, in which 2946 post-menopausal patients (T-score <–2; one or more vertebral fractures) were given 2.5 mg ibandronate daily, showed that after 3 years the relative risk of vertebral fractures was significantly reduced by 62% when compared to patients who received placebo. However, the effect of this therapy on hip fractures was not recorded at the time, probably because this was not one of the primary endpoints of the BONE Study. Nevertheless, as shown by post-hoc analysis, the risk of non-vertebral fractures was also decreased by 69% in 375 patients with an increased risk, i.e. T-score <–3.0. In this study, longer intervals between doses were also investigated. A patient friendly regimen for ibandronate, i.e. a monthly oral or i.v. administration, was then developed on the basis of the results of the BONE Study. The MOPS Study (Monthly Oral Pilot Study) of 144 post-menopausal patients was the first to apply the once-a-month tablet of 100 or 150 mg ibandronate. This dose was well tolerated and lead to a reduction in the biochemical levels of bone resorption markers to normal pre-menopausal values. Thereafter, the MOBILE Study (Monthly Oral Ibandronate in Ladies) comprising 1600 patients was initiated and this study, carried out over a 2-year period, demonstrated the efficacy of the once-a-month therapy of post-menopausal osteoporosis. European authorization for a monthly dose of 150 mg ibandronate (Boniva®) has already been granted, and patient preference for the once-monthly tablet has already been documented. In the head-to-head MOTION study, once monthly ibandronate was shown to be clinically comparable to weekly alendronate at increasing BMD after 12 months in both the lumbar spine and total hip. Efficacy of ibandronate in reducing the risk of fractures has been conclusively established in addition to its efficacy in a randomized

15

controlled trial. It should also be noted that ibandronate has the potential to be utilized for treatment of many diseases of bone from the prevention of osteoporosis to the therapy of osseous metastases.

15.11
Intravenous Bisphosphonates for the Treatment of Osteoporosis

Bisphosphonates are the current mainstay of the management of osteoporosis worldwide. Oral daily and weekly formulations have been linked to poor adherence, but nevertheless yielding a decrease in anti-fracture efficacy in real-life settings. The development of new, 3rd generation bisphosphonates with increased anti-osteoclastic potency and affinity to bone matrix allowed intravenous administration and intervals between administrations to be greater than 1 week or even 1 month. Intravenous administration of potent bisphosphonates can now be considered as an important component of the management of osteoporosis.

15.12
Ibandronate

The DIVA Study (Dosing Intra Venous Administration), a multicentric placebo-controlled study of 1400 patients with post-menopausal osteoporosis, demonstrated the efficacy of ibandronate in this setting. Ibandronate i.v. 2 mg every 2 months or *3 mg every 3 months* was fairly rapidly injected (20–30 s). Both were as effective as the 2.5-mg oral dose which had already proved its value in the reduction of fractures in the BONE Study. European authorization for the i.v. application has already been granted and this i.v. application constitutes an alternative to the monthly tablets.

15.13
Zoledronate

Zoledronate is possibly both a manufacturer's and a patient's dream come true – in the form of a single annual infusion of 5 mg for the prevention and treatment of osteoporosis. As shown in the HORIZON study, a single intravenous infusion of 5 mg zoledronic acid

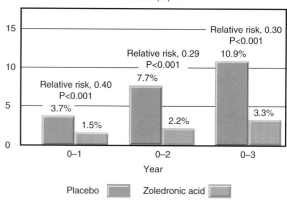

Patients with New Vertebral Fracture (%)

Fig. 15.9. Incidence of morphometric vertebral fractures during the 3-year study period (HORIZON Pivotal Fracture Trial)

significantly decreased bone turnover and improved bone density at 12 months in post-menopausal women with osteoporosis. The risk of morphometric vertebral fracture was reduced by 70% during a 3-year period, compared with placebo (Fig. 15.9). The risk of hip fracture was reduced by 41%, while non-vertebral, clinical and clinical vertebral fractures were reduced by 25, 33 and 77%, respectively. Adverse events, including long-term change in renal function, were similar in the two study groups, although transient renal changes were sometimes noted after the infusion of zoledronate. No cases of ONJ were reported or confirmed by the central adjudication committee. However, serious atrial fibrillation and transient post-infusion symptoms (pyrexia, myalgia, bone pain) occurred more frequently in the zoledronic acid group. Furthermore, an annual infusion of zoledronic acid within 90 days after repair of a low-trauma hip fracture was associated with a reduction in the rate of new clinical fractures and improved survival. Concomitant treatment with other osteoporosis therapies (other bisphosphonates, PTH or strontium) did not significantly affect the bone response to zoledronate. Increased mortality rates after hip fracture are well documented. Indeed, mortality in this study was about three times as high as that reported in the recently completed study of zoledronic acid in post-menopausal women (HORIZON study), and a relative reduction of 28% in the risk of death was observed in the zoledronic acid group. In a substudy of the HORIZON pivotal fracture trial, 152 patients underwent bone biopsy. Zoledronate reduced bone turnover by 63% and preserved bone structure and volume, with evidence of ongoing, active bone remodelling in

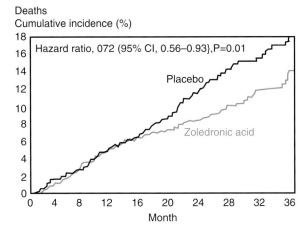

Deaths
Cumulative incidence (%)

Hazard ratio, 072 (95% CI, 0.56–0.93),P=0.01

Placebo

Zoledronic acid

Month

Fig. 15.10. Relative reduction of 28% in the risk of death in the zoledronic acid group (HORIZON Recurrent Fracture Trial)

99% of the biopsies examined. No significant difference in delayed union of fractured bone was observed between the two study groups. A post-hoc analysis suggests that first infusions of zoledronic acid given as early as 2 weeks after hip fracture reduce clinical fractures and mortality (Fig. 15.10). No adverse effects on fracture healing were observed, regardless of the timing of infusion. *A single annual i.v. infusion of 5 mg zoledronate* (Aclasta®) has now been authorized for post-menopausal women with osteoporosis. The most recent studies of zoledronate given once annually for 2 years showed that the BMD was maintained for another extra year after the second dose, i.e. 24 months instead of 12 months! This raised the possibility that zoledronate could be given even less frequently than once a year. These results graphically illustrate the journey of bisphosphonate therapy: from a daily dose of 10 mg to an annual dose of 5 mg! Data are not yet available for men or glucocorticoid-induced osteoporosis, but the same range of dosage could apply. It is advisable to begin therapy with a bisphosphonate prophylactically together with the glucocorticoid therapy, after a dual-energy X-ray absorptiometry (DXA) bone density measurement for baseline values.

15.14
Clodronate and Pamidronate

These two bisphosphonates have already proved their value in hypercalcaemia and in skeletal metastases. However, in most countries, they have not yet been authorized for therapy of osteoporosis; therefore, they should only be given within the setting of an osteoporosis centre and only after the patients have been fully informed and given their written consent to the treatment.

15.15
Recommendations for Intravenous Therapy

This has now gained a high degree of compliance, especially with patients who are already taking a number of other drugs orally. Additional advantages are 100% bioavailability and no gastrointestinal side effects; moreover, the effects on bone density and fracture rate are comparable to those of oral therapy. The following dosages and time intervals are currently used:

> - **Clodronate (Ostac®, Lodronat®, Bonefos®)**
>   600 mg Infusion every 3 months
> - **Pamidronate (Aredia®)**
>   30 mg infusion every 3 months
> - **Ibandronate (Bonviva®, Boniva®)**
>   3 mg infusion or injection every 3 months
> - **Zoledronate (Aclasta®)**
>   5 mg infusion annually

The administration of bisphosphonates at intervals of 3 months is based on the observation that a single intravenous dose inhibits resorption of bone for several weeks; zoledronate 5 mg i.v. every 12 months results in the same increase in bone density as a bisphosphonate taken orally daily, weekly or monthly.

15.16
Duration of Therapy with Bisphosphonates and Long-Term Studies

The optimal *duration* of bisphosphonate therapy is 2–5 years, depending on the initial severity of osteoporosis and the subsequent increase in bone density. Three phases are recognized:

15

- *Repair* (up to 12 months)
- *Rebuilding* (6–36 months)
- *Maintenance* (24–60 months)

Bisphosphonate therapy is a matter of years – this must be explicitly explained to each patient and re-emphasized at the start of and during therapy. The highest rate of increase in bone density occurs during the first 12 months when the resorption lacunae are repaired and refilled with bone. During the rebuilding and maintenance phases, the increase is less since the trabecular structure and width are being restored. It is assumed that repair of the trabecular bone network, plus the increase in bone density during the first year of therapy, are together responsible for the rather re-markable decrease in fracture rate which occurs dur-ing this period. An increase of more than 3% in bone density under alendronate therapy showed about the same decrease in fracture risk as an increase of 3% in bone density. Similar correlations were observed in patients on risedronate therapy: an additional decrease in fracture risk was not observed with bone density increases above 3%. Annual increases in bone den-sity of up to 10% are possible but do not necessarily imply a proportional decrease in fracture risk. Under risedronate therapy, markers of bone resorption show similar relationships. For example a decrease in uri-nary NTX of more than 40% did not lead to a further reduction in fracture risk.

There is relatively less increase in bone density dur-ing the phases of repair and maintenance because the increase in mineralization is now in the foreground. On cessation of bisphosphonate therapy in post-meno-pausal women, there is a moderate decrease in bone density during the first year, more pronounced in the lumbar spine than in the hip; this does not occur in men. On completion of 1–3 years of treatment, results of annual measurements of BMD will determine when bisphosphonate therapy should be resumed. Some studies have already shown that the positive effect on mineral density of both cortical and trabecular bone as well as fracture reduction is maintained for 1 year after cessation of bisphosphonate therapy. This should be checked by BMD measurements in each patient.

Long-term follow-up studies: Previous fears of a "frozen, poor-quality bisphosphonate bone" liable to microfractures ("cracks") have not been confirmed. There is no evidence that remodelling might be turned off completely leading to frozen bone and in-creased bone fragility with the doses used clinically. Some studies in dogs have shown that treatment with very high doses of bisphosphonates have caused in-creased microcracks. However, biomechanical and bone strength were preserved, so the relevance of increased microcracks is unclear, and results of long-term clinical studies of bisphosphonates to date have allayed these fears. Clinical studies of alendronate and risedronate conducted for more than 7–10 years have demonstrated that bone density consistently in-creased by approximately 0.7% per annum. Therefore, over a 10-year period bone density increased by an average of 13%. This indicates that apparently there is no time limit for therapy with bisphosphonates – the one important factor is the state of the patient's skeleton and this should be regularly monitored. The FIT Long-Term Extension study (FLEX) found that BMD decreases slowly on cessation of alendronate and bone remodelling gradually increases. Recent clinical studies have concluded that increased mi-crodamage accumulation may occur in patients on prolonged alendronate therapy. These data suggest that clinicians might consider a "drug holiday" after 5 years of alendronate in lower-risk patients. Frac-ture healing in patients on long-term bisphosphonate therapy does not seem to be a problem, although there are only a few studies which have addressed this im-portant issue.

15.17
A Summary of Results Achieved to Date

- Over a period of approximately 1–3 years 70 mg of alendronate are incorporated into the bones. With such a minute amount of bisphosphonate, when the skeleton contains 2,000,000 mg of hydroxyapatite, physicochemical damage is excluded for all practi-cal purposes. The same holds true for other modern bisphosphonates. Moreover, disturbances of miner-alization do not occur with these bisphosphonates.
- Under therapy with risedronate, patients have dem-onstrated a significant reduction of vertebral and non-vertebral fractures after a period of only 6 months. At 1 year after discontinuation of 3 years'

treatment with risedronate, the risk of new vertebral fractures remained lower in these patients compared to that in the control patients.

- After 7 years of therapy with alendronate or risedronate, the bone mass still increased by about 1% a year, indicating that a basic positive bone balance remained unchanged. However, a "drug holiday" after 5 years of alendronate therapy is advisable to avoid any possible microdamage accumulation, at least in low-risk patients.
- Bone biopsy findings showed that, after 7 years of therapy with alendronate or risedronate, the trabecular architecture and lamellar structure of bone were both preserved and that microfractures were absent.
- The number of normal hydroxyapatite crystals increased, thereby rendering the bone more resistant to compression.
- In contrast, fluoroapatite crystals, which are incorporated into the mineral phase of bone during fluoride poisoning, though denser than hydroxyapatite crystals, are brittle and shatter easily.

The following parameters can be used to estimate *success of therapy*:

- Decrease in collagen breakdown products in urine and TRAP in serum. These biochemical markers of bone resorption provide the earliest information on the effects of therapy.
- Increase in biochemical markers of bone formation: alkaline phosphatase
- Increase in BMD (DXA of lumbar spine and hip)
- Decrease in fracture rate (vertebral and extra-vertebral)
- Decrease in osteoporotic bone pain
- Increase in quality of life and mobility
- Decrease in duration of hospitalization
- Decrease in mortality (28% under zoledronate!).

After 3–6 weeks of therapy, a decrease in markers of bone resorption should occur. If such markers have not been reduced by 30–40% after 2–3 months of oral therapy, the patient should be questioned as to whether and in what form the drug was ingested, and appropriate measures taken according to the circumstances. Subjective parameters such as pain, mobility and quality of life can only be accepted as secondary criteria.

Resistance to therapy does appear to occur in some patients when the usual parameters such as BMD remain the same as those of the control group not on bisphosphonate therapy. The patients described so far were elderly, obese and with type 2 diabetes. The lack of response was seen especially in vulnerable regions, such as the hip, femoral neck and forearm.

BMD should be measured annually during therapy with a bisphosphonate, although, as shown in large studies of bisphosphonates, the risk of fractures may be decreased even in the absence of a measurable increase in density. In the absence of increased BMD after 1 year of therapy, four possibilities should be considered:

- Medication was not taken: Telopeptides (markers of bone resorption) should be checked.
- Medication was not taken according to instructions: Discussion with patient for information and clarification.
- Possible 'non-responder' when therapy was indeed taken: change to intravenous administration of nitrogen-containing bisphosphonates.
- Possibly the case is not that of primary but rather secondary osteoporosis: for example an undiagnosed primary malignant disorder may be present. Investigations, including MRI and bone biopsy, must be carried out as quickly as possible.

Even when there is no direct correlation between increase in bone density and decrease in fracture risk under antiresorptive therapy, the measurement of bone density (DXA) is still the most practical and quantifiable parameter for estimation of fracture risk, both within the framework of diagnostic evaluation as well as monitoring of therapy. In addition, results of DXA measurements have worldwide acceptance which simplifies comparison of results of trials. Results of two large meta-analyses of vertebral fractures have conclusively demonstrated that the reduction of 24–54% in risk of fractures under bisphosphonate therapy is unequivocally due to the increase in bone density. This relationship is even more pronounced with respect to non-vertebral fractures. These meta-analyses also indicate that bisphosphonates increase bone density not only by inhibition of osteoclastic activity, but also by their influence on osteoblasts and osteocytes (inhibition of apoptosis). The bisphosphonates improve the micro-architecture of bone, and thereby also decrease the risk of fractures. This graphically illustrates the close correlation between bone density, strength and micro-architecture.

Moreover, studies of bone biopsies have shown that the increase in bone density is closely connected to the improved micro-architecture of trabecular bone. This was demonstrated by Recker et al. by means of micro-CT and histomorphometry. Their results provide a convincing argument for DXA measurement in the evaluation of effects of bisphosphonate therapy on bone. These and other studies have demonstrated increases in trabecular thickness, as well as in numbers and connections, i.e. "the nodes" of the trabecular network while the porosity of cortical bone was also decreased. These micro-CT studies have clearly demonstrated improvement and preservation of the trabecular micro-architecture under bisphosphonate therapy. It should be mentioned that, although increases in bone density usually occur under therapy, lower values have also been registered by DXA. This apparent paradox has been observed especially in hip measurements after 6 months of teriparatide therapy: decreases in DXA values occurred together with increases in bone surface areas. In contrast, measurements with quantitative computed tomography (QCT) were able to register an increase in bone density. Under teriparatide therapy measurements may show a decrease in density, but bone volume and strength are increased – therefore, this is only an apparent paradox, which can be explained by the fact that DXA measurements underestimate the increase in density only in the presence of an increase in bone surface.

In practice, the success of antiresorptive therapy depends on regular and consistent administration, i.e. patient compliance. However, as shown in one study, this is attained by only a small percentage of the patients. With the introduction of the once weekly tablet, there was a 60% increase in compliance; therefore, a further improvement is to be expected with the monthly tablet. The once-monthly and possibly annual tablets (or i.v. administration) are expected to work wonders with compliance. Few studies have actually been carried out on compliance with long-time intervals. One such study did show that a demonstrable increase in bone density contributes to better patient compliance with the therapy. The results of a comprehensive study on adherence to oral bisphosphonates among 101,038 new bisphosphonate users demonstrated that age and type of fractures were two important factors in the determination of adherence. The results also showed that adherence was correlated with time, as there was a tendency for adherence to decrease from 1 to 3 years of therapy: a cogent reason for regular doctor–patient interaction and monitoring.

15.18
Meta-analyses of Antiresorptive Substances

According to the principles of evidence-based medicine, randomized studies and meta-analyses have the highest priority. However, classification and comparison of drugs pose methodological problems which are easily overlooked and/or underestimated. Meta-analyses provide data for comparative studies. However, reliable comparison between two drugs is only possible in "head-to-head" studies, as outlined previously. Frequently, significant findings are: (1) only revealed in sub-groups, (2) obtained after retrospective evaluation, (3) require re-definition of the inclusion criteria and (4) require utilization of specialized statistics. Nonetheless, a team of experts (in methods of evidence-based medicine) has recently undertaken the task of comparing the efficacy of various antiresorptive agents to decrease fracture risk in spite of all the difficulties involved. These studies were commissioned by The Osteoporosis Methodology Group (OMG) and the Osteoporosis Research Advisory Group (ORAG). The experts confirmed that the most reliable method is undoubtedly the "head-to-head" study. This implies that estimation of the nine most important antiresorptive agents alone would require 36 such studies! In addition, extremely high numbers of patients would be needed to recognize significant differences between two drugs! However, the ORAG analyses did show that there are differences between the drugs in degree and location of fracture reduction. The results demonstrated that after 1 year of therapy, alendronate and risedronate achieved significant reduction in fractures of both hip and spine. A recent review, sponsored by the Agency for Healthcare Research and Quality (AHRQ) analysed 76 randomized trials and 24 meta-analyses. The results outlined the benefits in fracture reduction as well as the adverse side effects of the various classes of pharmacotherapies for osteoporosis.

The significance of a decline in BMD during and after therapy with oral bisphosphonates was investigated by means of comparison of the results of numerous clinical trials. The conclusion was reached that patients who experienced a decrease in BMD had a higher fracture risk profile to begin with, than those whose BMD did not decrease. This emphasized the significance of the fracture risk profile! However, there is as yet no consensus on the criteria for an inadequate response including, among others, risk profile, compliance and duration of the treatment, and obviously criteria must be internationally established and complied with before conclusions can be drawn and comparisons made. Another study assessing the response to therapy for osteoporosis also emphasized the significance of the personal profile of the patients concerned: age, co-mobidity/ies, medications, nutrition, vitamins, gastrointestinal function, other lifestyle factors which could impinge on the effects of therapy and thereby also contribute to the lack of response. Many factors contributing to an inadequate response and a high rate of incident fractures in post-menopausal women with osteoporosis were identified in the Observational Study of Severe Osteoporosis (OSSO) in which 1885 women were investigated. Some elderly patients with severe, low turnover osteoporosis or adynamic bone disease failed to respond to first-line therapy with bisphosphonates, but did react to therapy with teriparatide.

Finally, there are always reports of new therapies, but many are still in the experimental stages, and have not yet been tested in clinical trials. However, one in particular should be mentioned, as it is a conjugate of a bisphosphonate: an osteotropic alendronate–beta-cyclodextrin conjugate which was developed as a bone-target delivery system. In an animal model, it was found to be a strong local anabolic agent as evidenced by the new bone formation at the injection site. Such a drug would be suitable for local application in fracture repair, possibly also in localized osteonecrosis of the femur and perhaps even of the jaw bone. Clearly, more studies are required.

16.1
A Brief Overview of SERMs – New Selective Antiresorptive Agents

In the last decade, more and more oestrogen-like substances have been developed and introduced into clinical practice. These drugs bind to the oestrogen receptors (ERs alpha and beta) throughout the body. For example *tamoxifen* had long been given to women with a history of breast cancer, after the initial chemo- and radiotherapy and surgery. It acts as an oestrogen antagonist on breast tissue but as an oestrogen on other organs and tissues in the body, namely bone, liver and fat. Tamoxifen inhibits growth of any residual breast cancer cells remaining in the body if they still have oestrogen receptors. However, due to adverse effects, tamoxifen has been replaced by the *aromatase inhibitors*, for example anastrozole.

16.2
Raloxifene – Utilization of Physiological Effects on Bone

The positive effect on bone has been further developed in raloxifene, a selective oestrogen-receptor modulator (SERM) of the second generation which has no effect on breast or uterus. Raloxifene was originally investigated as a treatment for breast cancer. Uterine bleeding, breast tenderness and water retention are not observed with raloxifene. However, "hot flushes" and leg cramps occurred in about 30% of previously asymptomatic patients, because raloxifene blocks all oestrogen receptors remaining in the body and thereby also the effects of the small amount of oestrogen that might still be produced. Leg cramps, especially nocturnal, can be treated by supplements of magnesium which is freely available; the recommended amount is 300 mg daily. An international clinical trial, the MORE study, showed that the risk of a vertebral fracture in patients taking raloxifene is half that of a control group. After 3 years, raloxifene 60 mg daily increased the BMD by 2–3% at the hips and spine and reduced the risk of new fractures by 30–50%. New clinical vertebral fractures were reduced by 68% after 1-year of therapy with raloxifene. The risk of breast cancer is significantly reduced (60–70%) in women taking raloxifene. This effect was mainly due to a 90% reduction of oestrogen-receptor-positive breast cancer. The RUTH trial is evaluating this positive effect.

The SERMs exert their effects by binding with high affinity to the oestrogen receptors (ERs) of which two different subtypes have so far been identified (ER-alpha and ER-beta) (Fig. 16.1). These receptor subtypes appear throughout the body with a predominance of ER-alpha expression in the reproductive tissues and a predominance of ER-beta expression in non-reproductive tissues. The structural features of each SERM differ so that unique ligand-induced changes take place in the ERs, which are thought to be the likely basis for tissue-selective pharmacology. For example, raloxifene operates as an oestrogen agonist in bone but as an antagonist in the breast and uterus. The mechanism by which SERMs inhibit bone resorption is likely to be the same as that of oestrogen, i.e. by blocking production of cytokines that promote osteoclast differentiation and

R. Bartl, B. Frisch, *Osteoporosis,* DOI 10.1007/978-3-540-79527-8_16,
© Springer-Verlag Berlin Heidelberg 2009

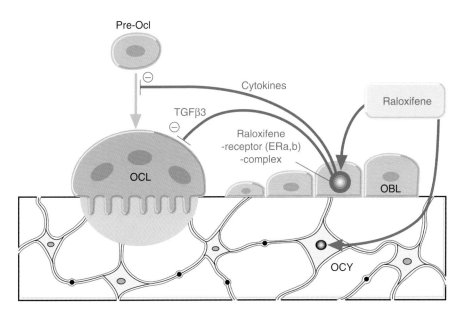

Fig. 16.1. Mechanisms of action of raloxifene on osteoblast (*OBL*), osteoclast (*OCL*) and osteocyte (*OCY*)

by stimulating TGF-beta3 that suppresses osteoclast activation, while osteoclastic resorption is inhibited by modulation of the OPG-RANKL system. Raloxifene decreases serum levels of OPG and RANKL, so that these levels can be compared to levels of the markers of bone resorption. TGF-beta3 also decreases expression of IL-6 which stimulates bone resorption. Raloxifene probably also acts on osteocytes, which participate in regulation of the maintenance of bone. This physiological pathway of action leads to a completely normal bone structure without mineralization defects or increased numbers of microcracks. Studies of the pharmacokinetics of SERMs have shown considerable differences in their bioavailability. Hepatic, but not renal, impairment affects their metabolism and there is a possibility of interaction with other agents such as warfarin and aromatase inhibitors. The main contraindication of raloxifene therapy is a previous history of thromboembolism, since studies have shown an increased incidence of thromboembolism in patients treated with raloxifene. One trial has shown that raloxifene improves renal function in postmenopausal women with diabetes. Raloxifene also reduces the levels of various plasma lipids and increases that of adiponectin; it slows the progression of atherosclerosis. The effects of raloxifene in postmenopausal women with chronic kidney disease (CKD) were investigated in a multicentre randomized, 3-year controlled trial of 7705 postmenopausal women with osteoporosis. Adverse effects in each category of kidney function were the same in the treatment and control groups. The bone mineral density (BMD) at the spine and the hip was increased and the risk for vertebral fractures in the patients with CKD was reduced in the patients on raloxifene therapy.

In summary, SERMs now constitute a new approach to therapy and have been approved for the prevention and treatment of postmenopausal osteoporosis while decreasing the risks of cardiac and circulatory disorders without the unwanted side effects and risks associated with hormone replacement therapy. Raloxifene is considered to be suitable for older women, but its possible side effects must be taken into account and the patients must be informed. In a recent study, SERMs have also been tried in men and the results are awaited soon. Recommended dosage: 60 mg raloxifene (Evista®) orally daily, without restrictions as to when the drug should be taken, but preferably with supplements of vitamin D and calcium. Raloxifene is the treatment of choice for postmenopausal women, especially women with one or more of the following factors:

- High risk for breast cancer or cardiovascular diseases
- High risk of vertebral fractures
- Modest degrees of osteopenia in the postmenopausal period (age 55–65)
- Osteoporosis diagnosed by DXA in the postmenopausal period (age 55–65)

A recent study was undertaken to investigate the efficacy of raloxifene and tibolone on a number of parameters in postmenopausal women, as a substitution treatment instead of the hormone therapy which is no longer recommended. Tibolone was chosen because it is a synthetic steroid with oestrogenic, progesterogenic and androgenic activity. The maintenance of skeletal muscle strength, BMD, body composition, balance, cognitive function and various psychological attributes were registered at baseline and monitored at regular intervals, i.e. 3, 6, 12 and 24 months. Results of a final follow-up measurement at 30 months are awaited. Results of the international Compliance with Raloxifene (CORAL) study of 1497 postmenopausal patients emphasized the fact that the effectiveness of therapy was related to the excellent cooperation of the patients. Raloxifene also provides additive beneficial effects on bone turnover when given together with alendronate and teriparatide.

Other aspects of raloxifene therapy have also been investigated, in addition to those on bone. These studies include the Raloxifene Use for the Heart Trial, and the Multiple Outcomes of Raloxifene Evaluation, which demonstrated a reduction in the risk of certain breast cancers in patients on therapy with raloxifene. These effects were later confirmed by results of other investigations. Raloxifene, also in combination with tibolone, modulates inflammatory markers such as C-reactive protein, Il 6, TNF-alpha and other markers. Moreover, in vitro studies have demonstrated that raloxifene is effective against endothelial cell dysfunction induced by oxidative stress.

Currently available and approved drugs for the therapy of osteoporosis inhibit bone resorption. Their great clinical value lies in reducing the activity of the osteoclasts and thereby increasing bone mineral density (BMD) and reducing fracture risk. But new bone is not produced and reduction of fracture risk, although highly significant, is rarely more than 50% of the baseline risk level. A different therapeutic approach is osteoanabolic therapy, with stimulation of new bone formation, for which fluoride, strontium ranelate, growth hormone (GH), insulin-like growth factor, the statins and parathyroid hormone (PTH) are the main candidates in humans for short-term administration. However, it should be mentioned that continuously elevated calcium and PTH levels as in *primary* hyperparathyroidism (pHPT) affect insulin sensitivity and result in increased insulin secretion, but the administration of recombinant human PTH (rhPTH) in the doses given in osteoporosis does not affect glucose homeostasis.

17.1
Osteoanabolic Action of PTH – Paradoxical Effects Depend on Type of Administration

Parathyroid hormone (PTH): This hormone is a principal regulator of calcium homeostasis. It is a polypeptide with 84 amino acids. PTH stimulates release of calcium and phosphate from bone and synthesis of active vitamin D in the kidney which promotes calcium transport in the gastrointestinal tract. In addition, when given intermittently by injection, PTH stimulates osteoblastic proliferation and differentiation and new bone formation on all available osseous surfaces (Fig. 17.1) so that bone size is changed, while the number of osteoclasts and bone resorption remain unchanged. PTH has been shown to increase bone density, strength and connectivity by which it improves the microarchitecture of bone (Fig. 17.2). Indeed, it is the first treatment for osteoporosis that leads to the formation of new bone while preserving the bone's microarchitecture. However, the underlying molecular physiology accounting for the true anabolic effect of PTH remains unknown. It is also not known why intermittent low dose PTH administration differs so dramatically from continuous administration in its effect on bone cells. Recently, evidence has emerged that PTH reduces osteoblast apoptosis, prolonging osteoblast survival and potentiating its function of collagen synthesis. Studies on bone biopsies have confirmed these findings. Biopsies were taken before and after 18–36 months of therapy with PTH in both men and women. Results showed that PTH stimulates remodelling, resulting in an increased percentage of newly formed matrix but of lower mineral density. This would indicate that calcium and vitamin D supplements are required together with PTH.

The combination of PTH with calcitriol strengthens its anabolic effect and induces an increase of 10–30% in bone density after 1–2 years of treatment. The fracture rate is also significantly decreased. In one study, PTH (1-34-hPTH) was given subcutaneously as a daily injection of 500 IU for 1 year. In another trial, hPTH(1-34) was given i.m. once a week with similar results. Back pain, nausea and headache were

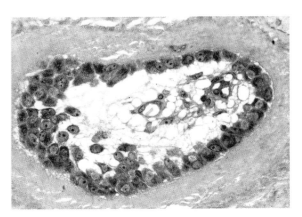

Fig. 17.1. Activation of osteoblasts and production of new bone under treatment with teriparatide

the most common side effects, but these occurred infrequently and in a dose-dependent manner. Less than 5% of the patients showed increased serum calcium levels, but the patients were asymptomatic. Moreover, there have been no reported cases of osteogenic sarcomas, and it is reasonable to assume that PTH is safe.

Teriparatide [rhPTH(1-34)] is the first of the bone-forming agents and has been approved in Europe and the US for treatment of postmenopausal osteoporosis and recently also of osteoporosis in men, with a treatment duration of 18 (Europe) and 24 months (USA). PTH stimulates bone formation and thereby induces a significant increase in BMD. Studies have already shown that age does not affect the efficacy or the safety of teriparatide. This PTH fragment is administered as a daily subcutaneous injection of 20 mcg dose. Adverse events include orthostatic hypotension, leg cramps, dizziness and injection-site reactions. Metabolic changes

may include hyper- and hypocalcaemia, hyperuricaemia or hypoparathyroidism. A major limiting factor with teriparatide is cost – approximately ten times the cost of bisphosphonate therapy. After completion of the 18-month course of teriparatide it appears that fracture protection persists when followed by an antiresorptive agent (e.g. alendronate). Indeed, the administration of an inhibitor of resorption (bisphosphonate or raloxifene) after treatment with PTH potentiates its skeletal benefit. Moreover, osteoporotic patients with previous long-term exposure to antiresorptive agents also showed positive effects on BMD and markers of bone formation under therapy with PTH. The bisphosphonates previously taken by the patients were alendronate, risedronate and etidronate.

Results of many studies have now been reviewed and these have demonstrated a significant reduction of vertebral and non-vertebral fractures in the treated patients, with or without prior antiresorptive therapy. Full-length PTH(1-84) is also available and provided significant protection against a first vertebral fracture in a high-risk population of postmenopausal women with osteoporosis. PTH(1-84) also provided significant protection against further fractures in women who had already experienced one osteoporotic fracture (TOP study). PTH(1-84) is administered as a daily subcutaneous injection of 100 mcg. The possible adverse side effects of the two formulations are similar; hypercalcaemia was observed in 14% of the patients treated with full-length PTH. More studies are needed to determine when and whether PTH monotherapy should be used and which patient population would benefit most from PTH or teriparatide. It is of interest that case reports of individual patients have shown that therapy with teriparatide can also enhance fracture healing.

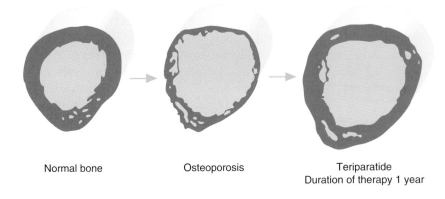

Normal bone   Osteoporosis   Teriparatide
                                     Duration of therapy 1 year

Fig. 17.2. Changes of cortical bone in osteoporosis and after treatment with teriparatide

Combinations with oestrogens also appear promising and are currently under investigation in clinical trials. The data obtained so far highlights two important points:

- PTH plus oestrogen has a greater effect on bone mass than either alone.
- Combination therapy has beneficial effects on the spine and the femur, the two most vulnerable areas for subsequent fractures.

It has already been shown that the combination of the anabolic PTH with an antiresorptive bisphosphonate or raloxifene is promising. This combination achieves a rapid increase in bone density and thus represents the most effective anti-osteoporotic therapy available today: for example, the use of PTH in combination with a modern bisphosphonate to treat glucocorticoid-induced osteoporosis. Studies have also recommended that treatment with teriparatide should be followed by therapy with an antiresorptive agent such as alendronate or zoledronate. Patients treated with raloxifene have shown a more rapid response to PTH than those treated with only a bisphosphonate. Other studies have shown that treatment with raloxifene after teriparatide prevented bone loss at the lumbar spine and increased BMD in the femoral neck in postmenopausal women with osteoporosis. New analogues of PTH and of "PTH-related peptide" are also being tested. A new PTH receptor (PTH2 receptor) has recently been described. Results of more studies now underway are awaited with interest.

PTH as an anabolic therapy for osteoporosis will soon play a major role, but some questions remain to be answered:

- Which patients are most likely to benefit from PTH?
- Is PTH only indicated in severe osteoporosis, with presence of fractures?
- How long should patients receive PTH?
- What is the best sequence for combination therapy?
- Is there a more rapid response to PTH following therapy with raloxifene?
- What is the precise mechanism of PTH's anabolic action on bone?

However, at least partial answers to these questions have been suggested by the results of some of the many trials with PTH therapy that have been published in the last year or so. It has been shown that teriparatide offers an effective therapeutic option for patients who are unresponsive or intolerant to antiresorptive treatment. It is now evident that women with severe osteoporosis, especially those who did not benefit from therapy with antiresorptive agents, are candidates for PTH. Elderly patients as well as patients with deformities, limited mobility, chronic or intermittent back pain and anxiety and depression improved after therapy with teriparatide. Osteoporotic patients with co-morbidities are also candidates for PTH therapy. A study of elderly patients with severe involutional osteoporosis recorded the favourable quality-of-life changes these patients underwent on therapy with PTH which included the following: 96.5% of the patients were protected from new fractures, the BMD increased by about 12% in the vertebral column and 11% in the femur, consumption of NSAIDS was reduced by about 80% and the overall quality of life was improved during the 18 months of therapy and the next 6 months of follow-up (according to the Quality of Life Questionnaire of the European Foundation for Osteoporosis, the QUALEFRO).

Strontium Ranelate

Strontium is a divalent cation that is closely chemically related to calcium. Strontium ranelate contains two atoms of stable strontium and an organic moiety (ranelic acid). Strontium increases pre-osteoblast replication, osteoblast differentiation, collagen type 1 synthesis and bone matrix mineralization (Fig. 18.1). In low doses strontium increases the density of the spongy bone. It reduces resorption and stimulates formation of bone, leading to a gain in bone mass and improved bone mechanical properties (Fig. 18.2). In other words, strontium uncouples the activity of the osteoclasts and osteoblasts, in favour of bone formation! Ongoing investigations of its activities have revealed other actions, whose overall effects include improvements in bone geometry, cortical bone thickness, trabecular bone morphology among other effects on bone quality, all of which enhance the strength of the bones. This has been confirmed in human trials with increased bone-specific alkaline phosphatase (a marker of bone formation) and decreased C-terminal peptide (a marker of bone resorption). The increment in bone density is comparable to that achieved by fluoride: up to 20%.

It is expected that strontium ranelate may have potential value in the prevention and treatment of bone loss. In the SOTI study, a 49% reduction in risk of new vertebral fractures was seen in the first year, and a 41% reduction over 3 years. Bone histomorphometry has shown normal lamellar bone and normal mineralization. In the TROPOS study there was a reduction of 19% in major fragility fractures. In a subgroup analysis of patients at high risk of hip fracture there was a risk reduction of 36%. The results of the prevention PREVOS and the treatment STRATOS investigations of strontium for the prevention of bone loss and the therapy of osteoporosis have now been published. The decrease in fracture rates observed with strontium ranelate is similar to that described for oral bisphosphonates. A recent study has shown that strontium ranelate also safely reduces the risk of vertebral fractures in women with osteopenia with or without a prevalent fracture. However, strontium following anabolic therapy is no more effective in reducing bone turnover markers than calcium/vitamin combined.

Strontium was well tolerated and the most common adverse events were nausea and diarrhoea, which are usually reported at the beginning of treatment. An increase in the incidence of venous thromboembolism (VTE) has been reported, but a causal relationship between VTE and the use of strontium ranelate has not been established. Effective doses

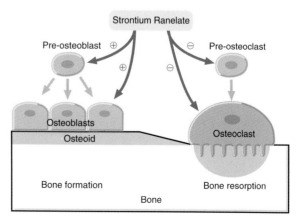

Fig. 18.1. Strontium ranelate has two distinct effects: (*a*) an increase in formation of bone and (*b*) a decrease in resorption of bone

R. Bartl, B. Frisch, *Osteoporosis,* DOI 10.1007/978-3-540-79527-8_18,
© Springer-Verlag Berlin Heidelberg 2009

18

Before strontium ranelate

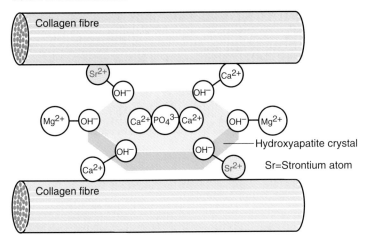

After strontium ranelate

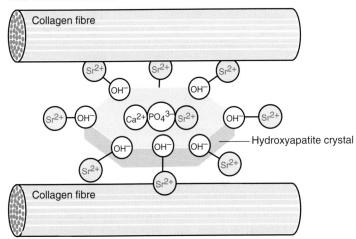

were 1 g daily for prevention and 2 g daily for therapy. The absorption of strontium ranelate is reduced by food and milk and the drug should be administered therefore between meals. Ideally, it should be taken at bedtime, preferably at least 2 h after eating. No dosage adjustment is required in relation to age or moderate renal impairment. However, in vitro stud-

ies have revealed a complicated dose-dependent action of strontium on bone cells and further studies are needed for clarification.

Strontium, with a higher atomic number than calcium (38 versus 20), will absorb more X-rays and therefore results in an overestimation (up to 50%) of the increase in bone density using DXA methods.

Calcitonin and Fluoride

Calcitonin is a polypeptide hormone produced by the parafollicular C cells of the thyroid. It inhibits the osteoclasts by binding to specific receptors on the cell surface. Calcitonin can be given as a subcutaneous injection or in nasal-spray form. However, use of calcitonin is limited because of its side effects such as feelings of heat and nausea with injection, and mucosal irritation with the nasal spray. However, the drawbacks of frequent injections and the high costs if nasal application preclude the long-term use of calcitonin as a first-line therapy of osteoporosis. The most valid indication for calcitonin today is the acute, intractable pain caused by a vertebral fracture, although even here its use is limited because of the superior results of intravenous bisphosphonates. On the other hand, calcitonins are physiological peptides which can be metabolized and therefore are not retained in the body. Toxic effects have not been reported. Calcitonins are therefore suitable for children and during pregnancy and breast-feeding. Calcitonins target the active osteoclasts and thereby reduce resorption, but have little effect on osteoblasts, so that there has been speculation that it could lead to a continuously positive bone balance. Efforts are currently underway to produce an oral formulation to improve patient acceptance and compliance, which would enable clinical trials of its efficacy. Consequently, calcitonin may not yet be a "drug of the past".

On the contrary, a recent trial of 126 male and 130 female patients on maintenance dialysis were treated with salmon calcitonin, 50 U three times weekly by subcutaneous injection for 18 months. The calcitonin was well tolerated and effectively increased the BMD of the treated patients.

Fluoride is still used in some countries for the treatment of osteoporosis because of economic considerations, but its role in the prevention of fractures has not been confirmed in clinical trials. The recommended dose ranges from 20 to 200 mg sodium fluoride daily (elementary fluoride constitutes half of this amount): There is general agreement that fluoride stimulates osteoblastic bone formation and thereby increases bone mass. But mechanical resistance of the newly formed bone is poor and it is even liable to fracture easily. Fluoride is incorporated into the crystal instead of the hydroxyl group in hydroxyapatite, thereby changing crystal size and conformation, which in turn produces poor quality woven bone (Fig. 19.1 a,b). A high dosage of fluoride results in increases in bone density, but vertebral fractures are not significantly reduced. Moreover, especially with high doses, there are serious adverse reactions:

- Gastrointestinal side effects: epigastric complaints, vomiting and diarrhoea.
- Lower extremity pain syndrome (LEPS): pain in the hips, knees and ankles. The cause may be delayed microcallus formation in the affected areas of these bones.
- Iatrogenic fluorosis: severe cases can be identified on X-rays as overgrowth and thickening of the bone (Figs. 19.2 and 19.3). This may be due to incorrect treatment. The patient sometimes increases the dose without medical advice because of continuing complaints and pain. However, it is not known whether there is an individual tendency to develop fluorosis.
- Exostoses and calcium deposits in the ligaments.

R. Bartl, B. Frisch, *Osteoporosis*, DOI 10.1007/978-3-540-79527-8_19,
© Springer-Verlag Berlin Heidelberg 2009

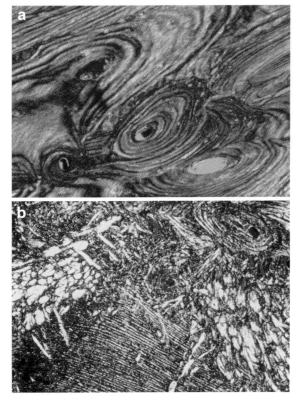

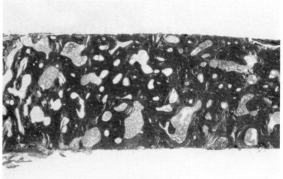

Fig. 19.3. Iliac crest biopsy of a patient with fluorosis showing marked osteosclerosis of the whole biopsy

Fig. 19.1a, b. Bone quality under therapy. (**a**) Normal lamellar bone under long-term therapy with bisphosphonates. (**b**) Altered lamellar bone structure with topographic disorganization

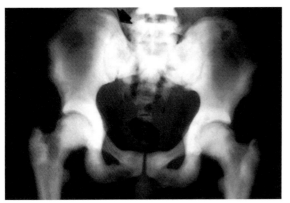

19.2. Iatrogenic fluorosis with thickening of bone

The latest clinical trials indicate that much lower doses (e.g. 15 mg daily) should be given over 3–4 years and always together with vitamin D and calcium. It is not known whether intermittent fluoride has any advantages over continuous administration, and the long-term effects have also not yet been clarified. Slow-release sodium fluoride at a lower dose (50 mg/d) appeared to be associated with reduction of fracture risk in one study, but confirmation of these results is not yet available. These and other questions will probably be answered when results of the present ongoing studies become available. In the meantime, a recently published meta-analysis has shown that in subgroup analyses a low fluoride dose was associated with a significant reduction in fracture risk. Daily dosage is an important issue for the anti-fracture effect of fluoride, but not for the occurrence of lower extremity pain syndrome. However, because of the various side effects and the availability of other efficacious agents, fluoride treatment is presently not recommended and also not approved by the FDA for the treatment of osteoporosis.

Combination and Sequential Therapies

20

When the response to a medication is inadequate or ineffective, the doctor in charge will either change the drug or substitute it with another with a different mechanism of action in order to achieve a satisfactory therapeutic result. In this context, the example of the treatment of established high blood pressure is relevant. The patient usually receives several medications with different mechanisms of action in order to decrease the blood pressure to the desired level on the one hand, and to minimize the side effects on the other. Although it would appear that this strategy is also applicable to the treatment of osteoporosis, some specific problems have arisen, particularly with monitoring the therapy. In clinical practice, the parameters currently widely applied for monitoring the efficacy of osteoporosis therapy – bone density and markers of bone remodelling – are in fact not reliable when it comes to evaluating the efficacy of therapy – that is, specifically, reduction in the rate of fractures.

Various studies have demonstrated that patients on therapy may definitely have a reduction in fracture risk even in the absence of a demonstrable increase in bone density. Moreover, changes in levels of markers of bone resorption under antiresorptive therapy do not always correlate with the fracture risk. In addition, there are considerable differences between the effects of the various antiresorptive agents. For example, there may be little change in markers of resorption and/or bone density under therapy with raloxifene, but accompanied nevertheless by considerable reduction in risk of vertebral fractures and even the occurrence of a fracture does not automatically indicate a "non-responders". It is clear, then, that fractures may occur in patients with manifest osteoporosis in spite of the fact that the therapy is effective; however, the doctor in charge has a tendency to prescribe an additional medication when there is no measurable increase in density or a new fracture occurs. Obviously, these considerations raise the question as to whether therapy with two antiresorptive drugs, or with a combination of antiresorptive/osteoanabolic medications, is preferable. Studies carried out so far with this combination therapy investigated bone density and bone remodelling markers, but unfortunately not the reduction in fracture risk – the decisive clinical parameter!

Combination of two antiresorptive agents results in a more pronounced decrease in bone resorption which induces a greater increase in bone mineral density (BMD), than either drug alone. But studies of patients on this type of combination therapy utilized bone density measurements and bone remodelling markers as parameters and not, unfortunately, the reduction in fracture risk – a decisive clinical criterion! The combination of selective oestrogen-receptor modulators (SERMs) and bisphosphonates also provides an additive increase in BMD, but again, the use of this combination remains questionable in terms of fracture reduction and also from a pharmaco-economic perspective. There are data for combinations of raloxifene with bisphosphonates, but again without information on the reduction of fracture risk.

If hormone replacement therapy (HRT) is used for a limited period of time for the management of climacteric symptoms, concomitant use of bisphosphonate may provide a further reduction in bone turnover and an additional increase in BMD. Studies have shown that such a combined-treatment group had a significantly greater increase in spinal and femoral

R. Bartl, B. Frisch, *Osteoporosis*, DOI 10.1007/978-3-540-79527-8_20,
© Springer-Verlag Berlin Heidelberg 2009

neck BMD than the increase in BMD seen by either oestrogen or alendronate alone. A greater effect on BMD also occurred with combined oestrogen and risedronate, than with either one alone. According to McDermott, adding a bisphosphonate to ongoing HRT should be considered in four clinical scenarios:

- Patients who sustain a fracture without an identifiable cause.
- Patients who show reduced BMD without an identifiable cause.
- Patients with persistently elevated NTX (CTX) without an identifiable cause.
- Elderly patients with BMD hip T score <−2.5, who have an increased risk of hip fracture.

In patients previously treated with HRT, several trials have examined the effect of adding parathyroid hormone (PTH) and have shown significant increases in spinal BMD, suggesting that the prior exposure to the antiresorptive HRT does not blunt a subsequent response to PTH. Therefore, patients pre-treated with inhibitors of bone resorption who have not achieved a full therapeutic response are good candidates for treatment with anabolic agents.

Another important question is whether the combination of a *bisphosphonate and PTH* would provide a therapeutic advantage, but results of trials reported so far have not provided any evidence of synergy between bisphosphonates and PTH, either in postmenopausal women or in men. Consequently, if therapy with PTH is contemplated, it should be given alone and not together with a bisphosphonate. However, the administration of an antiresorptive agent after treatment with PTH maintains or even potentiates the skeletal benefit which accrued during prior PTH therapy. Black et al. (2005) have demonstrated that increases in BMD during 1 year of treatment with PTH appear to be rapidly lost after therapy is stopped (Fig. 20.1). However, treatment with alendronate immediately after the discontinuation of PTH, further increased the BMD in the following year. Therefore, treatment with

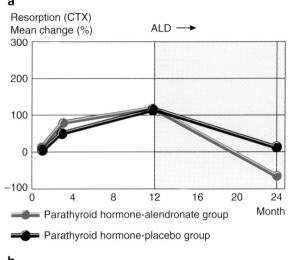

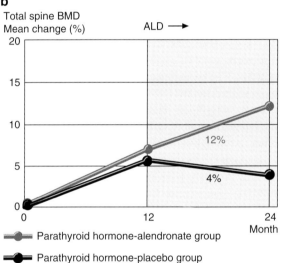

Fig. 20.1a, b. Treatment with alendronate (*ALD*) immediately after the discontinuation of parathyroid hormone (*PTH*). Resorption marker (CTX) (**a**) and bone mineral density (BMD) of the total spine (**b**)

PTH should be followed by antiresorptive therapy to consolidate the gains made during treatment with PTH.

Future Directions

Leptin: This is a hormone with many diverse functions. It is produced by fat cells, acts as a "saturation hormone" and influences glucose metabolism and the production of sex hormones. It has long been known that sex hormone deficiency stimulates bone resorption while overweight inhibits it. This underlies the speculation that bone mass, body weight and sexual glands are regulated by a common mechanism in the brain. Attempts are currently underway to influence the level of leptin or its receptors and thereby develop a novel way to treat osteoporosis.

Growth factors: These are produced primarily by cells in the bone marrow and regulate proliferation, function and interactions of bone cells. There are various regulators of bone formation, such as parathormone, insulin, growth hormone and cortisone, which all function by stimulation of growth factors in particular bone cells. In one clinical trial, bone formation was increased simply by the administration of one of these factors. It is anticipated that in the not-too-distant future, individually "tailored" growth hormones will be administered for the different types of osteoporosis. Prostaglandins also modulate metabolism of bone. PGE2 has a distinctly anabolic effect on trabecular bone – presumably by stimulation of proliferation and differentiation of the precursors of osteoblasts.

Vitamin D3 analogues: novel analogues have been synthesized and examined for their action on bone. In vitro studies showed that such analogues act on osteoblasts to suppress RANKL-dependent formation of osteoclasts, so that they could be considered as potential candidates for the therapy of pathologically increased resorption.

Statins: These are given for lowering concentrations of fat and cholesterol in the blood. Women who were treated with statins showed a higher bone density and a lower fracture risk than comparable women who had not been treated with statins. Animal studies have shown that statins shorten the life span of osteoclasts and thereby inhibit resorption of bone. Should this positive action of statins on bone be confirmed, then statins could become an effective drug for the prevention of arteriosclerosis and osteoporosis. But statins have one disadvantage: they act on the liver and therefore will never replace the bone-specific bisphosphonates in the treatment of osteoporosis, although the mechanism of action of the two drugs is similar. When administered orally, the statins are almost totally cleared during their first passage through the liver. It is still unclear how the statins reach the bone and how they affect bone turnover. It is also still a mystery how the statins can stimulate bone formation while the bisphosphonates, utilizing the same pathway, inhibit bone resorption. Nevertheless, in the future, specific statins selected for their high affinity to bone may be useful agents for the prevention or treatment of osteoporosis. The indications for such agents will be varied and numerous if they benefit both the skeleton and the cardiovascular systems.

Tetracyclines (chemically modified tetracyclines, CMTs): These prevent bone resorption by inhibition of matrix metalloproteinases, as well as induction of apoptosis in osteoclasts. The possible applications and risks of these agents are being tested in clinical trials.

Shorter acting antiresorptives: Denosumab, cathepsin K inhibitors, integrin-antagonists and prostaglandins: These newer antiresorptive agents may alter

R. Bartl, B. Frisch, *Osteoporosis*, DOI 10.1007/978-3-540-79527-8_21,
© Springer-Verlag Berlin Heidelberg 2009

osteoclast function with a much shorter biologic half-life and bone residence time than the bisphosphonates. They have short duration of activity and are not stored in human tissue.

Denosumab is a specific, high affinity, human monoclonal antibody to RANKL, and as such is a representative of "targeted" therapy (Fig. 21.1). It has demonstrated potent inhibition of bone resorption and increases in bone mineral density (BMD) with a twice yearly subcutaneous injection. Phase III trials with fracture incidence as end point are ongoing and the results are awaited with interest. Denosumab also interacts with immune cells and therefore could have systemic effects which could secondarily influence bone metabolism. Its efficacy in malignancy-induced bone loss has already been demonstrated, and initial studies of denosumab in rheumatic disorders are also promising. Integrin and prostaglandins may also offer means of inhibiting osteoclast-mediated bone resorption.

Cathepsin K is an osteoclast-mediated product that is required to participate in the degradation of type I bone collagen. Anti-cathepsin K (odanacatib) is already in phase III clinical development programs for the investigation of its potential as an inhibitor of bone resorption. Results of a 12-month phase IIB study with odanacatib, 50 mg once weekly, demonstrated a significant increase of 3.4% in lumbar spine BMD, reduction of 57% in sCTX and of 18% in sBSAP (bone-specific alkaline phosphate). This modest decrease in bone formation could be used to differentiate cathepsin K in-

hibitors from other antiresorptives and combinations with osteo-anabolic agents. Cathepsin K inhibitors could also be used for preventing or treating osteoarthritis and metastatic bone disease. They can be taken orally once a week. The potential therapeutic utility of using integrin inhibitors to interfere with integrin-mediated events in osteoporosis and other metabolic and metastatic bone diseases is both exciting and promising. Osteoclast adhesion involves several integrins and, therefore, integrin antagonists may be a logical mechanism-based approach to therapy of osteoclastic bone resorption in osteoporosis and bone metastases.

Future directions: In all the current pharmacologic approaches to osteoporosis, whenever decreases or increases in the activity of one cell line are induced, the changes in the same direction occur in the "coupled" cell lines. Thus, whenever an antiresorptive agent reduces bone resorption by inhibiting differentiation and/or function of osteoclasts, there will also be a reduction in osteoblast function. Likewise, whenever osteoblast function is increased, there will be an increase in osteoclast function. This linkage limits the current therapies for osteoporosis. Future agents which could "uncouple" these activities, even temporarily, would enable unopposed bone formation, thus attaining greater increases in BMD and more directed modulation of bone architecture to improve bone strength. Pharmacologic intervention in the control of osteocytes, the most abundant cells in bone, is a further interesting and promising target in bone research.

ANGELs (activators of non-genomic oestrogen ligands) is another new paradigm of biology that is being investigated and may prove to be an entirely new approach to modulation of skeletal tissue.

Oxytocin promotes osteogenesis at the expense of adipogenesis, and animal experiments have shown that administration of oxytocin to ovariectomized mice reversed bone loss and reduced marrow adiposity. Application in humans is under investigation, both as a serum marker for osteoporosis and as a potential therapy.

Many other potential points of possible intervention in the complex mechanisms in control of skeletal metabolism are under investigation. To give but a few examples: different polymorphisms in steroid hormone receptors, delivery systems for bone morphogenetic proteins to induce the generation of new bone in special circumstances and injection of autologous mesenchymal stem cells – such as osteogenic cells – to augment healing processes in bone.

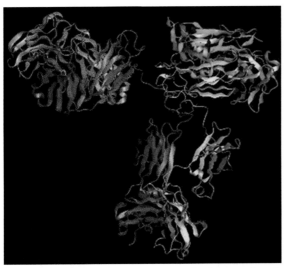

Fig. 21.1. Three-dimensional structure of a denosumab molecule

22.1
Adherence to Treatment

Non-adherence to medical treatment or lack of perseverance over time is a worldwide health problem in all chronic conditions, especially asymptomatic ones. It has been estimated that only 50% of patients comply with long-term therapy. A large proportion of patients discontinued treatment with bisphosphonates, and a majority of these did not even renew their first prescription. Adherence, although enhanced by less frequent dosing, was suboptimal in all of its aspects, i.e. acceptance, persistence and compliance (Fig. 22.1). Furthermore, risk of non-adherence increases with increased duration of treatment. In osteoporosis and osteopenia, non-adherent patients have smaller decreases in rates of bone turnover, smaller increases in bone mineral density (BMD) and a greater risk of fracture. Patients may be encouraged to adhere when presented with results of measurements of BMD or bone turnover indicating the positive effects of therapy. Compliance is also increased by utilization of simplified and user-friendly treatment modalities such as tablets given weekly or monthly, and infusions given every few months or annually. When discussing adherence or non-adherence, three definitions are usually used in the literature:

- Persistence: indicates for how long the drug is taken.
- Compliance: indicates the proximity to the treatment recommendations as given in the official product information.
- Primary non-adherence: when the patient has never taken the prescribed drug.

Studies have shown that the regular analysis of markers of bone turnover as well as annual dual-energy X-ray absorptiometry (DXA) tests to monitor bisphosphonate therapy increase persistence. Therefore, measurements of markers after a few months of therapy may provide useful information on efficacy of the therapy and improve persistence. One large study was designed to compare adherence rates between patients with one or more of seven different conditions. The results showed that adherence rates for osteoporosis medications were among the lowest (36.8%). Younger patients (<60 years) had poorer adherence than older ones, and as co-morbidities increased, adherence among subjects with osteoporosis decreased. A population-based study carried out in Canada (Perrault 2008) found that only 2% of women with prior fractures were on long-term therapy with antiresorptive drugs. However, results of a recent investigation in Denmark in 2008 showed that persistence has improved, both in men and women. One large scale study of 4994 postmenopausal women in 33 states in the US (the Prospective Observational Scientific Study Investigating Bone Loss Experience) has been initiated to evaluate the impact of characteristics of patients and their doctors on compliance and persistence with osteoporosis medications. Results are awaited at the end of 2008.

22.2
Monitoring Treatment

Patients who are not on drug therapy should be checked and evaluated at regular intervals, taking into consideration the baseline values established at diagnosis,

R. Bartl, B. Frisch, *Osteoporosis*, DOI 10.1007/978-3-540-79527-8_22,
© Springer-Verlag Berlin Heidelberg 2009

as well as the patient's individual risk factors. Bone density (DXA) should be checked every 1–2 years (Fig. 22.2). A documented decrease in height of more than 2 cm or acute back pain could be symptomatic of a fracture. In such cases, immediate radiological investigation is required, as are further measures as indicated by the results. Since the goal of drug therapy in a patient with osteoporosis is to increase bone strength and so decrease the fracture risk, the efficacy of osteoporosis-specific agents is monitored by means of changes in BMD and biochemical markers (BCM) of bone turnover, although neither is a perfect indicator of response to therapeutic interventions. Patients on drug therapy should initially be checked every 3–6 months for the first 2 years and subsequently at 6–12 months.

To evaluate the efficacy of the therapy administered, measurements of bone density are only partially valid, but nevertheless should be checked every 2 years. A lack of increase in bone density does not necessarily imply reduction of fracture risk (Fig. 22.3). However, in some medical centres, annual DXA measurements are preferred for the following reasons:

● To encourage regular intake of the tablets
● To emphasize the necessity of long-term therapy measured in years
● To motivate the patient by demonstrating the increase in bone density.

Psychology has always been an important intrinsic factor in the success of medical treatment. The patient's

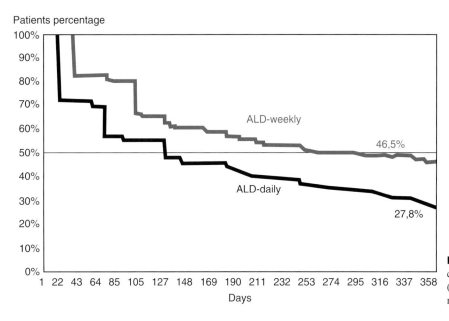

Fig. 22.1. Evidence of better compliance with alendronate (*ALD*) weekly versus alendronate daily

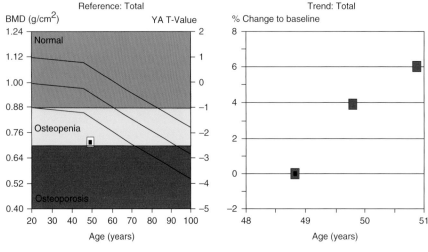

Fig. 22.2. Continuous increase of bone mineral density (*BMD*) of the lumbar spine (L1–L4) under bisphosphonate therapy. Annual monitoring using DXA measurement

Percent reduction in vertebral fracture risk

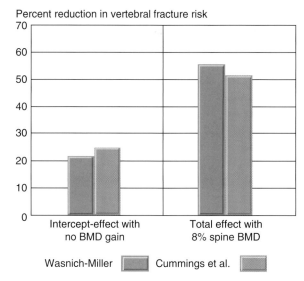

Wasnich-Miller ▨ Cummings et al. ▨

Fig. 22.3. Two meta-analyses showing the relationship between change vs. no change in vertebral bone mineral density (*BMD*) and reduction in vertebral fractures (Data from Wasnich R, Miller P [2001] Antifracture efficacy of antiresorptive agents is related to changes in bone density. J Clin Endocrinol Metab 87:1586–1592; Cummings S, Karpf D, Harris F et al [2002] Improvements in spine bone density and reduction in risk of vertebral fractures during treatment with antiresorptive drugs. Am J Med 114:281–289)

preferences must always be taken into consideration if at all possible, in particular type and frequency of administration. With long intervals, the following are advised: regular communication between patient and doctor, possibly reminders of when the next dose is due and, as indicated above, blood tests for bone turnover markers or BMD measurements of crucial bone areas, e.g. hip or vertebra, to encourage patients by demonstrating progress. The details of the long-term monitoring of patients on antiresorptive and osteoanabolic therapy are outlined below. When dealing with the assessment of response to therapy, racial and ethnic differences may occasionally be observed due to the polymorphisms in the vitamin D receptor (VDR) and in the oestrogen receptor-alpha (ER-alpha) loci, which may vary in different populations.

22.3
Monitoring Antiresorptive Therapy

It is now recognized that the increase in bone strength induced by antiresorptive treatment is only partly due to the increase in bone density. The reduction in the

rate of fractures is also dependent on additional parameters, but these cannot as yet be accurately assessed by the application of current methodology. These factors include:

- Increase in extent of mineralization
- Reduction in the rate of osseous remodelling
- Repair and refill of the resorption pits
- Stabilization of the trabecular microstructure
- Changes in cortical bone remodelling
- Changes in bone geometry.

Meta-analyses of large randomized trials have retrospectively investigated the relevance of bone density and the levels of markers of bone remodelling in the reduction of vertebral and non-vertebral fractures. Two meta-analyses concluded that 24–54% of the reduction in vertebral fractures was due to the increase in bone density, while the reduction in non-vertebral fractures was attributed almost entirely to the increase in bone density. The observations also indicated a close correlation between the increase in bone density and the decrease in markers of bone remodelling; changes in bone turnover markers have been confirmed as reliable and significant indicators for the assessment of response to therapy. Obviously, reduction in bone remodelling can also lead to changes in microarchitecture as well as in bone strength, but neither of these is necessarily manifested by changes in bone density. After treatment with alendronate, increases in BMD at both the joint and hip were associated with reductions in the risk of non-vertebral fractures. However, for patients treated with risedronate or raloxifene, changes in BMD did not reliably predict the degree of reduction in vertebral (raloxifene) or non-vertebral (risedronate) fractures. In these cases, the monitoring can be accomplished by using the parameters of antiresorptive therapy. Recent up-to-date studies have demonstrated that changes in biochemical markers of bone remodelling under therapy more sensitively reflect the decrease in fracture rate as a result of the antiresorptive therapy. However, to what extent these investigations will be applicable in routine practice is still an open question. One important advantage of the application of osseous markers in monitoring is that "non-responders" can be recognized after only 1–3 months of therapy. The LSC (least significant change) is 25% for markers of bone formation, and 40–65% for those of bone resorption. When the resorption markers decrease by about one-third of the initial value (i.e. at diagnosis) the following assumptions can be made:

- The patient has taken the medication.
- The medication has been adequately resorbed.
- A biological effect on the bone has occurred.

In clinical trials, the "response" rate to bisphosphonates proved to be more than 90%.

22.4
Monitoring Osteo-anabolic Therapy

When the bones to be measured have enlarged under osteo-anabolic therapy, the actual increase in bone mass (bone mineral content, BMC) is not demonstrated in the results of a DXA measurement, since this is based on the following equation: BMD = BMC/Area (g/cm^2). Consequently, the relatively lower density indicated by the DXA measurement is not a result of loss of bone mass, but is due to enlargement of the ossified area measured. The clinical relevance of this apparently paradoxical effect was demonstrated in a study with teriparatide. A head-to-head comparison of the density of the forearm was carried out using the results of DXA and *peripheral quantitative computed tomography* (pQCT) measurements. While on therapy with teriparatide, the forearm was enlarged as shown by pQCT as well as by three-dimensional analyses of bone biopsies. In contrast, lower values were obtained with DXA measurements. Nevertheless, bone strength was increased and the fracture rate of the forearm was reduced. Moreover, similar results were obtained on measurements of the hip bones. The increase in osseous remodelling stimulated by parathyroid hormone (PTH) therapy first results in endosteal bone formation together with "trabecularization" of the cortical bone. Shortly thereafter, subperiosteal bone formation leads to enlargement of the contour of the bone as well as an increase in bone mass. During the first year of therapy, this structural change is reflected in the DXA measurement as a reduction in bone density (BMC/Area), while the pQCT measurements more accurately reflect the positive effects of PTH therapy. However, when correctly interpreted, DXA can still be considered the "Gold Standard" even for monitoring the effects of osteo-anabolic therapy. Increases in BMD account for approximately one-third of the vertebral fracture risk reduction with teriparatide. A larger proportion (up to 74%) of the antifracture efficacy of strontium ranelate might be explained by changes in BMD of total hip. BMD monitoring in patients treated with osteo-anabolic agents appears to be more informative than results of monitoring when patients were treated with antiresorptive substances.

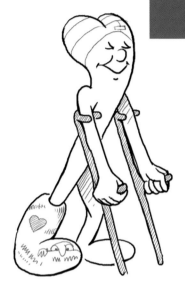

23.1
Fragility Fractures

The US National Osteoporosis Foundation estimates that currently 25 million Americans are affected by osteoporosis and are at heightened risk for skeletal fractures, especially spinal and hip fractures. The number of individuals who will suffer from osteoporosis and fractures will rise as the worldwide population of people over 60 years of age increases from about 540 million to more than 1 billion by the year 2020. Even with the emergence of highly efficacious treatments for osteoporosis, such as modern bisphosphonates, fractures are only reduced by about 50%, leaving the other 50% to suffer the consequences. Not only are osteoporotic fractures debilitating, they also have a high mortality rate. Swedish studies have concluded that more than 1% of all deaths are causally related to hip fractures. It has been estimated that

about 25% of people over 50 years of age who suffer a hip fracture die within 1 year of that fracture, most in the first 3–6 months. Improved therapeutic interventions to accelerate and ensure healing are needed. Fractures can occur at many sites in the skeleton, but are most frequent in the hip, spine and wrist. Associated clinical complications include pain, disability, deformity and postural changes, particularly with vertebral compression fractures. These so-called fragility fractures result from low-level trauma that would not normally cause bone to fracture. In the US alone, osteoporosis is responsible for over 2 million fractures annually: 700,000 vertebral fractures, 300,000 hip fractures and 250,000 wrist fractures. Simple activities such as bending over to pick up a piece of paper or sneezing can cause a fracture in a patient with osteoporosis. Though vertebral fractures are the most common, hip fractures have particularly high morbidity and mortality rates (20–25%). Fractures are more common in females than cancers of the breast, uterus and cervix combined. The estimated lifetime risk of a fragility fracture after the age of 50 is 40% for women and 13% for men. One out of six women will suffer a hip fracture during her lifetime.

In conclusion, the burden of osteoporosis for 2005 was estimated at >2 million incident fractures, with direct medical costs of about $17 billion in the US. Non-vertebral fractures accounted for 94% of costs and 73% of fractures. Almost 30% of fractures and a quarter of the total cost are borne by men. By 2025, annual fractures and costs are projected to grow by 50% and will surpass 2 million fractures and $24 billion, respectively.

In collaboration with Christoph Bartl MD, Department of Orthopaedic and Trauma Surgery, University of Ulm, Germany

23

23.2
Fractures and the Healing Process

In osteoporotic patients, a minor trauma may cause extensive injury to bone with displacement, haemorrhage and clot formation; or it may affect only a small number of trabeculae without spectacular displacement or pain. Minute breaks or cracks ("microfractures") occur chiefly in weight-bearing bones, especially the vertebrae, usually after marked bone loss as seen in osteoporosis. Sometimes only a single trabecula is involved, as demonstrated in bone biopsies. However, in iliac crest biopsies recognition of cracks may be difficult. It should be mentioned that these cracks are the result of the daily "wear and tear" as the body gets older, and not of a specific external trauma or fall. Major fractures are always accompanied by bleeding, and subsequent organization of the clot is an integral part of the unique and highly complex healing process (Fig. 23.1a,b). Bone, bone marrow, periosteum, surrounding muscles, nerves and blood vessels each contribute to the healing process. Fracture healing may be considered to be complete when:

- The fracture line is no longer seen on radiology
- Histology demonstrates restoration of the anatomical architecture
- The bone strength has recovered its mechanical strength

In brief, the following is the main sequence of events in fracture healing – both in normal and in osteoporotic bones (Fig. 23.2):

Intensity

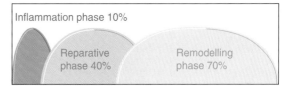

Fig. 23.2. Durations of the inflammatory, reparative and remodelling phases in fracture healing

- *Inflammatory phase*, with an immediate and intense inflammatory reaction to the necrotic material: haemorrhage, vasodilatation and exudation of plasma. During the next few days, the haemorrhagic area undergoes organization. Interestingly, it has been shown that this tissue has osteoblastic potential. The necrotic tissue is removed by phagocytosis and lysosomal breakdown.
- *Reparative phase*, this is characterized by the formation of callus, a complex tissue composed of fibrous, cartilaginous and osseous elements, derived from and produced by the surrounding mesenchymal cells. This matrix, or early callus, consists of collagen and proteoglycans. At about the same time, within a week, blood vessels begin to proliferate, bringing nutrients, hormones and growth factors. The progression of soft, fibrous callus to hard, bony callus (woven bone) occurs by mineralization of the matrix (osteoid) and by enchondral ossification. Within 3–6 weeks the new bone has acquired a trabecular pattern, which may be observed in bone histology.
- *Remodelling phase*, this is characterized by conversion of the woven bone to lamellar bone over a period

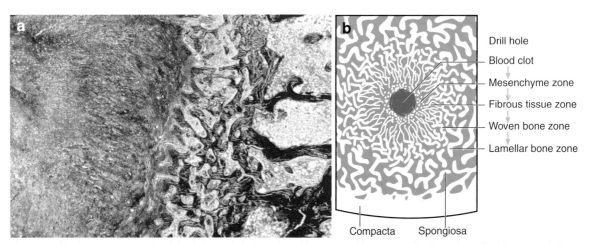

Fig. 23.1a,b. Sequence of repair of the hole made in bone by taking a bone biopsy. (**a**) Histology, from the blood clot (*left*) to the lamellar bone (*right*), Gomori staining. (**b**) Schematic representation of the sequence

of months or even years. Under bisphosphonate therapy, there may be some delay in bone remodelling, but not at the cost of the quality and strength of the final lamellar bone. The repaired bone slowly regains its original shape and strength. Resorption of the callus is primarily due to the osteoclasts which in turn are controlled by mechanical and electrical factors, responsible for the stimulation of cellular proliferation and activity, as well as morphological changes.

Studies of an osteoporotic rat model have provided evidence of *altered fracture healing in osteoporotic bone*, which may have important implications in evaluating the effects of new treatments for osteoporosis on fracture healing. In the osteoporotic, ovariectomized rat, histomorphological analyses revealed a delay in healing of callus with poor development of mature bone. Meyer et al. (2008), also in a study of female rats, showed that both age and ovariectomy impaired the normalization of mechanical properties and the accretion of mineral by the fracture callus during healing of osteoporotic fractures. In contrast, it has been shown that direct application of ultrasound may accelerate the healing process by stimulating bone formation.

23.3
Effects of Drugs and Lifestyle on Fracture Healing

Antiresorptive agents are widely used for the treatment of osteoporosis in postmenopausal women. However, inhibition of bone resorption secondarily suppresses bone formation, which results in a substantial reduction in bone turnover, as confirmed by a 90% reduction in activation frequency after 2 years of alendronate treatment in women. Furthermore, bisphosphonates have a high affinity for mineral and their skeletal half-life in bone is very long – about 12 years in humans. Since patients with osteoporosis are prone to fractures and because bisphosphonates, oestrogen and selective oestrogen receptor modulators (SERMs) suppress bone remodelling, animal and clinical studies are required to investigate the effects of these antiresorptive agents on the healing of fractures. Animal experiments had previously shown that high doses of etidronate interfered with the healing and mineralization of fractures. This does not apply to the modern *aminobisphosphonates (third generation)*,

which can be taken without increased risk by patients with osteoporotic fractures. In addition, animal experiments have shown that, under therapy with the modern bisphosphonates:

- Both the formation of callus and its calcium content were increased, which could be attributed to the inhibition of bone resorption.
- The process of callus remodelling from the irregular woven bone to the well-organized lamellar bone may be delayed under long-term therapy with bisphosphonates. The consequence may be a normal radiological disappearance of the fracture line and a normal restoration of the anatomical architecture, but a delayed mechanical recovery of bone strength.
- Long-term continuous treatment with bisphosphonates did delay the process of fracture healing, especially under high doses, but did not impair the long-term recovery of the bone's mechanical integrity.

However, recent clinical studies have reported on the increased prevalence of subtrochanteric fractures in patients taking *bisphosphonates for the long-term treatment of osteoporosis*. Non-traumatic, non-pathologic fractures of the femoral shaft with a simple transverse pattern and hypertrophy of the diaphyseal cortex in patients taking alendronate have been described. On the basis of these studies, the authors recommended that patients having sustained a fracture should stop taking alendronate and that patients receiving long-term treatment should be carefully monitored.

Although the effects of PTH are also associated with bone resorption, the response of osteoclasts to parathyroid hormone (PTH) is mediated through osteoblastic activity – so that the characteristic effects of PTH are anabolic. Several recent reports have examined the effects of PTH on fracture healing and all showed significant increases in both histological and mechanical properties of the callus with a positive effect on fracture healing.

Cytokines and small molecular mediators such as prostaglandins play key roles in cellular immune function, but also in the initiation of the process of fracture repair. One of the best studied examples, showing the crucial role of these factors during repair of bone, concerns the role of cyclo-oxygenase-2 (COX-2). In animal studies in which the effects of a non-selective non-steroidal anti- inflammatory drug (NSAID) were compared to those of a *COX-2 selective drug*, greater impairment of fracture healing occurred under treatment with the COX-2 than with the NSAID.

Beta-blockers: these have also been studied in relation to skeletal health. Several studies have demonstrated that the sympathetic nervous system has a catabolic effect on bones. Indeed, functional adrenergic receptors are present in osteoblasts and osteoclasts, and sympathetic nerve fibres have been demonstrated in bone tissue. Therefore, the nervous system may well be a co-regulator of osseous metabolism and thus influence the healing of fractures.

Smokers as well as *individuals with chronic and heavy alcohol consumption* are not only more susceptible to falls and fractures, but also to delay in healing of fractures. Moreover, it has been reported that the maturation of the regenerating bone is abnormal and non-union or mal-union is more frequent in these patients. Smokers themselves assess their outcomes after surgery much less favourably than non-smokers. The detrimental effects of alcohol include: suppression of bone formation by osteoblasts, changes in the composition of the ossifiable matrix and decreased ability of osteoblasts to respond to signals that normally trigger bone formation.

To summarize: bisphosphonates do not prevent initiation of fracture healing or formation of callus, but continued use of bisphosphonates may impede remodelling of the callus, possibly due to bisphosphonate concentration in the bone. Mild suppression of bone turnover with oestrogen or raloxifene, however, has no significant effects on the repair of a fracture. In patients with severe osteoporosis and/or multiple fractures, anabolic agents are preferable as first-line therapy followed by bisphosphonates. It should be borne in mind that other factors, (as outlined above) including drugs such as NSAIDs or COX-2 inhibitors, as well as smoking and heavy consumption of alcohol, may significantly delay the process of fracture healing. Patients may need to be alerted about the risk imposed by NSAIDs if taken during the period of fracture healing.

23.4
Risk Factors for Osteoporotic Fractures

Many, if not the majority, of "fragility fractures" occur as a result of falling, and approximately 5% of older patients require hospitalization, either short or longer term (Table 23.1). Contemporary estimates suggest

Table 23.1. Main causes of falls in the elderly

General deterioration
• Poor postural control
• Weakness
• Abnormal gait
• Poor vision
• Slow reaction time
• Anxiety and agitation
• Fear of falling
Specific diseases and drugs
• Cerebrovascular disease
• Parkinson's disease
• Arthritis
• Cataracts and retinal degeneration
• Blackouts
• Urge urinary incontinence
• Sedatives
• Hypotensive drugs
• Alcohol
Environmental causes
• Low-level lighting
• Slippery surfaces
• Uneven pavements
• Lack of assistance devices in bathrooms
• Loose rugs
• Bad weather, wind and rain
Tripping

that about 50% of vertebral fractures and more than 95% of distal forearm and hip fractures occur as a direct result of trauma.

The *most common risk factors for falls* identified in 16 large studies are (Tables 23.2 and 23.3):

- Muscle weakness
- History of falls
- Impairment of balance and motion
- Lack of devices for protection and assistance in walking
- Visual impairment or defective eyesight (poorly compensated)
- Arthritis
- Psychological factors such as depression
- Cognitive impairment
- Age >80 years

Table 23.2. Risk factors for osteoporotic fracture

Non-modifiable:

- Personal history of fracture as an adult
- Maternal history of fracture
- Caucasian race
- Poor vision
- Advanced age
- Female sex
- Late menarche
- Dementia
- Poor health/frailty

Potentially modifiable:

- Parkinson's disease
- Low body weight
- Oestrogen deficiency
- Testosterone deficiency
- Vitamin D deficiency
- Low dietary calcium intake
- Excess alcohol consumption
- Impaired eyesight despite adequate correction
- Recurrent falls
- Inadequate physical activity
- Glucocorticoid therapy
- Various medications

Table 23.3. Osseous and extraosseous factors that may affect fracture risk

Skeletal factors: Increased bone fragility

- Bone configuration
- Bone microarchitecture
- Bone density
- Bone quality

Extraskeletal factors: Increased risk of trauma

- Increased propensity to fall
- Environmental hazard
- Loss of protective responses

In the OFELY study, seven independent predictors of fragility fractures in postmenopausal women were identified, reflecting different potential mechanisms. In order of decreasing importance, they were:

- Previous fragility fractures

- Low bone mineral density (BMD) (Fig. 23.3)
- Insufficient physical activity
- Reduced grip strength
- Older age groups
- Maternal history of fractures
- Patient history of falls

These items should be included in the clinical assessment of risks for osteoporotic fractures in postmenopausal women.

Five main *intrinsic factors lead to weakening of bone*:

- Reduced bone mass (density)
- Discontinuities in microarchitecture of bone
- Disturbance of mineralization ("osteo-poromalacia")
- Increased, unregulated bone turnover ("secondary hyperparathyroidism")
- Increased tendency to fall, for whatever reason

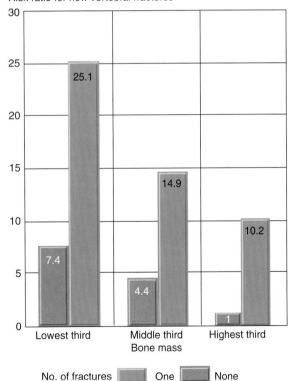

Fig. 23.3. Relationship between prevalent vertebral fractures and bone mineral density on the risk for subsequent vertebral fractures (modified from Ross P, Davis J, Epstein R et al. [1998] Pre-existing fracture and bone mass predict vertebral fracture incidence in women. Ann Intern Med 114:919–923)

About a third of older persons fall at least once a year, but only about 5% of these falls result in a fracture. Taller and thinner patients are more likely to sustain a fracture on falling than shorter, plumper ones. Wrist fractures usually involve a fall onto an outstretched arm. Therefore, it appears that the orientation of the fall is an important factor in determining the kind of fracture. Forces in the spine or ribs generated by activities such as lifting, stepping down or coughing may also be sufficient to cause a vertebral or rib fracture. Other factors such as degenerative disc alterations and the distribution of body weight influence biomechanical forces in the spine and thereby the risk of vertebral fractures. The elderly are more liable to fall due to:

- Reduced muscle mass and strength
- Slowing of reflexes
- Loss of equilibrium
- Impaired vision
- Impaired coordination
- Hypnotics, sedatives and psychotropics
- Alcohol
- Obstacles such as loose mats, cables, wires and small pieces of furniture etc.

Fractures of the wrist or vertebrae are early manifestations of postmenopausal osteoporosis, while those of the hip are more common in the later stages of age-related osteoporosis (Fig. 23.4). Generally, the lower the bone mass, the less likely the trauma is to cause a fracture, for example coughing or rolling over in bed. The risk of fractures (for the rest of their lives) in 50-year-old women and men (percentages in brackets are for men) are:

- Proximal femur 18% (6%)
- Vertebral column 16% (5%)
- Distal radius 15% (3%)
- Any location 40% (13%)

In the course of a lifetime, women lose 35–50% of trabecular bone and 25–30% of compact bone, in the absence of preventive measures (Fig. 23.5). If an osteoporosis-associated fracture has occurred, the following steps should be taken:

- Alleviate the pain.
- Accelerate fracture healing by appropriate surgical, non-surgical and other supportive measures.
- Restore mobility as quickly as possible.
- Exercise the muscles.
- Prevent future fractures.
- Improve bone mass and skeletal stability.
- Nerve root injections given to patients locally before operative or other therapy are effective in reducing pain.

Rehabilitation: This is indicated in patients with manifest osteoporosis. Successful rehabilitation may take months, but usually no longer than a year. Each patient

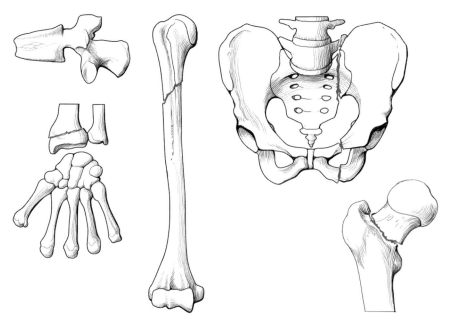

Fig. 23.4. Skeletal sites commonly involved in osteoporotic fractures

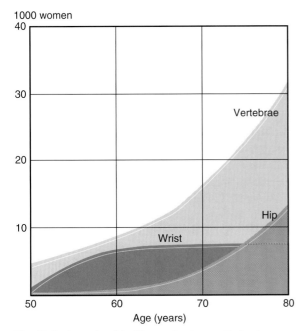

Fig. 23.5. Age-related incidence of osteoporotic fractures

should receive guidance as outlined previously. As mentioned above, early mobility and muscular exercise are important aspects of rehabilitation. Studies have shown that early mobilization, as well as its duration, influences the regeneration of muscles traumatized by the cause of the fracture, and that contractile activity in particular contributes to the restitution of skeletal muscle mass.

23.5
Management of Osteoporotic Fractures

The specific goals of the orthopaedic management of osteoporotic fractures are: (a) early surgical management, (b) rapid mobilization and (c) a return to normal activities as soon as possible. Adherence to these guidelines will avoid undesirable consequences.

General guidelines for the management of osteoporotic fractures are the following:

- Elderly patients are best treated by rapid fracture management. Surgical intervention should be minimized in order to reduce surgery time, blood loss and stress. Indeed, a delay of more than 2 days before surgical intervention proved to be an important

predictor of mortality within 1 year of the time of fracture.
- Surgical intervention should achieve stable fracture fixation to enable a return to weight-bearing status within days.
- The primary cause of implant failure after fracture fixation is the impaired healing capacity of osteoporotic bone.
- Calcium, vitamin D and protein supplementation should be administered in the peri- and postoperative periods. Bisphosphonates and/or raloxifene can be given as required.

23.6
Prevention of Further Fragility Fractures with Specific Drugs

As discussed above, the risk for subsequent fractures in patients with a low-trauma fracture is increased within the first 6 months; therefore, initially agents with a rapid effect are preferred. Treatment with risedronate, alendronate or zoledronate has been shown to decrease the incidence of additional vertebral fractures during the first year by 40%. In one post-hoc analysis, *risedronate*, a bisphosphonate with a rapid suppression of osteoclastic activity, decreased the risk for clinical vertebral fractures by 6 months. In other studies with risedronate and alendronate, there was a significant decrease in hip fracture risk at 18 months, which was sustained for 3 years. Teriparatide also decreased vertebral fractures significantly by 18 months. Although prescribing practices have changed substantially over the last 10 years, and the proportion of patients with hip fractures treated for osteoporosis has increased, it still remains low, with less than one third receiving specific therapy.

23.7
Fracture Sites and Their Clinical Significance

Osteoporosis causes symptoms when a bone fractures. It is important to realize that bone loss itself does not cause pain or disability. Fractures of the hip, spine, wrist and proximal humerus are the most common, although they also occur in other parts of the skeleton, particularly in the pelvis, ankle and ribs. Although any fracture can have a devastating impact on the affected individual, hip fractures are by far the most important from the perspective of public health.

23.7.1
Hip Fractures

Hip fractures account for most of the medical costs, as they are responsible for about 65% of the total costs of osteoporotic fractures. More than 300,000 patients annually in the US alone sustain a *fracture of the proximal femur*; 25% are men with an average age of 80 years. One out of every six Caucasian women (15%) will suffer a hip fracture in her lifetime. The two important types of fractures of the proximal femur are the *intertrochanteric* (50%) and the femoral neck (also 50%) (Fig. 23.6). The mean age is about 80 years and half of the patients live alone. Hip fractures are rare below 50 years of age. In more than 90% of patients, hip fractures are caused by a fall. The type of fracture depends on several factors including the angle and manner of falling, as well as the patient's neuromuscular and protective responses to the fall and its impact. Hip fractures have very serious consequences, most require surgical intervention and the patients are frequently left with a disability:
- Nearly 20% will die within the first year.
- Nearly 25% require a long-term nursing facility or in-home care.
- Nearly 50% never fully recover their mobility.

Risk factors for the first hip fracture have been well characterized and include:
- Previous fracture at any site
- Advanced age
- Low body weight
- Low BMD

Various treatments are available to reduce fracture risk, but only about 5% of women are treated properly after the occurrence of the first hip fracture, with the specific intention of avoiding another one.

About 20% of beds in orthopaedic wards are still occupied by patients with fractures of the proximal femur. Femoral neck fractures in the elderly patient are most commonly treated by hemialloarthroplasty or total hip replacement, while intertrochanteric fractures are best treated with an intramedullary fixation device in combination with a compressive screw (Fig. 23.7). These fixation devices allow an early return to full weight-bearing and help avoid complications (e.g. screw cutting out) and non-union of the fracture (Fig. 23.8). During rehabilitation special attention must be paid to:
- Coordination of movement
- Muscle training
- Avoidance of risks of tripping and falling

Hip fractures are nearly always painful and require hospitalization and *surgery*. The mortality rate immediately after the hip fracture is increased for both women and men; it decreases during the next 5 years, but remains higher than that of the general population. Patients also have a significantly higher relative risk for a second fracture in the future. On a more optimistic note, the results of a prospective randomized trial (Lyles

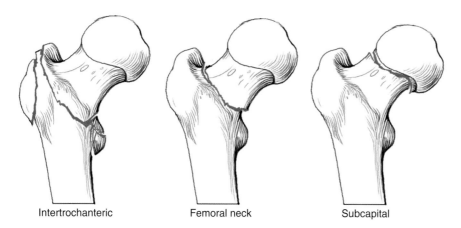

Intertrochanteric   Femoral neck   Subcapital

Fig. 23.6. Types of femoral fractures

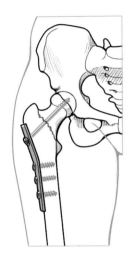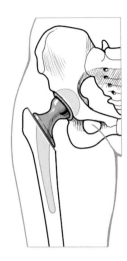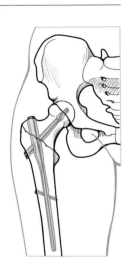

Fig. 23.7. Common surgical procedures for the repair of hip fractures

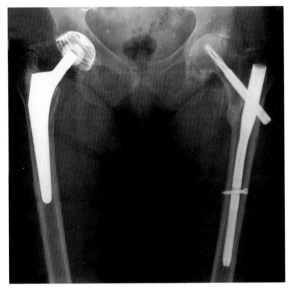

Fig. 23.8. Stabilization of an intertrochanteric fracture using an intramedullary hip screw and total prosthetic replacement

et al. 2008) showed a reduction of 35% in new clinical fractures and of 28% in mortality in the 2 years after the fracture, achieved by a single infusion of zoledronic acid given within 3 months of the first fracture. In addition, fracture union was not delayed by the bisphosphonate.

23.7.2
Vertebral Fractures

Vertebral fractures are often asymptomatic and therefore not diagnosed. Indeed, only about one-third of the vertebral fractures seen on radiographs of the spine come to clinical attention, as these X-rays were not requested due to back pain. The greatest risk factor for compression fractures is an underlying osteoporosis, with multiple myeloma and metastatic cancer, especially of breast, high up in the differential diagnosis of painful vertebral compression fractures. The correct diagnosis requires lateral radiographs of both the thoracic and lumbar spine. Vertebral fractures are very common in older women; they are found in radiographs in 5–10% of women at 55 years, rising to 30–40% by 80 years. The cortical shell of a vertebral body contributes only about 10% of the resistance to compressive loads. Thinning and microcracks in trabecular bone occur with age. Although these heal with callus formation, excess accumulation of microcracks results in critical weakening which in turn leads to vertebral compression and to fracture. Spinal fractures may result from falling, but more commonly they occur spontaneously as a result of common everyday movements such as coughing, lifting, bending or turning. Vertebral fractures occur in many different circumstances, and approximately 50% cannot be attributed to an identified loading effect. Vertebral fractures most commonly involve the midthoracic region (T7–T8) and the thoracolumbar junction (T12–L1) (Fig. 23.9). In contrast, fractures of the upper thoracic spine (T2–T6) are more likely to be due to metastatic disease or multiple myeloma. MRI can help to distinguish benign from malignant disease; however, it cannot distinguish between traumatic and osteoporotic fractures.

23

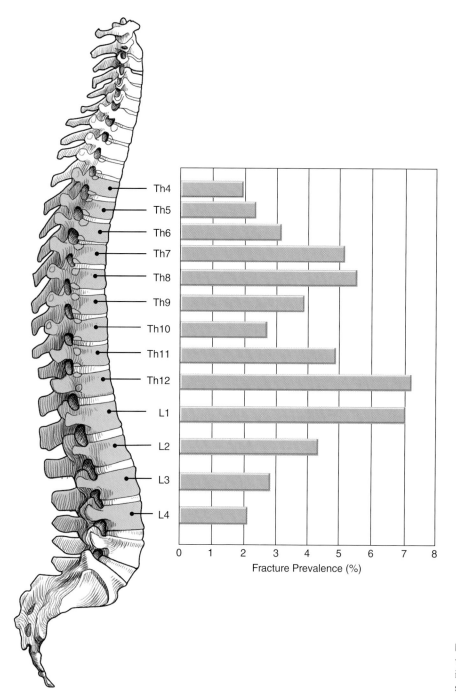

Fig. 23.9. Frequency of vertebral fractures according to their location in the spine

There is great variability in the symptoms caused by spinal fractures. Some patients experience very little or no pain when the fracture occurs, whereas others feel severe pain. The reason for this difference is not known. Although some affected individuals become pain-free after a few months, others may be left with long-lasting pain or discomfort. Patients with vertebral fractures experience aggravation of pain during physical activities such as bending and rising up and even standing up straight. Spinal fractures do not usually cause back pain radiating down the legs, which is more typical of radiculopathy due to disk problems.

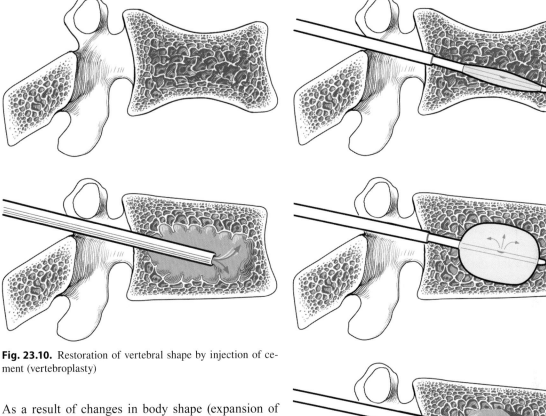

Fig. 23.10. Restoration of vertebral shape by injection of cement (vertebroplasty)

As a result of changes in body shape (expansion of the waistline and prominence of the abdomen), many patients have trouble finding clothes that fit. The long-term effects of vertebral fractures are still underestimated: many result in chronic back pain and limitation of activities. Multiple vertebral fractures can deform the thorax and seriously restrict pulmonary function.

The *repair phase* lasts 2–4 months, during which the use of orthopaedic appliances and corsets should be limited to as short a time as possible. Their purpose is alleviation of pain, avoidance of kyphosis and preservation of pulmonary function. Specialized bandages and supports may be utilized according to the instructions of the orthopaedic specialist. Rehabilitation strategies which increase the strength of spinal muscles will reduce the load on vertebral bodies and thereby decrease the risk of fracture in mechanically incompetent bone. Research into the risk of vertebral fractures, found a four- to six-fold increase with a 2 SD decrease in the BMD of the lumbar spine. One symptomatic vertebral fracture causes a two-fold increase in hip fractures, while two or more vertebral fractures result in a 12-fold increase in new vertebral fractures.

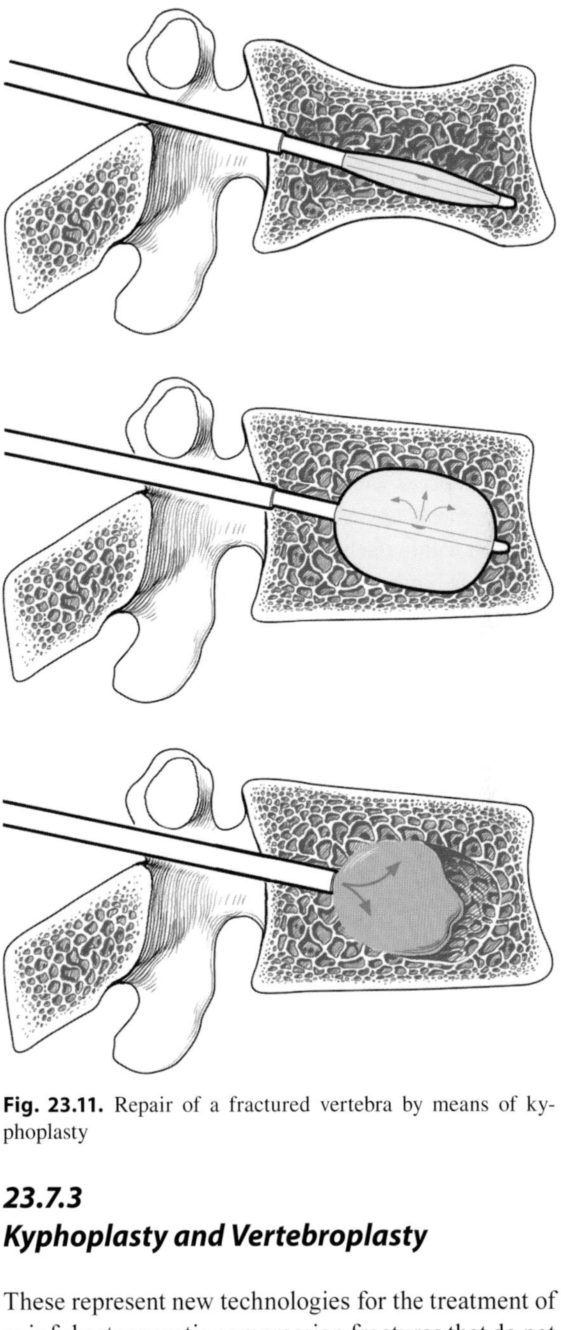

Fig. 23.11. Repair of a fractured vertebra by means of kyphoplasty

23.7.3
Kyphoplasty and Vertebroplasty

These represent new technologies for the treatment of painful osteoporotic compression fractures that do not respond to conventional treatment. Vertebroplasty is the term for the percutaneous injection of polymethylmethacrylate (PMMA), by means of one or two bone biopsy needles, into the fractured vertebra (Fig. 23.10). After hardening, the PMMA stabilizes the restructured vertebral body. Kyphoplasty involves inserting a bone tamp/balloon into the vertebral body under image guidance (Fig. 23.11). When inflated with PMMA

23

and radiocontrast medium (for visualization), the bone tamp compacts the cancellous bone, re-expands the vertebral body and elevates its endplates. Both techniques have a high rate of use and acceptance.

Unilateral transpedicular augmentation is less time-consuming than the bilateral procedure and would be preferable if it provided the same mechanical support as the bilateral procedure.

There is 95% reduction in pain and significant improvement in function following treatment by either of these percutaneous techniques. Kyphoplasty improves height of the fractured vertebra and reduces kyphosis by over 50% if performed within 3 months of the fracture, but later on, there is less improvement in height. Complications occur with both methods mainly due to leakage of cement, less in kyphoplasty because the cement is confined within the balloon (Figs. 23.12 and 23.13). Cement emboli may occur in vertebroplasty. There is also a potential for other significant complications: pulmonary, gastrointestinal, vascular, spinal cord and cauda

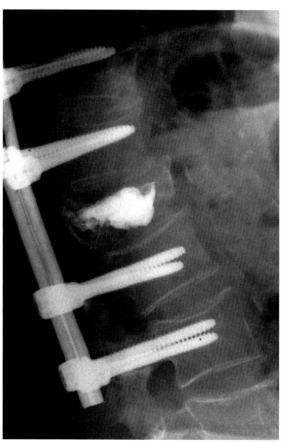

Fig. 23.13. Compression fracture with involvement of the posterior wedge. Surgical stabilization by kyphoplasty

equina injuries. In some cases, collapse because of new compression fractures has been observed in adjacent vertebral bodies, as well as in those above and below the vertebroplasty. However, as pointed out in a recent study, the rate remains low and vertebroplasty retains its position as an effective procedure for these patients.

23.7.4
Distal Forearm Fracture (Wrist Fractures)

Colles´ fracture (named after the Irish surgeon who first described them) is a fracture of the distal radius with or without involvement of the radiocarpal joint. It is the most frequent fracture before the age of 75 years, occurring mainly in women around the time of the menopause. Wrist fractures are usually sustained outdoors and especially in icy conditions. Most of

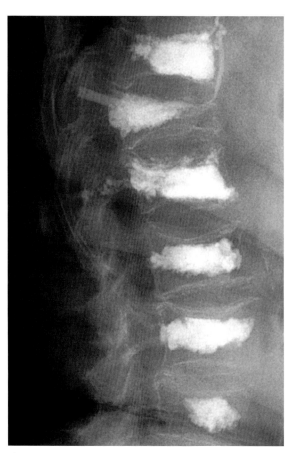

Fig. 23.12. Kyphoplasty of multiple fractured vertebral bodies

these wrist fractures occur after a fall on the outstretched arm. Wrist fractures are painful and require out-patient treatment at a hospital, although elderly patients may need to be hospitalized. Fractures are treated by closed reduction and a plaster cast which is kept in place for 6 weeks. However, fractures with metaphyseal or radio-carpal joint involvement require surgery with open reduction and plating. To date it is not clear whether it is better to treat an elderly patient with casting or with surgical fixation in order to achieve a postoperative condition which will enable the patient to cope with the activities of daily living (Fig. 23.14). The fractured ends of the bone(s) are sometimes displaced and must be manipulated into place and stabilized before a cast or splint is applied. A fracture of the radius in patients between 40 and 60 years of age is always a sign of osteoporosis and calls for immediate measurement of bone density. A cast is retained for 6–8 weeks, during which time active and passive exercises of the fingers, hand, upper arm and shoulder should be carried out regularly to preserve their motility and function and to prevent further onset or deterioration of osteoporosis. A significant complication, after either conservative or surgical therapy, may arise in the form of algodystrophy. In these patients, there is often persistent pain, tenderness, swelling and stiffness of the hand that may last for years after the injury. A fracture of the radius in patients older than 50 years of age raises the question of an underlying osteoporosis and calls for immediate measurement of bone density. As previously outlined, osteoporotic patients are also at a higher risk of additional fractures at any site. Studies have shown that mortality after a distal radial fracture is not increased,

but there is a significant impairment of health-related quality of life.

23.7.5
Proximal Humerus Fractures

The most common osteoporotic fracture of the upper arm is that of the proximal humerus; fractures of the shaft or the supracondylar elbow are less common. Most proximal humerus fractures occur after a fall onto the shoulder with the arm adducted. The majority are nondisplaced, impacted fractures (fractures at the surgical neck) that can be treated conservatively with a sling and permit early functional rehabilitation. Displaced fractures or complex fractures require surgery with open reduction and plating, nailing or minimal invasive pinning, or even hemiarthroplasty if the fracture is complex with involvement of the joint. Elderly patients should start physiotherapy as soon as possible to prevent loss of movement in the postoperative period. Fractures of the proximal humerus are associated with an increased risk for future spinal and hip fractures in both women and men, and with an increased mortality immediately after the fracture, but this declines during the subsequent 5 years.

23.7.6
Other Fractures

These include fractures of the pelvis, the distal tibia or fibula and the ribs, all composed predominantly of trabecular bone. Fractures around the knee (supra-

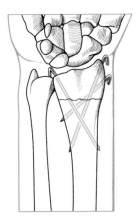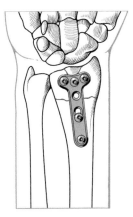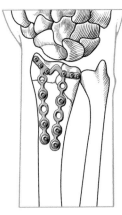

Fig. 23.14. Common procedures for the repair of wrist fractures

23

condylar fractures of the distal femur or fractures of the tibial plateau) carry a high risk for postoperative degenerative joint disease and arthrofibrosis. Pelvic fractures of the superior and inferior rami and the sacral ala can be debilitating and very painful and the mortality associated with pelvic fractures is similar to that of hip fractures: 20% at 2 years and 50% at 5 years. Nondisplaced fractures are usually treated conservatively. Elderly patients with pelvic fractures require special health care resources and are usually hospitalized for long periods of time.

The National Osteoporosis Foundation has established *guiding principles for the treatment of patients with osteoporotic fractures*:

- All patients presenting a low-energy fracture should be screened for osteoporosis.
- All patients should be placed on 800 IU of vitamin D and 1200–1500 mg of elemental calcium (preferably calcium citrate) daily.
- Before discharge, all patients should be started on alendronate (70 mg per week), risedronate (35 mg per week), ibandronate (150 mg once monthly) or a modern intravenous bisphosphonate (ibandronate 3 mg every 3 months or zoledronate 5 mg once annually). Intravenous administration is the route of choice if the patient has a history of gastrointestinal dysfunction.
- In severe osteoporosis with multiple osteoporotic fractures, osteoanabolic drugs such as teriparatide (20 µg s.c. daily) or parathormone (100 µg s.c. daily) can be used alternatively.
- Within 6 weeks following discharge, all patients should undergo a dual-energy X-ray absorptiometry (DXA) scan and a metabolic work-up to rule out secondary causes of osteoporosis. For monitoring, a DXA scan should be performed every year.

23.7.7
Improving Quality of Life After Osteoporotic Fractures

This is best achieved by focussing not only on prevention and treatment but also on ways to deal with the personal and social consequences of the disease, such as pain, depression, loss of self-esteem and social isolation:

- Acute pain can be treated with bed rest for 2–3 days, analgesics, heating pads, massage and back support.
- Treatment of chronic pain includes strengthening of the back extensor muscles with an exercise program and/or weight-bearing according to the individual patient's ability, as well as support for the back.
- Various devices (including single or double canes) to assist in maintenance of balance, gait and walking, and, importantly to prevent falls
- Patients who have suffered osteoporotic fractures often feel anxious, helpless and depressed due to lifestyle limitations, changes in appearance and difficulties in functioning independently at home, especially if living alone. Therefore, patients should be informed of the social amenities available and directed to support groups which bring patients together and provide useful information.

An increasing drain of maternal reserves mineralizes the foetal skeleton. In total, the developing foetal skeleton gains up to 33 g of calcium and about 80% of this is deposited during the third trimester when the foetal skeleton grows rapidly. This high demand for calcium is largely met by a doubling of maternal intestinal calcium absorption, mediated by calcitriol and other hormones, which is usually enough to meet the daily calcium needs of the foetus without long-term consequences to the maternal skeleton. The increased calcium absorption early in pregnancy may stimulate the maternal skeleton to prepare for the peak foetal demands that occur later in pregnancy (Fig. 24.1). Subsequently during lactation, sufficient calcium must be supplied in the breast milk to enable skeletal growth of the infant. Calcium homeostasis in human pregnancy and lactation is illustrated in Fig. 24.1.

The female body has several *compensatory mechanisms* to supply the increased demand for calcium during pregnancy and lactation, so that problems only arise if the calcium depots (in the bones) are not full to begin with. Indeed, fragility fractures in pregnancy may be a consequence of pre-existing low bone mineral density (BMD) and increased bone resorption. Therefore, supplements of calcium and vitamins are recommended and should be taken from the beginning of pregnancy. However, pregnancy per se is not a risk factor for osteoporosis. But risk factors are incurred if the pregnant woman is subjected to bed rest and/or is treated with muscle relaxants and/or sedatives. In some cases even corticosteroids are given. In these situations, a massive withdrawal of calcium from the bones is unavoidable, and should be compensated at the very least with adequate supplements of calcium and vitamin D. During pregnancy, there is normally a slight decrease in bone density, but this loss is soon replaced after birth. However, it should be remembered that during lactation about 500 mg calcium is excreted daily into the milk, which should be balanced on a daily basis by increased ingestion of appropriate foods and supplements. In reality, very few women suffer from osteoporotic fractures during (and as a result of) the pregnancy itself. The vast majority of women can be assured that the changes in bone and calcium metabolism during pregnancy and lactation are normal and without adverse consequences in the long term.

Results of a study comparing the bone status in young "primiparas" (young women immediately after the birth of their first child) with that of young "nulliparas" (young women who had not yet been pregnant and given birth) showed that the values of quantitative ultrasound (QUS) measurements were significantly lower and the bone markers higher in the primiparas in the early postpartum phase than in the nulliparas. Since later measurements were not given, definitive conclusions cannot be drawn. Possibly such early examinations were not previously recorded and the deficiency very quickly rectified, with no lasting adverse effects.

The *maternal status of vitamin D during pregnancy* has lately attracted some attention, and the suggestion has been put forward that this may affect intra-uterine skeletal mineralization, growth and development of muscles, as well as possibly even having a more sustained influence in childhood and later. These possibilities raise the question of early determination of the pregnant woman's vitamin D level and administration

R. Bartl, B. Frisch, *Osteoporosis*, DOI 10.1007/978-3-540-79527-8_24,
© Springer-Verlag Berlin Heidelberg 2009

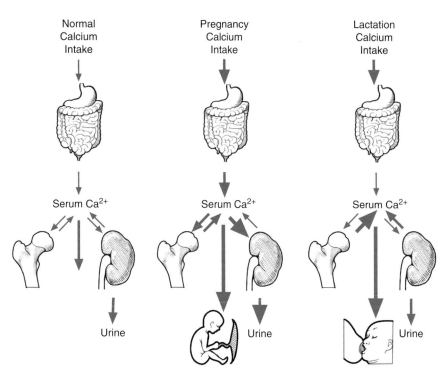

Fig. 24.1. Calcium homeostasis in normal women compared to that during pregnancy and lactation (modified from Kovacs C, Kronenberg H [1997] Maternal–fetal calcium and bone metabolism during pregnancy, puerperium and lactation. Endocr Rev 18:832–872)

of supplements as required. However, few investigations of possible benefits and adverse reactions of such supplements in pregnant women and on the foetus have been published. One such study from the UK was carried out on a group of pregnant women whose vitamin D concentrations were measured in late pregnancy. A total of 466 (78%) children were examined at birth, 440 (74%) at 9 months and 178 (30%) at 9 years of age. The results showed that maternal concentrations of vitamin D >75 nmol/l did not influence the new born child's body size, psychological health or cardiovascular system. A low incidence of atopic disorders was observed, which requires confirmation. However, results of another study from Australia showed that maternal vitamin D deficiency increased the risk of lower birth weight and neonatal vitamin D deficiency. Low maternal levels of vitamin D may increase the risk of preeclampsia, a cogent reason for determination of the level of vitamin D at the beginning of pregnancy. Longitudinal studies of women have found a relationship between a history of preeclampsia in pregnancy and insulin sensitivity and vasodilatory functions, as well as impaired insulin sensitivity later in life.

The pregnant woman is also subject to many general musculoskeletal disorders and injuries as well as specific conditions that may affect non-pregnant women at that age. A crucial factor in the determination of therapy for these conditions is the protection and preservation of the pregnancy itself. As pointed out in various reviews, most orthopaedic issues in pregnancy can be controlled conservatively, and surgical interventions postponed until after delivery.

If a fracture has occurred in a pregnant woman it is advisable not to breast feed or at least to shorten the nursing period as much as possible. Though bisphosphonates are not yet authorized for premenopausal women, they should be considered when confronted by manifest, severe premenopausal osteoporosis, together with the ancillary measures already outlined. In addition, the patient must be fully informed about the use of bisphosphonates, the beneficial effects and the possible, though rare, adverse side effects, the indications and contraindications, and how and when they should be taken. In these patients, questions concerning residual bisphosphonates within the bones and subsequent pregnancy and lactation are still open. It is quite possible that osteoporosis in pregnancy and lactation is more frequent than recognized simply because it is only recognized when an unexpected fracture occurs. Nevertheless, a few studies of osteoporosis during pregnancy and lactation have been reported, including one in which three cases of severe vertebral fractures were described. The patients were treated with bisphosphonates. So far, adverse effects on the infants have not been reported. Only one patient with painful lumbar and thoracic vertebral fractures was treated with osteoanabolic therapy, and had a good response. Intravenous bisphosphonate therapy during lactation has also been used in cases of severe osteoporosis with vertebral fractures which had developed during pregnancy. In another somewhat unusual case, a 30-year-old woman developed moderate back pain during the last month of her first pregnancy. The pain worsened after delivery and eight vertebral fractures were seen on radiology. The total T-score of the lumbar vertebrae 2–4 was –4.7. Therefore, when back pain occurs during pregnancy and/or lactation, osteoporosis should be considered in the differential diagnosis.

Transient osteoporosis of the hip, a subtype of the "bone marrow oedema syndrome" is a rare, self-limiting form of local pregnancy-associated osteoporosis. Some hypotheses to explain this painful condition include femoral venous stasis due to the gravid uterus, reflex sympathetic dystrophy, ischaemia, trauma, viral infection and immobilization. These women present unilateral or bilateral hip pain and/or hip fracture in the third trimester, together with bone marrow oedema demonstrable on MRI. The symptoms and MRI findings usually resolve within 2–6 months postpartum.

Longitudinal studies of women have found a relationship between a history of preeclampsia in pregnancy and subsequent insulin sensitivity and vasodilatory function, as well as impaired insulin sensitivity later in life.

With respect to *HIV in pregnant women*, programmed therapies have been developed and the effects studied in women before, during and after pregnancy, as well as during the period of lactation. Results showed that cell-free and, to a lesser extent, cell-associated HIV-1 RNA levels in breast milk were suppressed by the antiretroviral treatment used to prevent mother-to-child transmission. But there was no significant reduction in the reservoir of infected cells and these could contribute to the transmission of HIV-1 to the breast milk. The maternal viral load also played a part. In this connection, it is worth mentioning that there were no serious adverse effects on the foetus when bisphosphonates were given to lactating women. No bisphosphonate was detected in the breast milk collected for 48 h after an infusion of pamidronate.

Osteoporosis in Men

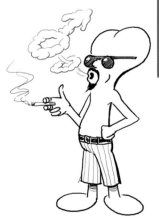

A near-perfect example of sexual equality in nature! Osteoporosis does not discriminate! Men are as vulnerable as women! It just strikes them about 10 years later. And not only the trabecular network, but also the cortical bone which further increases the fracture risk.

25.1
Clinical Evaluation of Osteoporosis in Men

Ageing in men is accompanied by a steady decline in levels of gonadal steroids and of growth hormones which largely determine the decrease in bone mineral density (BMD). The concept of the "andropause", i.e. the natural age-related decline in testosterone levels in men, is beginning to be understood and to be accepted by health care professionals and by the general public. Many studies have now been carried out on the effects of hypogonadism in men and its consequences, not only osteoporosis, for example the Partial Androgen Deficiency of the Ageing Male (PADAM) study and the Late-Onset Hypogonadism (LOH) study. A recent review from Finland, the Turku Male Ageing Study (TuMAS), also summaries the results of investigations into the connections between testicular endocrine function and the physical, psychological and sexual symptoms of ageing. The consequences of ageing usually also affect the bones,

directly or indirectly. One of the presumed universal consequences of ageing is telomere shortening, which is directly correlated with chronological age as well as with some ageing phenotypes. Studies in healthy men aged 71–86 years have demonstrated the connection between longitudinal bone loss and shortened telomeres.

However, there is insufficient awareness of the benefits of *testosterone replacement therapy*, which has already proved its value in the relatively short term, while the long-term results are awaited. Moreover, so far little attention has been paid to the direct effects of gonadal steroids and the effect their decline has on bone and its metabolism in elderly men. Age is recognized as the most important risk factor for male osteoporosis, which occurs about 10–15 years later than in women, that is, at about 60–65 years of age, with an acceleration of bone loss after 70 years apparently due to unbalanced remodelling, which also results in deterioration of the microarchitecture of the bone. It should be noted that a high proportion of men (approximately 60% in some studies) no longer have optimal secretion of androgens from 60 years of age, though levels start to decrease much earlier. Studies have indicated that the majority of men with androgen deficiency do not receive treatment, despite adequate access to medical care, as shown in the results of the Boston Area Community Health Survey. It should also be emphasized that the beneficial effects of testosterone therapy on bone density, obesity, insulin resistance and coronary angina have already been documented in clinical trials.

Decline in other factors associated with ageing may also contribute to osteoporosis. A decrease in muscle mass ("sarcopenia") is common even in healthy people over 60 years and increases with age and influences the status of the bones. Directed efforts to prevent muscle loss should emphasize sustained physical activity from childhood throughout life as the years pass, including appropriate exercises.

It is only in recent years that osteoporosis in men has been recognized as a major public health problem, the extent of which is increasing steadily, also as a result of the increase in numbers of elderly people in the population, and with a corresponding increase in cost. For example, the cost of osteoporosis in men for the year 1999 in France was calculated, according to hospitalizations caused by 21,857 fractures, at a total cost of 198 million Euro. In Britain, the cost has been estimated at a quarter of a billion pounds annually (perhaps more by now). Moreover, men with hip fractures have higher morbidity and mortality rates than women. This is graphically highlighted by a recent report on "Outcomes and secondary prevention strategies for male hip fractures", which draws the conclusion that men with hip fractures had received inadequate evaluation and treatment for osteoporosis. But the situation has begun to change for the better, as more data are published and public awareness increases. It should be emphasized that, particularly since the beginning of the 21st century, there has been a steady stream of reports from trials and studies of all aspects of osteoporosis in men. Clearly, only a few of the key publications can be considered in this chapter. The first large population-based study carried out in many countries in Europe, the European Prospective Osteoporosis Study (EPOS), has confirmed the frequent occurrence of vertebral fractures in men and their increase with age. Criteria for the densitometric diagnosis of osteoporosis in men have been recommended and published, as have up-dated guidelines for osteoporotic screening in men (2008) by the American College of Physicians. These also include the key risk factors: advanced age, low body weight, physical inactivity, prolonged corticosteroid use, previous osteoporotic fracture, androgen deprivation therapy and, of course, the comorbidities which are fundamental to some of the risk factors.

A recent study reviewed the main risk factors of 2035 males >50 years who all presented with fractures. In these patients, the main risk factors associated with osteoporosis were: smoking, excess alcohol, low body mass index and family history of osteoporosis. In all, 58% of the patients with hip fractures had osteoporosis, but only 18% of patients with fractures of the ankles. Other risk factors in patients with hip fractures were immobility and loss of height. Clearly, all the patients would have benefited from early institution of preventive measures.

According to recent estimates, 20% of all cases of osteoporosis occur in men. The estimated number of men with osteoporosis in the US is now put at 5 million (2003). Osteoporosis is present in 6% and osteopenia in 47% of males over age 50. However, there are ethnic and racial differences in the bone structure of some bones, for example the thicker cortical bone in the proximal femur, as well as in BMD, which are more prominent in older men. These differences may also account for the lower fracture rate among black and Asian men. The clinical picture of established osteoporosis in men is comparable to that in women, with kyphosis due to wedge fractures of the thoracic column, protuberance of the abdomen and transverse skin folds over the dorsal trunk. The male:female ratio of hip fractures has been calculated to be 1:3 and the vertebral fracture ratio even approaches 1:2. Four *diagnostic steps* are recommended:

- Exclusion of other bone disorders with diminished bone mineral content (osteomalacia)
- Quantification of the degree of osteopenia [dual-energy X-ray absorptiometry (DXA) of lumbar spine and proximal femur, and possibly additional sites as indicated in the individual patient]
- Evaluation of the clinical stage of osteoporosis (from preclinical and uncomplicated to advanced with complications)
- Exclusion of secondary osteoporosis, in addition to the primary, involutional, age-related osteoporosis.

In young men especially, transient osteoporosis of the hip must be distinguished from avascular necrosis, which is done by the distinctive, typical MRI findings in the former condition. Establishing the correct diagnosis avoids unnecessary surgery and other inappropriate measures.

The percentage of men with secondary osteoporosis is around 50% – higher by 10% than that in women. Consequently men, especially the older age groups, should be carefully screened to reveal any additional underlying causes for the osteoporosis. The Osteoporotic Fractures in Men Study (MrOs), the first US "men only" study, deals extensively with risk factors.

Other recent studies (2008) examined the efficacy of osteoporosis risk assessment tools in large cohorts of Caucasian and Chinese men, the OST and MOST studies. The tools included body weight and quantitative ultrasound index for screening and their efficacy was confirmed in this study.

Important *risk factors* include:

- Heavy smoking: Recently, the Tromso study (2008) demonstrated that smoking in men reduces BMD at the hip and forearm and increases the fracture risk.
- Hypogonadism: The effects are directly related to time of onset (at about 60 years) and duration. Age-related (>73 years) decrease in measurable free testosterone levels are accompanied by clinical symptoms including erectile dysfunction, prostatism, changes in cognitive functions, inability to perform daily activities and osteoporosis.
- High alcohol consumption: The precise mechanism of the negative effect of alcohol on bone has not yet been elucidated, but it appears to be on bone formation. However, other deleterious lifestyle factors undoubtedly also contribute to reduced BMD and fractures which occur in chronic alcohol abusers.
- Dietary factors: Studies have shown that the consequences of eating disorders in men, i.e. the various sub-types of anorexia nervosa and binge eating, can be as bad if not worse than in women as predicted by the duration of the condition, low body mass index (BMI) and severe osteoporosis. Duration of the disorder(s) is also an important factor in the consequent osteoporosis. Moreover, as pointed out previously, undernutrition in early life may also predispose accelerated ageing and its accompanying dysfunctions.
- Weight loss: A low BMI and weight loss in middle-aged men, before and continuing into the andropause, are strongly and negatively related to BMD of the hip.
- Stress and anxiety: These states could be classified as primary or secondary, for example together with depressive states. But there is one important difference, the age of the patients, as the patients with stress fractures are usually young and may be male military personnel. Investigation of 32 young military personnel patients and 32 healthy controls showed only that the patients had a decreased bone turnover and calcaneal stiffness, but no other pathological or biochemical cause for the fractures was found.
- Prostate cancer: This poses a major risk factor for osteoporosis, especially when the patient is on androgen deprivation therapy. BMD should be measured before starting therapy, which should be initiated as quickly as possible after diagnosis to prevent spread and skeletal metastases. Various non-hormonal therapies have been advocated to improve patients' quality of life and, possibly, survival.
- Renal disorders: Older men with reduced renal function are at increased risk of osteoporosis and hip fractures.

The most frequent cause (about 30%) of osteoporosis in men is testosterone deficiency and it is a risk factor for hip fractures. The level of testosterone in the blood must always be determined, since some patients do not suffer from sexual dysfunction and appear to have normal testes in spite of decreased levels of testosterone. Specific causes of *hypogonadism* include:

- Klinefelter syndrome
- Prolactinomas
- Kallmann syndrome
- Prader-Willi syndrome
- Male Turner syndrome (Noonan syndrome)
- Haemochromatosis
- Status post orchitis
- Castration.

Symptomatic late onset hypogonadism (SLOH) may be particularly troublesome due to physical and mental effects, including fatigue, lethargy, reduced physical and mental activities, reduced muscle and bone mass, anaemia, increased sweating and decreased sense of well-being, among other symptoms. These patients require very inclusive examinations (PSA, haemoglobin etc.) before specific therapy, especially with androgens, is advised. Men with low testosterone levels may have a variety of physical manifestations such as increased weight and fat mass, especially abdominal. The biochemical changes include higher glucose, insulin and triglyceride levels. BMD is decreased, which is due to an increase in resorption of bone as well as a decrease in its formation and thereby a rapid loss of bone. Moreover, it has been demonstrated in several studies that oestrogen deficiency also plays an important part in causing osteoporosis in men by the following mechanism: a high serum level of the sex hormone-binding globulin lowers the levels of both testosterone and oestrogen in the blood, reducing the availability of androgen for synthesis of oestrogen by aromatization in peripheral tissues. It is a deficiency of oestrogen rather than androgen which is responsible for the increased bone resorption – even in men. This has been confirmed by data from the Framingham Study, which demonstrated that low hip BMD in elderly men is correlated with low serum oestradiol levels rather than with testosterone deficiency. Indeed, oestrogen action is clearly essential for the normal development of bone in young males, and also exerts important effects on bone in adults. Therefore, selective oestrogen receptor modulators (SERMs) may also have applications in men at risk of bone loss. A short-term trial of raloxifene in older men revealed reductions in bone markers even in men with the lowest oestradiol levels. Long-term trials are needed to show the effectiveness and safety of raloxifene and in which male populations they may be most useful. An increase in serum leptin also reduces bone formation and thereby BMD. It has been postulated that the age-related difference in serum parathyroid hormone (PTH) levels and in bone resorption between men and women is due to the fact that there is more residual testosterone in men than oestrogen in women. An increase in serum leptin also reduces bone formation and thereby BMD.

25.2
Special Features in Men

There are differences in frequency and fracture site between men and women. Boys have fractures of the extremities more frequently than girls. However, this is readily explained by: (a) the fact that boys are more active in sports than girls, particularly aggressive and contact sports, and by (b) the stronger physical force of young men. The diameter of the vertebral bodies and of the long bones is greater in men than in women and this constitutes an important defence against fractures. The frequency of femoral neck fractures in men decreases during the period of 35–60 years of age and only begins to rise again after 70 years. Two main factors determine the differences in the condition of the skeleton between men and women. The first is the peak bone mass and the second is the late and slow decline in testosterone. Due to their greater physical activity and higher calcium intake, young men have a peak bone mass 25% greater than

that of young women. Moreover, the age-related bone loss that begins at around 30 years of age is slower in men: 0.3% annually compared to 0.8% in women. Testosterone levels in men decline slowly with age so that the "andropause", as it is now called, is not due to a sudden decrease in sexual hormones as in women. Women may lose up to 40% of their trabecular bone during their lifetime but men only about 14%. The comparatively low incidence of osteoporosis in men can be explained by:
- A higher peak bone mass at maturity
- Greater diameter of the long bones and vertebral bodies
- A low rate of bone loss in later life
- Men do not undergo the sudden hormonal decline equivalent to the menopause
- The andropause is characterized by a later, gradual decrease
- Men on average have a lower life expectancy, but this is changing (fortunately).

25.3
Prevention and Treatment in Men

Prevention of osteoporosis in men starts with the investigation of calcium intake and blood levels of testosterone, which can be given as needed in gels, patches, tablets or by i.m. injections, for example 250 mg testosterone enanthate i.m. every 3–4 weeks or testosterone patches 2.5 mg daily, though not of course to patients with carcinoma of the prostate. An International Consensus Document (see Stanworth and Jones 2008) has recently been published and provides guidelines on the diagnosis, treatment and monitoring of late-onset hypogonadism in men, as well as the utilization of the various testosterone preparations currently available. Isolated hypogonadotrophic hypogonadism (IHH) which may occur in severely obese men, possibly because of increased oestradiol production, can be treated by an aromatase inhibitor, such as letrozole at low dosages (2.5 mg weekly) to begin with. However, it is important to take into account that men may be subject to fractures at higher bone densities than women, and that men have higher mortality rates than women after hip fractures. Although the level of vitamin D does not automatically decline with age in healthy men, hypovitaminosis D is prevalent and therefore supplements are recommended. The following program can be applied for the prevention of osteoporosis in men:

- Daily intake of 1000 mg calcium and 1000 IU vitamin D
- Regular physical activity, adapted to each patient
- No smoking!
- Moderate alcohol consumption only
- Monitoring of testosterone levels and treatment as required
- Monitoring additional disorders and medications which possibly affect the bones
- Avoidance of falls and use of hip protection devices especially in elderly men.

25.4
Therapy of Osteoporosis in Men

The same guidelines apply as for women: adequate calcium, vitamin D and exercise should be encouraged. If the testosterone levels are found to be low and there are no contra-indications, intramuscular, subcutaneous or transdermal testosterone will increase bone mass. As demonstrated in clinical trials, the aminobisphosphonates are equally effective, safe and well-tolerated in men as in women! Alendronate, risedronate and zoledronate have been approved and are considered the bisphosphonates of choice for os-

teoporosis in men, as already demonstrated in prospective studies (Fig. 25.1). However, fractures of the femoral shaft have occurred after long-term, i.e. >6-year therapy with alendronate. Therefore, careful monitoring is required. It is worth emphasizing that a low BMD is associated with a higher risk of fractures and mortality in men and therefore adequate and early prevention is even more important.

In spite of the efficacy of antiresorptive therapy, it is clear that anabolic agents to stimulate bone formation could also play a significant part in prevention and therapy of primary osteoporosis in men. In this context, several reports have suggested that PTH, especially as low-dose intermittent therapy, results in significant increases in BMD in male osteoporosis. However, results of long-term studies have not yet been published. Another novel treatment is short-term administration of growth hormone together with testosterone which appeared to have a favourable effect on BMD, but long-term results of this combination are still awaited. Finally, more attention has been paid in recent years to replacement therapy in men; several options are under investigation and results should be published soon. These options include SERMs, calcitonin and PTH alone or in various combinations. SERMs have already been used to maintain BMD in men during androgen deprivation therapy. A different approach to replacement therapy recently advocated is transdermal oestrogen, which avoided or substantially reduced unwanted side effects and proved effective at a tenth of the cost of

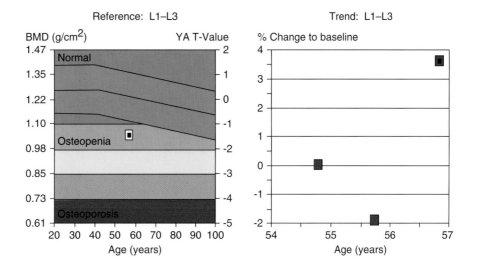

Fig. 25.1. Monitoring of bone mineral density (BMD) (L1–L3) before and during therapy with bisphosphonates

conventional hormone therapies, in men with androgen deprivation due to prostate cancer. Androgen deprivation therapy (ADT) in men with prostate cancer has a considerable impact on muscle, fat and bone mass. Measurements were made at baseline and after 36 weeks of ADT in a cohort of men aged 44–88 years with non-metastatic prostate cancer. At 36 weeks, there were significant decreases in whole body and regional lean mass as well as in bone mass, while whole body and regional fat mass increased in the older men with prostate cancer. Strategies must be advised by the attending doctor and implemented by the patient to minimize the occurrence of sarcopenia, osteoporosis and obesity.

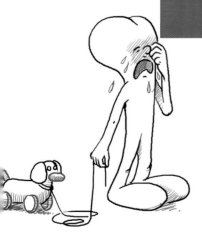

During growth, the shape, architecture and strength of the bones are modulated by three major processes: growth, modelling and remodelling. Modelling is of particular interest as it appears that bone is much more capable of responding to external loads during growth than at any other time. Remodelling also occurs during growth, but is limited and does not participate in active growth, i.e. to accrue bone. Information on the pattern of bone mineral deposition is illustrated in Figs. 26.1 and 26.2, showing the plots and velocity curves of total body bone mineral content during growth. The authors of these longitudinal studies of boys and girls have also shown that, on average, 26 % of adult total bone mineral was accrued during the 2 years around peak bone mineral content velocity, at average ages of 12.5 years for girls and 14.1 years for boys. Furthermore, it is of interest that true bone density does not increase with size or age and reported increases in BMD with age are a reflection of growth and an increase in size rather than an increase in bone mineral per unit volume. The crucial importance of food in childhood to achieve optimal physical and cognitive development has long been acknowledged, as has the recognition that the promotion of children's health will help to reduce diet-related risks of many adult diseases, including degenerative and cardiovascular disorders, type 2 diabetes, cancers, obesity and osteoporosis.

Consequently, nutrition guidelines for children from 2 to 11 years have just been published: the Position of the American Dietetic Association.

26.1
First Clarification – Hereditary or Acquired?

Though osteoporosis rarely occurs in children, it may do so and cause severe pain, multiple fractures and lifelong limitations of movement and locomotion unless adequately treated. Osteoporosis in children is often not diagnosed until after one or two fractures have occurred or if low density is suspected on radiographs (Table 26.1). Consequently, increased awareness is just as important, if not more so, than for adults, as any decrease in bone density during childhood and adolescence which remains uncorrected will have a negative impact on peak bone mass with increased risk of osteoporosis later in life.

Osteoporosis in children has not yet been officially defined. The WHO *definition* is based on values for adults. However, recommendations for paediatric densitometry have now been published. In practice, however, the diagnosis is based on a bone density measurement (Fig. 26.3):
- More than 2 SD below the average value of a child of similar age with healthy bones
- Number of pathologic fractures.

Musculoskeletal complaints are relatively frequent in children, accounting for about 20 % of visits to the doctor. This is not surprising taking into account that

26

BMC TG in g

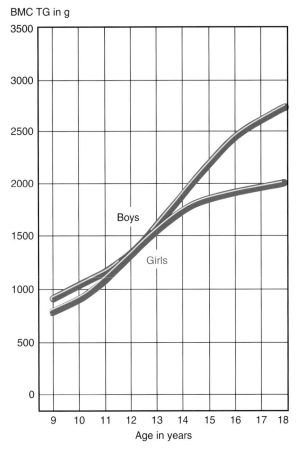

Fig. 26.1. Total body bone mineral content for boys and girls according to age (modified from Baily [1996])

BMC TB velocity in g per year

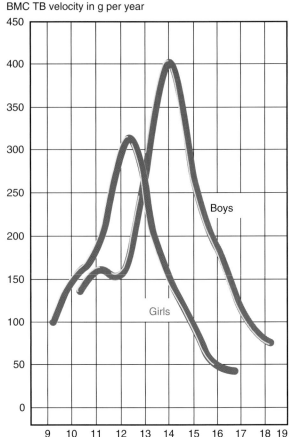

Fig. 26.2. Velocity curves depicting sex and age differences in timing and magnitude of peak bone mineral accrual (modified from Baily [1996])

bone is a very active organ metabolically and maintains homeostasis of calcium and phosphorus, so that an imbalance may result in many osteological and other metabolic disorders.

The *differential diagnosis* includes rheumatic disorders, infections, metabolic bone disorders, neu-

Table 26.1. Investigation for underlying disease in childhood osteoporosis

• Complete blood count and ESR
• Renal and liver function (serum)
• Glucose (serum, urine)
• TSH (serum)
• Calcium, phosphate (serum)
• Alkaline phosphatase (serum)
• Vitamin D and PTH (serum)
• Fasting urine calcium
• X-ray skull and lumbar spine
• Bone turnover markers
• Bone/bone marrow biopsy (when indicated)

ropathies and specific orthopaedic conditions, among others. All may be associated with osteopenia/osteoporosis. The first steps in diagnostic evaluation include family history, physical examination and elementary laboratory tests.

The major causes of osteopenia/osteoporosis in children, both congenital and acquired, are listed below in alphabetical order (this list is not exhaustive):

● Acute leukaemias, lymphatic and myeloid: Long-term survivors of cancer are at risk for low bone mineral density (BMD) and must be given preventive treatment.

● Anorexia nervosa and binge eating.

● Anticonvulsant therapy.

● Asthma bronchiale: the effects of long-term corticosteroid use on BMD have been evaluated in the Childhood Asthma Management Program (CAMP) study.

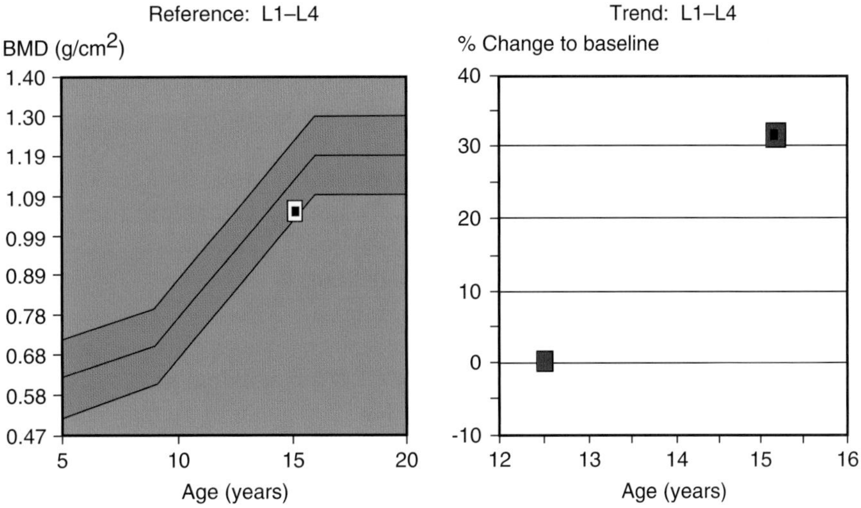

Fig. 26.3. Dual-energy X-ray absorptiometry measurement of bone mineral density (*BMD*) in a 15-year-old child with osteoporosis. Marked increase of BMD after therapy with a bisphosphonate for approximately 3 years

- Biliary atresia.
- Cerebral palsy: early preventive therapy in children 1–6-years old is especially indicated.
- Chronic hepatic disorders.
- Chronic renal insufficiency.
- Crohn's and celiac diseases: >40% of children with celiac disease have reduced BMD, and >75% if the diagnosis is delayed.
- Congenital autoimmune disorders, especially those treated with glucocorticoids.
- Glucocorticoid therapy.
- Cushing's syndrome.
- Cyanotic congenital heart disease.
- Cystic fibrosis: especially with lower BMD in the early stages. Early recognition and preventive therapy indicated.
- Diabetes mellitus: children with diabetes are liable to accelerated tooth eruption, so special attention to oral health is required.
- Drugs: metabolic and endocrine adverse consequences may occur as a result of anti-psychotic agents. Therefore, children must be carefully monitored, with attention to size and weight according to sex and age.
- Glycogen storage disorders.
- Growth hormone deficiency.
- Homocystinuria.
- Hypogonadism (e.g. Turner's and Klinefelter syndromes).
- Idiopathic hyperphosphatasia.

- Hypoparathyroidism.
- Infections and their consequences if chronic, e.g. hepatitis C with metabolic risk factors.
- Juvenile chronic arthritis.
- Juvenile Paget's disease.
- Malabsorption syndromes.
- Malignancies such as sarcomas: rhabdomyosarcoma is the commonest sarcoma in children.
- McCune Albright syndrome: characterized by the classic triad of fibrous dysplasias, skin manifestations which may appear shortly after birth and precocious puberty. All require therapeutic attention, including the musculoskeletal conditions which are frequently treated by bisphosphonates.
- Neurofibromatoses.
- Obesity.
- Organ transplantations: in the past, children who underwent organ transplantations had a highly elevated prevalence of fractures, so that today, pre-transplant evaluation of BMD, risk factors and preventive programs are initiated before the transplantation and continued in particular thereafter when the risk factors are even greater due to immunosuppressive therapy, short- or the longer-term immobilization, as well as nutritional and other factors. Screening for additional fractures is also carried out regularly. One recent investigation, a controlled study of a resistance and aerobic exercise training program started in the hospital after the transplantation, clearly demon-

strated the physical and overall health benefits of regular training.

- Renal disorders: for example decreased activity of renal 1 alpha-hydroxylase results in decreased intestinal calcium absorption, increased parathyroid hormone (PTH) levels and high turnover renal osteodystrophy with subsequent growth failure, hypercalcaemia, cardiovascular and other complications. Therapy must be very carefully adjusted, taking all these aspects into consideration. In practice, changes in mineral and skeletal metabolism characterize chronic kidney disease (CKD). CKD in growing children is particularly detrimental in view of its potentially adverse effects on the skeleton. Many reviews of therapy of chronic and acute CKD have been published, including effects on mineral metabolism and the cardiovascular system. Skeletal changes, including visible alterations of the head and face, known as Sagliker syndrome due to secondary hyperparathyroidism (HPT), can be very severe in CKD, if not prevented by early therapy. Once they are established, reversal is well-nigh impossible, as emphasized in a recent international review of the possible changes and deformities, and the necessity of early preventive therapy (Sagliker et al. 2008).
- Rheumatic disorders: Central nervous system (CNS) involvement in numerous such disorders has recently been documented and the manifestations, diagnoses and therapies outlined (Buzova 2008).
- Spinal cord injury.
- Thalassaemia.

Clearly, it is not practical to deal with all or even most of the conditions listed above, though many have been studied. However, a recent systematic review of juvenile idiopathic arthritis (IJA) should be mentioned. The short- and long-term data available indicated that children with IJA had lower BMD and more fractures than those without. Bisphosphonates are considered a promising therapy, but sufficient evidence-based data are not yet available.

Acute immobilization decreases bone formation and increases bone resorption. Additionally, bone growth is severely impaired in prolonged immobilization, due to a lack of mechanical stimulation. Further important *mechanisms* of osteoporosis in children include:

- Inadequate production of collagen type I (congenital disorders)

- Prolonged immobilization (fractures or neurologic disorders)
- Inflammatory cytokines (chronic rheumatic disorders)
- Deficiency of vitamin D (nutrition and gastrointestinal disorders)
- Neoplastic diseases of the bone marrow (oncologic disorders).

Glucocorticoid therapy is an integral part of the treatment of many disorders, and therefore the BMD of the children should always be checked before the initiation of therapy and the relevant prevention program initiated. The conditions include: renal glomerular diseases, dermatomyositis, inflammatory bowel diseases, juvenile rheumatoid arthritis, post organ transplantation and Duchenne muscular dystrophy. Therapy with glucocorticoids and immunosuppressive drugs is given for example for oncological disorders and transplantations. However, it should be stressed that the causes of osteoporosis in children with cancer are multifactorial. Several reviews have stressed that more awareness is required of the adverse effects of cancer treatment in long-term survivors, especially in view of the fact that, fortunately, increasing numbers of childhood cancer patients are surviving and require close monitoring so that timely application of preventive measures is facilitated. The Bone1 and the Bone11 studies have been designed and initiated precisely for this purpose: Bone1 for identification of survivors and estimation of reduced BMD, as well as risk factors for osteopenia/osteoporosis; Bone11 for nutritional counselling and estimation of the effects of supplements of vitamins and calcium on the markers of bone remodelling in serum and urine. The accumulated data is expected to provide the baseline for further studies in the management of survivors. In the meantime, the Children's Oncology Group (2008) has provided guidelines for the long-term follow-up of survivors of childhood and adolescent cancers and given recommendations for the diagnosis and management of osteopenia/osteoporosis.

Paediatric patients with *HIV infection* face a lifetime of anti-viral treatment with all the attendant side effects and toxicities, which must also be treated and managed, among them osteopenia and osteoporosis with the consequences thereof. Moreover, beneficial changes in IGF-1 and lean body mass, but not in linear growth, have been noted in children under anti-retroviral therapy, which has also been associated with increases in lipid measurements and in insulin resistance. These changes were presumed to be associated with immune restitution and levels of insulin-like growth factor (IGF)-1. HIV infection-associated proteinuria in children with kidney disease can be ameliorated and progression of the renal disease prevented by initiation of highly active antiretroviral (HAART) therapy.

Insufficient physical activity, not caused by a neurologic deficit, but by the general physical condition as well as psychological aspects could be responsible for sedentary habits which in turn account for a low BMD, for example sedentary habits in children with haemophilia. These children may be somewhat apprehensive because of the risk of bleeding.

Adolescent athletes: According to the literature, about a quarter of teenage girls are liable to develop amenorrhea, in spite of increased physical activities. This hypogonadism has a negative impact on bone metabolism, which is particularly detrimental at this age, during the time of accrual of the peak bone mass, so that preventive measures are mandatory.

Treatment of childhood osteoporosis includes *general measures* such as:

- Adequate pain relief in children with vertebral fractures.
- Orthopaedic procedures to fix fractures of the long bones.
- Physiotherapy with rehabilitation to improve muscle strength.
- Occupational therapy if necessary.
- Protection of the spine.
- Periods of bed rest in paediatric illness should be minimized to avoid immobilization osteoporosis, for which immediate therapy should be considered if long periods of rest (matter of months) are anticipated.

Literature on the *medical treatment* of childhood osteoporosis is limited and still not evidence-based, but some studies have been reported and the following recommendations made:

- *Calcium and vitamin D* supplementation is recommended although there is little evidence of benefit in the studies available. Nevertheless, a recent study from the UK emphasizes the fact that the majority of teenage boys and girls fail to meet the UK Government targets for calcium intakes. Most probably this applies to many other countries as well. The importance of this lies in the fact that 90% of the peak bone mass is attained by the age of 18 years in girls and 20 years in boys. Attention has now been drawn to the fact that hypovitaminosis D is worldwide in children and young people. Studies have shown that it is even prevalent in healthy infants and toddlers! Moreover, today when obesity is considered almost a global epidemic due to its prevalence in many developed and so-called under developed counties, attention must be paid to the nutritional requirements of obese children, who frequently suffer from hypovitaminosis D. These children are at increased risk of developing impaired glucose metabolism with the complications that this implies, including effects on the bones. The good news is that it has been conclusively demonstrated that vitamin D can safely be given to children in high doses (14,000 IU) once a week. Moreover, as mentioned earlier, it has been confirmed that poor nutrition in early childhood may accelerate ageing and predispose to various age-related disorders. Therefore, a first priority is the provision (and of course the ingestion) of an adequate well-balanced diet from a very young age onwards.
- *Calcitriol* has been investigated in several small studies with improvement (though not significant) in symptoms, fracture risk and BMD.
- *Growth hormone* is a powerful anabolic agent and it is well established that children with growth hormone deficiency benefit from growth hormone therapy.
- *Calcitonin* is known to inhibit bone resorption and some small studies have shown that bone pain may disappear and radiographic signs of osteoporosis may improve under intranasal administration of calcitonin.
- *Bisphosphonates* have also been investigated in childhood osteoporosis and there have been several encouraging studies in idiopathic juvenile osteoporosis (IJO) and osteogenesis imperfecta. Concern has been expressed about potential adverse effects on the growing skeleton, though so far these have not appeared and sequential bone biopsies showed normal, lamellar bone without development of osteomalacia. There were also

no adverse effects on fracture healing or growth rate. Indeed, nitrogen-containing bisphosphonates are a treatment option in childhood osteoporosis, but randomized controlled studies are required. Although not yet approved by the FDA for use in children, nitrogen-containing bisphosphonates demonstrated benefits to the children treated, with no serious adverse effects. Indeed, bisphosphonates are the first agents to give paediatricians the opportunity to treat bone disorders of childhood effectively. It is important to realize that *spontaneous improvement* without any medical treatment may also occur. Thus, for some children with osteoporosis, it may be appropriate to monitor their progress over time – "watch and wait" – particularly if they appear to have stopped breaking their bones. This would also depend on the cause and circumstances of the child's daily life.

26.2
Idiopathic Juvenile Osteoporosis, Idiopathic Juvenile Arthritis, and Other Conditions

In the absence of a primary causative condition, the diagnosis of *idiopathic juvenile osteoporosis* (IJO) is made. IJO is a transient, non-hereditary, rare form of childhood osteoporosis without extraskeletal involvement. In the absence of fractures the term "osteopenia in childhood" would be more appropriate. It is important to exclude other possible causes of vertebral collapse such as acute leukaemia.

The *aetiology* of IJO has not yet been elucidated. A decrease in osteoblastic reactivity has been reported, and consequently the skeleton no longer adequately adapts to the increased mechanical loads during growth. Spontaneous remissions are the rule and with onset before puberty (mostly between age 8 and 12 years of age).

Differential diagnosis: Osteogenesis imperfecta (OI) is the commonest congenitally determined condition with osteoporosis which must always be carefully excluded (Table 26.2). Osteoporosis-pseudoglioma syndrome is a very rare congenital disorder with severe osteoporosis and blindness.

The *clinical picture* presents three different manifestations:
● Fractures of the extremities, especially of the trabecular bones, occasionally with an early onset, even early post natal, pain in the ankles and knees, with fractures of the lower extremities.
● Fractures of vertebral bodies with backache, kyphosis, decrease in height and difficulties in locomotion (walking, running).
● Evidence of low bone density (dual-energy X-ray absorptiometry, DXA) without pathologic fractures.

The *diagnosis* of IJO is made by exclusion of OI and of diseases causing secondary osteoporosis. It should be emphasized that IJO is strictly a diagnosis of exclusion and that malignancies in the marrow must be considered. Diagnosis requires X-rays of the lumbar spine in two planes. When OI is suspected, X-rays of the long bones are also required to check for the characteristic metaphyseal compression fractures. The long bones are usually of normal width in IJO, the cortex might

Table 26.2. Differential diagnosis between idiopathic juvenile osteoporosis (IJO) and osteogenesis imperfecta (OI)

	IJO	OI
Family history	Absent	Often positive
Onset	Late childhood	Birth or soon after
Duration	1–4 years	Lifelong
Clinical finding	Abnormal gait metaphyseal fractures, back pain	Abnormal dentition Blue sclerae Long bone fractures
Growth rate	Normal	Normal or decreased
Radiologic findings	Vertebral fractures "Neo-osseous osteoporosis"	Thin cortex of long bones
Bone biopsy	Decreased bone turnover	Increased bone turnover
Connective tissue defect	No	Collagen abnormalities

be thinned and metaphyseal fractures are common. On X-rays, the new bone formed in metaphyseal areas appears as a radiolucent band ("neo-osseous osteoporosis"). The onset of OI is usually much earlier in life. The children often have blue sclerae and abnormalities of collagen. Bone density should preferably be measured by DXA of the lumbar vertebrae and, if possible, a whole body measurement. For children weighing less than 30 kg, a special paediatric software program is required. The modern bone marker NTX is useful for differentiating OI and IJO.

There are no known biochemical characteristics, and alterations of bone markers are non-specific.

With the introduction of *bisphosphonates*, therapy of osteoporosis in children is now simple and effective. Several clinical trials have already provided evidence for an increase in bone density and a reduction in fracture risk in children treated with bisphosphonates. Previous fears that such therapy might interfere with the growth of the long bones have not been substantiated. In addition, the osteomalacia seen under therapy with the earlier bisphosphonates is no longer observed with the newer more potent aminobiphosphonates, which can be given orally or as infusions at 3–6 month intervals. Since randomized clinical trials in children have not yet been carried out, treatment should only be undertaken in paediatric centres, after consultation with the Ethics Committee and signed consent by the parents or guardians has been obtained. Calcium 500–1000 mg daily and vitamin D 500–1000 IU daily should also be given as basic therapy. Calcitriol – the active metabolite of vitamin D – could also be considered.

Patients with IJO can experience a complete recovery within a few years. Growth may be somewhat impaired during the active phase of the disease, but normal growth resumes thereafter. However, in some cases, IJO may result in permanent disability such as kyphoscoliosis or even collapse of the rib cage. Since children undergo spontaneous remissions especially when there is osteopenia without fractures, in these cases a policy of watch and wait is recommended to begin with.

Children with IJA often have quite considerable physical impairment. Some do not respond to medication and are then treated with immunosuppression followed by autologous haematopoietic stem cell transplantation, which can induce long-term remissions. However, they have long-term (9 years in one study)

impaired exercise tolerance, while functional ability and joint status were also decreased. These children require special attention and management to prevent long-term complications including osteoporosis.

26.3 Osteogenesis Imperfecta Must Not Be Overlooked!

This congenital condition should be considered in every case of severe osteoporosis occurring in infancy and childhood. A thorough family history and physical examination are important diagnostic aids. The spine frequently shows severe changes, but fractures occur primarily in the extremities (Figs. 26.4 and 26.5). Attempts to explain the pathophysiology of OI are being made by application of the still-evolving Utah

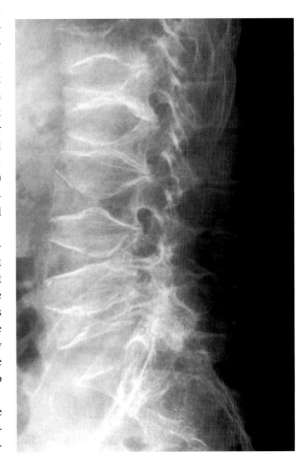

Fig. 26.4. Massive narrowing of all the vertebral bodies and ballooning of the intervertebral discs in a patient with osteogenesis imperfecta

26

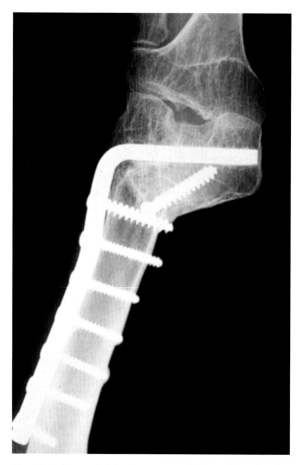

Fig. 26.5. X-ray of girl with osteogenesis imperfecta showing thin cortices and poorly mineralized bone. Note old, healed and new fractures with surgical stabilization

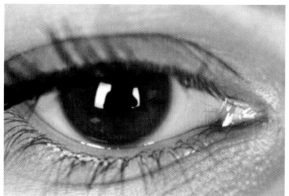

Fig. 26.6. Blue sclerae in a patient with osteogenesis imperfecta

- Anomalies of the heart valves and aorta, prolapse of the mitral valve, aortic insufficiency
- Deafness due to damage to the stapes in the middle ear
- Kidney stones and hypercalciuria
- Hyperplastic callus formation.

OI occurs in 1 of every 20,000 live births. There are approximately 15,000 patients with OI in the US. The condition varies from apparently typical osteoporosis to severe skeletal anomalies in childhood. Four *types* of OI are distinguished:
- Mild form with blue sclerae (Type I)
- Lethal perinatal form (Type II)
- Progressive deforming form (Type III)
- Mild form without blue sclerae (Type IV).

paradigm of skeletal physiology; however, results have not yet been widely publicized and accepted.

Various genetic mutations have now been related to different types of OI showing differences in clinical features. Different mutations of the genes for collagen type I occur. When even one of the amino acids is incorrectly incorporated into the collagen molecule, a defective molecular structure may result. As a consequence, the helical structure of collagen is altered which in turn leads to a fault in the quality of the bone as evidenced by lack of lamellar structure and susceptibility to breakdown by collagenases. In addition to bone, *other organs* that incorporate collagen type I are also affected, as shown by the following manifestations:
- Thin blue sclerae (Fig. 26.6), rupture of sclerae, keratoconus
- Anomalies of the teeth which appear brown and transparent and are liable to rapid shedding

Previous attempts at *therapy* with fluorides were unsuccessful, as were bone marrow transplants including replacement of stromal cells. Today, early administration of bisphosphonates is the therapy of choice, in severe cases by infusions every 3 months, otherwise orally. Recent studies have shown that oral alendronate therapy is safe and effective in children with OI, even very young ones.

Over the past 3 years we have treated 50 patients with aminobisphosphonates, both orally and intravenously. All showed the following impressive improvements in their conditions:
- Increase in bone density
- Increase in bone quality demonstrated in sequential biopsies
- Decrease in symptoms, especially bone pain

- Striking decrease in fracture rate (before therapy up to 12 fractures annually!)
- Bone healing was not impaired
- Despite decreasing bone turnover, aminobisphosphonates did not impair growth.

Calcium and vitamin D are given together with the bisphosphonates to improve the mineralization of the newly formed bone. Results of several clinical trials of bisphosphonates (pamidronate, zoledronate, neridronate) in children and adults with OI have now been published. BMD and physical activity increased markedly under treatment with bisphosphonates and the fracture rate decreased by 65%. After 4 years of treatment with pamidronate, bone mineral content, bone volume and volumetric bone mineral density were 54%, 44% and 65% higher, respectively, in treated than in untreated patients who were matched for age and type of OI. Patients with larger deficits in bone mass at baseline had a more marked gain of bone mass during therapy. An interesting effect of bisphosphonate therapy in young children is delayed eruption of teeth, previously described in animals. A study has confirmed that under bisphosphonate therapy, tooth eruption in children with OI was delayed for a mean period of 1.67 years.

It is noteworthy that long-term adverse side effects have not been reported. On the contrary, it has been claimed that, until the advent of realistic gene therapy, bisphosphonates appear to be the most efficient way of arresting the progression of OI and improving the quality of life of the patients, irrespective of type of collagen mutation, clinical severity and age at start of therapy. A recent review and update on the diagnosis, classification, pathophysiological mechanisms and current therapy has been published (Glorieux 2008).

The potential for direct replacement of collagen-producing cells in the bone marrow (stem cell therapy) has led to a limited number of studies in severely affected infants, with variable results.

In Summary: Treatment of childhood osteoporotic syndromes requires an *interdisciplinary approach* including orthopaedic surgeons, physiotherapists, occupational therapists, dentists, paediatricians and psychologists for immediate therapy, further information and support and to prevent and care for recurrent fractures. Appropriate organizations and support groups (e.g. Osteogenesis imperfecta Foundation) are very important for patients and their families.

26.4
Turner Syndrome and Charge Syndrome

Two other congenital disorders with very complex and distinctive features including retarded growth and development are Turner syndrome and Charge syndrome. These both require a multidisciplinary approach to therapy. Turner syndrome affects only female infants, girls and women, who all have a lifelong risk of osteoporosis. This risk must be managed according to age-related requirements, including appropriate dietary factors, e.g. calcium and vitamins, as well as hormones at the menarche, modified hormone replacement therapy (HRT) after the menopause and appropriate anti-osteoporotic therapy thereafter to prevent involutional osteoporosis. Similar considerations are applicable to patients with Charge syndrome regarding nutrition, hormones and, for both groups, the correct physical exercise and training to maintain the bones. In this connection, it is worth mentioning that abnormal growth in childhood could well be the first manifestation of as yet undetected disorders, for the possible presence of which the children should be thoroughly checked, for example according to the recommendations of the Dutch Consensus Guideline (DCG). The diagnostic procedure should include testing for celiac disease and Turner syndrome. Young girls with primary amenorrhea should also be checked for Turner syndrome.

26.5
X-Linked Hypophosphatemic Rickets

These children also require early growth hormone treatment, which improves serum levels of phosphate and vitamin D and normalizes parathyroid function. However, the degree of improvement in rickets should be checked by investigation of the mineralization of bone. If there is evidence of early skeletal deformities, these must be carefully followed.

26.6
Gaucher's Disease

Gaucher's disease is the most common lysosomal storage disorder. It is due to a deficiency of the enzyme glucocerebrosidase. The disease is divided into

26

sub-types, of which the non-neuropathic is the most common and has the greatest variability. Prominent clinical manifestations are hepatosplenomegaly, cytopenias, and skeletal disorders. Early recognition, diagnosis and therapy are essential to prevent disease progression, which includes irreversible skeletal deformities and other severe co-morbidities. Safe and efficient enzyme substitution therapy has been available for nearly two decades. The essential factor is early diagnosis and it has been shown that over 50% of affected children present symptoms well before the age of 10 years.

Immobilization Osteoporosis

Possible causes include spinal cord injuries, strokes, hospitalization (prolonged), post-fracture conditions and others.

27.1
Examples of Bone Loss

Insufficient physical activity is one of the most important overall risk factors for osteoporosis. This is especially true for young bed-ridden patients who can lose up to 30% of their bone density within a few months, while years are required for its replacement – that is for restoration of density as it was before, i.e. "restitutio ad integrum" (Figs. 27.1 and 27.2) (see also Bartl and Frisch, *Atlas of Bone Biopsy in Internal Medicine*). For example, when an arm is enclosed in plaster for 3 weeks after a fracture, the immobilized bones may lose up to 6% of their bone mass during this short period. A study of patients confined to bed has shown that, on average, trabecular bone decreases by about 1% a week. When physical activity is resumed, bone density increases by 1% a month – considerably slower than its loss.

Examples of causes of immobilization bone loss are:
- Damage to the vertebral bone marrow with deleterious effects on the bone
- Hemiplegia after cerebrovascular incidents
- Paraplegia of the lower half of the body
- Immobilization after fracture of the lower extremities (rapid bone loss especially in children)
- Immobilization after surgery on the legs or feet with subsequent reduced mobility for prolonged periods
- Immobilization due to muscular diseases or neurological disorders, e.g. multiple sclerosis.

In a recent study, 20 paediatric patients (age 1–16 years, bed-ridden due to cerebral palsy) were successfully treated with risedronate to prevent secondary osteoporosis. It has recently also been demonstrated that there is a significantly increased prevalence of osteoporosis in both men and women with *multiple sclerosis*. Consequently, bone density screening and appropriate measures, including bisphosphonates, need to be undertaken to avoid fractures in these patients. Shortly after the occurrence of paraplegia, bone loss can be so rapid and extensive that relatively minor efforts can cause fractures (for example transfer from bed to wheelchair, or the effort of pulling up tight supportive stockings and socks). After 1 year, 42% of paraplegic patients have osteoporosis of the femoral neck. The muscular spasms some patients undergo may have a positive effect on bone density, but such cramps are painful and patients prefer to avoid them by appropriate therapy. It is essential to emphasize that early initiation of physical training and activity is mandatory for all patients. Prophylactic initiation of bisphosphonate therapy does avert and reduce bone loss, but therapy must be continued to maintain bone in the long term.

Patients who already have osteoporosis and are immobilized for several weeks due to a fracture are likely to incur a further fracture during their mobilization period, unless preventive measures are taken as early as possible. The period of postoperative bed rest should be kept as short as possible and the bones protected by effective medication, e.g. bisphosphonates to prevent further loss of bone mass, physiotherapy, if at all possible, and attention to proper nutrition and supplements.

R. Bartl, B. Frisch, *Osteoporosis*, DOI 10.1007/978-3-540-79527-8_27,
© Springer-Verlag Berlin Heidelberg 2009

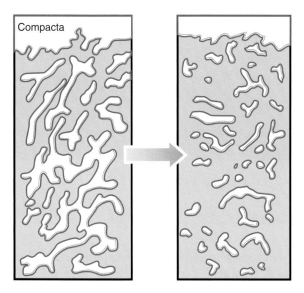

Fig. 27.1. Immobilization osteoporosis in a child after 17 weeks' of bed rest: marked reduction in volume of trabecular and cortical bone, documented in sequential iliac crest biopsies (from Bartl and Frisch [1993])

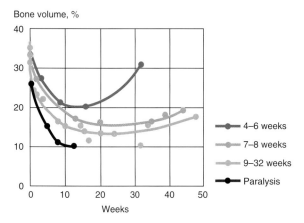

Fig. 27.2. Periods of immobilization and recovery of bone mass in children. Lack of recovery after paralysis (from Bartl and Frisch [1993])

27.2
Space Travel and the Force of Gravity

27.2.1
Weightlessness in Space Due to Lack of Gravitational Force

Astronauts undergo specialized and regular muscu-loskeletal training before and during space flight to counteract the absence of the force of gravity in outer space. In spite of this they lose about 1% of their bone density every month. A study of the bones of rhesus monkeys before and after a 14-day space flight revealed that they had sustained a 35% reduction in bone volume. In the conditions prevailing in outer space, astronauts are subject to a ten-fold higher bone loss than earth-bound osteoporotic patients. This dem-onstrates unequivocally that the earth's gravitational force is nature's way of preserving the skeleton. The mechanisms of bone loss in astronauts have been thor-oughly investigated and are used today as models for immobilization osteoporosis. Three main factors are recognized:

- Demineralization of bone
- Inhibition of osteoblastic activity
- Activation of osteoclasts.

Timely preventive measures, i.e. before and during the flight, are mandatory. Recommendations made so far include the following: supplements of calcium, vita-mins D and K, a bone anabolic agent and a long-act-ing bisphosphonate well before the flight, in addition to the specialized exercise training mentioned above. The most recent investigation in animals studied the efficacy of zoledronate and OPG.

27.3
Therapy of Immobilization Osteoporosis

The emphasis is on physical activity as early and as varied as possible, adapted to each patient's condi-tion and ability. The primary aim of medication is prevention; therefore, bisphosphonate therapy should be started as early as possible and in accordance with the results of bone density measurements. This is es-pecially important as the massive decrease in bone density which occurs immediately after the onset of paralysis (immobilization) should and can be prevent-ed. The following are recommended:

- Alendronate (Fosamax®) 70 mg weekly.
- Risedronate (Actonel®) 35 mg weekly.
- Ibandronate (Bonviva®) 3 mg injection monthly, later every three months.
- Zoledronate (Aclasta®) 5 mg infusion once a year.

(The first two only if the patient is able to sit up straight for at least 30 min after ingestion and there are cogent reasons for oral administration. Intravenous administration, as indicated above is definitely preferable!)

Investigations to identify the best preventive therapy for astronauts are still ongoing, including attempts at more targeted interventions. When established, these will undoubtedly also be adapted for immobilization osteoporosis here on planet earth.

28.1
Assessment of Secondary Osteoporoses

The first step in any assessment is the separation of "primary" or "idiopathic" from the "secondary" osteoporoses which have an underlying cause, i.e. a specific disease or disorder. "Primary osteoporosis" refers mainly to postmenopausal and age-related involutional osteoporoses, in spite of the fact that a number of factors contributing to their pathogenesis are already known. "Secondary osteoporoses" are responsible for about 20% of all osteoporotic fractures. Secondary causes of osteoporosis, i.e. as co-morbidities, are also frequent in older patients who already have primary involutional osteoporosis (Table 28.1). Physicians should consider the possible causes of secondary osteoporosis, particularly when patients present with any of the following:

- Unusual fractures
- Very low bone densities for their age
- Recurrent fractures despite adherence to effective therapy
- Abnormal basic laboratory tests (anaemia, hypo- and hypercalcaemia, elevated ESR)
- Unexplained bone pain
- Undetermined bone lesions on bone scan or X-ray (metastases, myeloma, malignant lymphomas, mastocytosis)

Osteoporosis is most likely to occur in the disciplines discussed below. Only conditions not dealt with in other chapters are included here. This list represents the major secondary disorders which may affect the bones.

28.2
Cardiology

Many reports have dealt with the connection between osteoporosis and cardiological conditions. For example, a recent study investigated the presence of osteoporosis in 198 patients undergoing coronary angiography because of chest pain. The results showed that 53 (27%) had osteoporosis, 79 (40%) had osteopenia and only 66 (33%) had normal bone mineral density (BMD) values. Moreover, 76% of the patients with osteoporosis and 78% of those with osteopenia had obstructive coronary artery disease. This would suggest that patients who come for angiography should also be checked for osteoporosis, especially in the older age groups. Another study investigated the level of vitamin D in 3299 patients sent for coronary angiography. The patients were followed for a median period of 7.75 years during which 95 patients died of cancer. The authors concluded that deficiency or insufficiency of vitamin D is associated with an increased risk of cancer in patients with cardiovascular disease, which itself also has a correlation with vitamin D deficiency. This was demonstrated in an investigation of 1739 people with a mean age 55 years, the Framington Offspring Study participants, all without cardiovascular disease. Initial levels of vitamin D were assessed and the participants followed-up for a mean period of 5.4 years, during which 120 participants with low levels of vitamin D underwent a first cardiovascular event. The authors concluded that more studies were required for confirmation and determination as to what influence on the cardiovascular system correction of the vitamin D deficiency might have.

R. Bartl, B. Frisch, *Osteoporosis*, DOI 10.1007/978-3-540-79527-8_28,
© Springer-Verlag Berlin Heidelberg 2009

28

Table 28.1. Diseases and surgery associated with an increased risk of generalized osteoporosis (alphabetical list)

Diseases
Acromegaly
Addison's disease
Amyloidosis
Ankylosing spondylitis
Anorexia nervosa
Chronic obstructive pulmonary disease
Congenital porphyria
Crohn's disease
Cushing's syndrome
Diabetes mellitus
Endometriosis
Gaucher's disease
Gonadal insufficiency
Haemochromatosis
Haemophilia
Hyperparathyroidism
Hypophosphatasia
Hyperthyroidism
Idiopathic scoliosis
Immobilization
Lactose intolerance
Lymphoma and leukaemia
Malabsorption syndrome
Mastocytosis
Metastatic disease
Multiple myeloma
Multiple sclerosis
Nutritional disorders
Osteogenesis imperfecta
Parenteral nutrition
Pernicious anaemia
Primary biliary cirrhosis
Rheumatoid arthritis
Sarcoidosis
Thalassaemia
Thyrotoxicosis
Surgery
Gastrectomy
Intestinal bypass
Thyroidectomy
Transplantation

Patients after surgery on the cardiac valves and on long-term anticoagulant therapy (depending on the anti-coagulant used) are particularly vulnerable to bone loss. Additional causes are insufficient physical activity or immobilization due to chronic cardiac insufficiency. Cardiac patients who are candidates for transplantation should also be checked for osteoporosis before and after in order that preventive therapy may be given and fractures avoided. Excessive alcohol consumption has also been related to cardiomyopathy and eventually to heart failure.

Atherosclerosis and osteoporosis are both multifactorial disorders related to the ageing process. There is accumulating evidence that progressive telomere shortening is involved in both cardiovascular and other cardiometabolic disorders. Vascular calcification has been linked to high levels of vitamin D and to aspects of bone remodelling. Patients with vascular calcification may also suffer from osteoporosis, which requires treatment for prevention of fractures. However, other studies have shown that high levels of vitamin D not only promote vascular calcification, but also constitute a risk factor for cardiovascular disease. There appears to be only a very narrow range of vitamin D levels within which vascular function is optimal and the risk of calcification and cardiac disease is avoided. Moreover, vitamin D deficiency, as mentioned above, is also a risk factor for cardiovascular disease. Patients with chronic renal disease may also derive benefit from vitamin D given for concomitant cardiac problems.

Hypercholesterolemia and dyslipidemia are linked to arteriosclerotic vascular diseases as well as to osteoporosis. Statins are usually prescribed for the disturbed lipid metabolism, but it should be noted that atorvastatin also increases vitamin D levels, so that these should also be checked. The patients are also advised to pay attention to diet, with reduction of fat intake if this is above recommended levels. Bisphosphonates are the therapy of choice for the osteoporosis. The type, dose and route of administration are decided according to the patient's requirements and preferences.

Some previous epidemiological studies and comprehensive reviews found that beta-blockers and thiazide diuretics apparently have a beneficial effect on fracture risk in older adults, but information on long-term effects was limited. Two large recent studies from the UK and the Netherlands did not find a causal relationship between therapy with beta-blockers and reduction in risk of fractures.

A population-based case controlled study on the relationship between atrial fibrillation and flutter, on the one hand, and bisphosphonates prescribed for and taken by women as therapy for osteoporosis, on the other, found no evidence for an effect of the bisphosphonates on cardiac rhythm.

28.3
Dermatology

Glucocorticoids are frequently required, for short- as well as long-term treatment in dermatology. European and US guidelines have been published, in particular for the prevention of corticosteroid-induced osteoporosis in dermatologic patients. The recommendations include calcium and vitamin D supplements and bisphosphonates when therapy for >3 months is contemplated. Supplements of vitamin A have also been recommended.

As protection against the constant challenges of microbial pathogens, the skin has developed antimicrobial peptides (AMPs) such as the cathelicidins, which have antimicrobial activity and stimulate host responses, i.e. inflammations, angiogenesis and cytokine release. It has now been demonstrated that vitamin D is directly involved in the regulation of cathelicidin activities, which could be significant in the treatment of various dermatologic conditions. Vitamin D analogues have been applied as therapy for the hyperproliferative skin disease psoriasis, as well as other infectious and inflammatory skin disorders. However, it should be borne in mind that the skin itself is an organ for vitamin D synthesis, as well as being a target for its application in autoimmune, infectious and inflammatory diseases of the skin, and to counteract the effects of glucocorticoids as mentioned above. Some investigators have regarded the human skin as "the largest peripheral endocrine organ".

28.4
Endocrinology

It should be clearly stated at the outset that numerous endocrine disorders are inexorably associated with the metabolism of the musculoskeletal system, and only a few can be mentioned here. Moreover, many of these disorders are also closely connected to other systems, which in turn are also correlated with the function of the bone cells.

- *Growth hormone deficiency*: Many studies have shown that there is considerable variability in individual patients' responses to therapy with growth hormones. Nevertheless, the long-term studies have demonstrated improvements in body composition, bone mass and density, as well as increases in muscle strength. However, women may also require some degree of oestrogen therapy to maintain BMD. Therapy with growth hormone is also effective in congenital disorders such as Turner and Prader-Willi syndromes. In addition, therapy with growth hormone has beneficial effects on the cardiovascular and other systems which themselves are risk factors for the bones. An interesting hypothesis has been suggested in connection with the GH–IGF-1 axis and longevity. Studies have shown that some patients with hormone deficiency survive to 75–78 years of age or even longer, in spite of dwarfism and marked obesity. The hypothesis is that the growth hormone deficiency is a major contributing factor in protection from cancer, a significant cause of death in older populations.
- *Hyperthyroidism*: Patients with thyrotoxicosis may have generalized osteoporosis because bone formation cannot keep up with resorption, in spite of the fact that both are increased in hyperthyroidism: a classic example of high turnover osteoporosis. The hypothesis had been put forward that in hypothyroidism the thyroid stimulating hormone (TSH) caused the effects in the skeleton, but recent animal studies have shown that they are due to lack of the thyroid hormone, T 3.
- *Primary hyperparathyroidism* (pHPT): Increased secretion of parathyroid hormone (PTH) due to adenomas, carcinoma, and congenital disorders such as Turner syndrome or parathyroid hyperplasia produces disturbances in calcium homeostasis with release of calcium from the bones. However, although there may be no or few clinical symptoms, the increase in bone turnover leads to a loss of both cortical and trabecular bone. Many studies have reported a decrease in BMD. The changes in vitamin D metabolism as well as increases in fibroblast growth factor (FGF)-23 also contribute to the decline in BMD, which increases the fracture risk.

The increase in bone turnover and bone resorption in particular is manifest in complex bone changes, affecting both cortical and trabecular bone throughout the skeleton, and may also affect the joints and even the vessels. But it must be pointed out that the skeletal changes in pHPT are very variable as documented in different studies. Primary HPT is another example of hormonally-determined generalized osteopenia/osteoporosis. However, in one study, measurements of total body calcium failed to demonstrate large overall deficits of bone mineral in pHPT. Indeed, there is a broad spectrum of histologic changes in pHPT. Experimental and in vitro studies have shown that intermittent PTH inhibits adipocytes and induces osteoblast differentiation of mesenchymal cells. In our biopsy study, 20% of patients, particularly those with kidney stones, had no morphologic abnormalities in the bone biopsy. In intermediate bone disease, usually characterized by vitamin D deficiency, histologic parameters such as bone resorption, osteoclasts and endosteal fibrosis were predominant ("dissecting fibro-osteoclasia"). While it has been suggested that the primary osteoclastic effect in parathyroid bone disease might result in widespread osteopenia, in our study the cortical and trabecular bone volume was maintained. Only in severe cases (10%) are the classical skeletal manifestations of pHPT seen: osteitis fibrosa cystica with marked bone loss, osteolytic destruction of the trabecular network ("brown tumours") and presence of multiple fractures. Studies on BMD and levels of vitamin D metabolites in 246 patients, age range 19–91 years, with pHPT showed that low vitamin D status together with high plasma 1,25(OH)(2)D were associated with increased bone turnover and decreased BMD in patients. The long-term beneficial results of parathyroidectomy, also in elderly patients, have been documented, including an increase in BMD and reduction in fracture risk. A combination of a calcimimetic and a bisphosphonate has been suggested for patients when curative surgery is contraindicated. Secondary hyperparathyroidism (sHPT) has been described in patients with renal disease on dialysis. A multicentre observational study (COSMOS) was recently initiated in Europe for the diagnosis, prevention and treatment of sHPT in patients on dialysis. The study will include investigation of numerous relevant parameters, including changes in bone mineral markers. The study is planned to run for 3 years, at the end of which results will be evaluated. sHPT has also been observed in congenital disorders, such as Turner syndrome.

- *Cushing's disease*: This endogenous form of hypercorticolism is rare, in contrast to glucocorticosteroid-induced osteoporosis, which is common, severe and progressive if not treated.
- *Diabetes mellitus*: "Diabetic osteopathy" occurs more frequently than is generally realized and is mainly due to inhibition of collagen production by osteoblasts occurring as a direct effect of insufficient insulin secretion and which impedes osteoblastic bone formation and leads to deterioration of bone quality. To address the question of the occurrence of diabetic osteomyelopathy as a distinct entity, we investigated iliac crest biopsies of 120 patients with manifest diabetes mellitus. Histomorphometry of the vascular system, bone and bone marrow was performed. In our study, diabetic microangiopathy was found in 82% of the biopsies. The marked inflammatory reaction of the bone marrow stroma correlated with serologic parameters of inflammation in these patients. This may significantly contribute to the bone marrow atrophy and the "anaemia of chronic disorders" in diabetes mellitus. Atrophic reduction of the trabecular bone was also significantly higher in the patients with diabetes mellitus, but bone remodelling was normal or only slightly decreased. Insulin-dependent patients had a lower bone loss than orally adjusted diabetics. These results demonstrate the occurrence of a more or less specific "diabetic osteomyelopathy" comprising degenerative changes of the bone marrow vasculature, degenerative reactions of the marrow stroma, marrow atrophy and osteopenia with slightly decreased bone remodelling and with changes in parameters of bone quality. An interesting observation has previously been associated with bisphosphonate therapy in type 2 diabetes (DM 2): significant reduction in intimal thickness, suggesting an anti-atherogenic effect of etidronate, the bisphosphonate used in this study. However, today only the modern aminobisphosphonates are given to these patients, and this effect has so far not been reported. Many studies have demonstrated an increased risk of fractures in patients with DM 2, but these patients did not have a decrease in BMD. The main causes were listed as other consequences of the diabetes such as visual impairment and imbalance, peripheral neuropathy,

orthostatic hypotonia, ischemic states of various organs including the legs and other conditions that predispose to falls, which were the immediate cause of the fractures. DM 2 has been associated with structural brain changes and accelerated cognitive decline. In patients with symptomatic arterial disease and DM 2, hyperglycaemia and duration of the DM 2 contribute to brain atrophy and deterioration of the patients' condition, including the state of the bones. DM 2 is frequently treated by rosiglitazone or by pioglitazone, which belong to the thiazolidinediones (TZDs). Studies have now demonstrated that these drugs increase bone loss and decrease bone formation, thereby increasing risk of fractures, so preventive measures must be taken or the patient advised to take other drugs.

28.5
Gastroenterology

Chronic disorders of the liver or the gastrointestinal tract (GI) (e.g. malabsorption syndromes, lactose intolerance, Crohn's disease, colitis ulcerosa, pancreatic insufficiency and primary biliary cirrhosis) frequently cause a combination of osteoporosis and osteomalacia ("osteoporomalacia") due to deficiencies of vitamins D, K and C. It should be mentioned that patients with Crohn's disease, even young adults, are subject to sarcopenia frequently related to osteopenia/osteoporosis. The changes which occur in patients with chronic disorders of the GI tract, as listed above, tend to worsen as the patients get older, so that regular screening for osteopenia/osteoporosis is recommended. It is noteworthy that sarcopenia is high even in young patients with Crohn's disease, and this increases the risk of bone loss. Gastric and intestinal surgery (e.g. Billroth I and II and small bowel resections) interfere with absorption and utilization of calcium and vitamin D and eventually may lead to osteopathy, in particular vertebral osteoporosis. Variations in intestinal absorption (with no obvious cause) may lead to hypercalciuria, and this has been linked with calcium nephrolithiasis, bone loss and idiopathic osteoporosis in some patients, including postmenopausal women. These cases are examples of the interwoven connections between gastrointestinal absorption, renal function and skeletal metabolism.

In all patients regardless of cause, administration of glucocorticoids and alcohol abuse increase the loss of bone. Large-bowel disorders are rarely associated with bone loss, since the process of absorption is generally completed in the small intestine. Celiac disease, in particular, has been associated with numerous disorders, which in turn affect the bones. Examples include: auto-immune inflammatory conditions and, in particular, some of the associated cytokines such as TNF-alpha and Il-1, diabetes, thyroid disease, secondary HPT, hypopituitarism and others. Each patient must be carefully assessed before appropriate therapy is given. However, the emphasis today is on early diagnosis and treatment, and appropriate nutritional and lifestyle interventions to prevent the development of the disorders listed above, all of which present a danger to the bones. It should be taken into consideration that bone loss in celiac disease already begins in childhood, if preventive measures are not taken early enough. The only effective measure able to keep celiac disease under control is lifelong adherence to a gluten-free diet.

A 2008 panorama on osteoporosis and inflammatory bowel disease lists the main pathogenic factors for osteoporosis as malabsorption and its consequent deficiencies, inflammation with increased cytokine production, hypogonadism and glucocorticoid therapy. However, bisphosphonates have proved to be highly effective in inflammatory bowel disease, as well as for the therapy of its complications such as the hypogonadal- and the glucocorticoid-induced bone loss. Research has shown that about 10% of all cases of gastric carcinoma are associated with Epstein-Barr (EBV) infection and it has been suggested that potentially useful therapeutic approaches could utilize viral–host interactions, including targeted radiotherapy.

28.6
Genetics

Studies of twins have shown that osteoporosis may be genetically determined – up to 50% – and many genes are involved. Peak bone mass is therefore to some extent genetically programmed and the subsequent degree of loss of bone density applies especially to trabecular (cancellous) bone. It has also been demonstrated that genes may have different effects on bones at different skeletal sites, and play a part in

28

overall bone development as well as in the degree of osteoporosis at these sites. Recently the connection between the genes for vitamin D receptors and bone density has been of particular interest and the subject of research, although the results of such studies have been somewhat contradictory. Clinically, osteogenesis imperfecta is the most important of the hereditary osteoporoses. Other congenital syndromes with an osteoporotic component are: Turner, Klinefelter, Ehlers-Danlos, Marfan and Werner.

Studies of the congenital premature ageing syndrome dyskeratosis congenita have identified mutations in the genes that encode the telomerase complex. Cells of these patients have very short telomeres and they age prematurely. The patients suffer from early greying of the hair, dental loss, osteoporosis and malignancies.

Recently it has been shown that bone may be influenced by the GH–IGF-I axis in intrauterine (genetically determined) and in postnatal life. This effect may continue into adulthood, suggesting a role for the GH–IGF-I axis in the programming of bone mass in women. Results for men are awaiting publication. With successful enzyme replacement therapy in Gaucher's disease, the infiltration decreases but the osteoporosis increases and should be treated prophylactically after measurement of BMD. Congenital syndromes with involvement of the muscles are also prone to lead to disturbances of bone remodelling and osteoporosis. It is also of interest that a polymorphism of the growth hormone receptor gene (exon-3 deletion, d3GHR) increases the response to recombinant human growth hormone (rhGH) in children, while in adults with growth hormone deficiency it contributes to the differences in efficacy of short-term rhGH therapy only. Patients with other rare congenital syndromes with partial growth hormone deficiency, such as type 1 trichorhinophalangeal syndrome, may not respond at all to growth hormone treatment.

Numerous studies have now accumulated on: genetics and disorders of bones and joints; congenital syndromes; genes involved in pathways of development and differentiation; osseous phenotypes; genes associated with onset of osteoporosis and various types of fractures; genes associated with skeletal metabolism and race, ethnicity and age in population studies; investigations into which single nucleotide polymorphisms may be involved in differences of response to treatment as well as their association with bones

and muscles in the metabolic syndrome. All these and more have made it clear that osteoporosis is related to multiple genes and many environmental factors. Some relevant studies are listed in the references.

28.7
Haematology and Storage Disorders

Diseases of the bone marrow have a direct influence on osseous remodelling and can cause severe osteoporosis. *Multiple myeloma*, by way of the osteoclast activating factors produced by the pathologic plasma cells, regularly causes osteoporosis or, more frequently, osteolytic skeletal lesions (skeletal related events, SRE). *Polycythaemia vera* (PV) and *chronic myeloid leukaemia* (CML) induce widespread osteoporosis by their expansive growth, but different histologic manifestations (Fig. 28.1). Changes in the bones also occur in myelofibrosis and during leukaemic transformation when increased levels of TNF-alpha and lactate dehydrogenase (LDH) are found. Not only the degree of cellularity, but also the different proliferating haematopoietic cell lines influence osseous remodelling. While in PV the trabeculae are attenuated

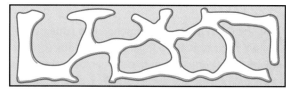

Normal compacta and trabecular bone

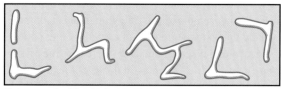

Osteoporosis, histologic type A

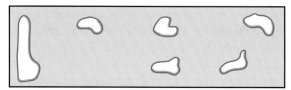

Osteoporosis, histologic type B

Fig. 28.1. Osteoporotic trabecular variants: type A in polycythaemia vera and type B in chronic myeloid leukaemia (from Bartl and Frisch [1993])

but with normal microarchitecture and connections, a coarsening of the trabecular network with fewer connections and correspondingly large marrow spaces is characteristic of CML. Similar changes are produced by congenital haemolytic conditions which cause extreme erythroid hyperplasia and osteoporosis.

Storage diseases such as *Gaucher's disease* (Fig. 28.2a,b) or *hereditary oxalosis* (Fig. 28.3a,b) also cause osteoporosis and/or osteolytic lesions by comparable mechanisms. On the other hand, malignant lymphomas and acute leukaemias are rarely accompanied by osteoporosis in the initial stages, but it does develop later on. The mode of spread of marrow infiltrations is a major parameter determining the pattern of osseous lesions. Processes with diffuse marrow infiltrations are characterized by systemic osteopenia in bones, while in patients with focal, nodular or patchy infiltrations local osteopenia or even circumscribed osteolytic lesions are found.

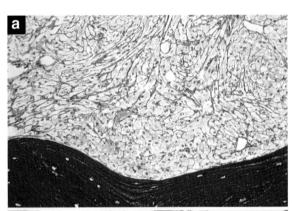

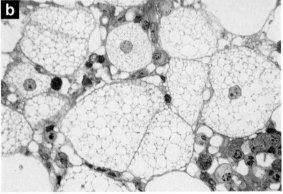

Fig. 28.2a, b. (a) Iliac crest biopsy of patients with Gaucher's disease, with complete replacement of haematopoiesis and severe osteoporosis in the DXA measurement (**b**) Higher magnification showing typical Gaucher cells of variable size, with characteristic "wrinkled tissue paper" appearance of cytoplasm, all Gomori staining

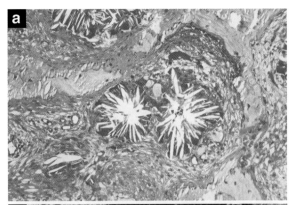

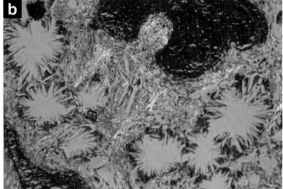

Fig. 28.3a, b. (a) Iliac crest biopsy of young patient with hereditary oxalosis, complicated by chronic renal failure, aluminium intoxication under haemodialysis, renal osteopathy and pancytopenia. (**b**) Multiple rosettes of calcium oxalate crystals in the intertrabecular marrow spaces surrounded by coarse fibrosis and newly formed woven bone (*top*). There is no residual haematopoiesis, Gomori staining, polarisation

For example, *systemic mastocytosis* is always accompanied by skeletal lesions, partly osteosclerotic, partly osteolytic, depending on the pattern of spread and topography of the mast cell granulomas (Fig. 28.4a–d). Moreover, mast cells, because of their ability to produce and secrete heparin and histamines, probably also play a part in the pathogenesis of primary osteoporoses. Systemic mastocytosis, especially during the early or indolent stages, usually requires a bone biopsy for diagnosis. Biochemical markers have now been tested and the following three chosen as probable indicators of mastocytosis: serum tryptase, urinary N(-)methylhistamine and N(-)methylimidazole. However, at this stage, a biopsy is still recommended for confirmation. Vitamin D participates in the regulation of development, differentiation, maturation and function of mast cells which play a critical part in various inflammatory disorders, some neoplasias

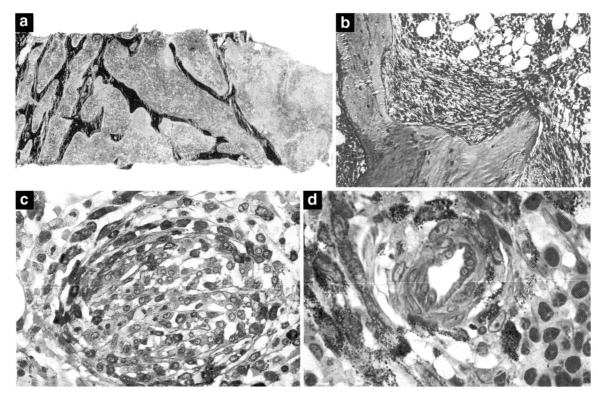

Fig. 28.4a–d. (**a**) Iliac crest biopsy of a patient with systemic mastocytosis, Gomori staining. (**b**) Higher magnification of round and spindle-shaped mast cells with variable granulation in a mast cell granuloma, endosteal orientation within a deep resorption bay, Giemsa staining. (**c**) Larger mast cell nodule (granuloma) with lymphoid cells in the centre, Giemsa staining. (**d**) Arteriole with mast cell infiltration, Giemsa staining

and which also directly and/or indirectly influence the metabolism of bone cells, as evidenced by the skeletal manifestations which almost invariably accompany mastocytosis. Animal studies have suggested that vitamin D or the more potent analogues could be effective therapeutic agents in disorders of mast cells.

Patients with *red cell anomalies* such as sickle cell disease commonly also have osteoporosis and osteomalacia, with decreased BMD values. Some patients also have vitamin D deficiencies, for which they must be appropriately diagnosed and treated, in addition to therapy with bisphosphonates, given according to markers of bone resorption and BMD values.

Patients with *haemophilia* may have low BMD and osteopenia/osteoporosis, which may have started in childhood and which leads to shorter height and lower weight than normal controls. Psychological factors, especially in childhood, such as apprehension and fear of bleeding may also be involved in restriction of some physical activities in individual cases. Other factors such as overall reduced physical activity and suscepti-

bility to infections may also stimulate bone loss during adulthood. Clearly, patients with osteopenia/osteoporosis must be evaluated and treated on an individual basis taking into account their medical history results of tests and the individual risk factor profile.

28.8
Infectious Disorders

In view of the fact that over 33 (in some estimates 43) million people worldwide are infected with HIV-AIDS, this now constitutes the most important infectious disease in which osteoporosis can occur. Recent reports have shown that HIV infection is an additional risk factor for osteoporosis and pathologic fractures. Changes in bone mineral metabolism, bone histomorphometry and bone density document the existence of a complex "AIDS osteopathy" comprising a mixture of osteoporosis, osteomalacia and secondary hyperparathyroidism. Immobilization, gastrointestinal infections, lipodystrophy, hepatitis and hormone deficiencies are all further risk factors for bone loss. Highly active antiretroviral therapy (HAART) has also been shown to accelerate bone loss in HIV-infected patients and is therefore a potent inducer of osteoporosis in these patients. The hypothesis that the systemic activation of T-lymphocytes leads to an osteoprotegerin ligand-mediated increase in active osteoclasts and loss of bone may in part explain the interaction of HIV infection and bone resorption. Risk factors such as nutrition, insufficient physical activity and other lifestyle influences also play a part in the skeletal changes listed above. With the widespread introduction of treatment to delay the progression of AIDS, early attention should be paid to these potential complications in order to avoid them as much as possible.

Other chronic infections may also influence the bones, especially when the patient's physical ability is impaired and long-term therapy is required, which may be the case in, for example, tuberculosis. The situation is worsened if drug resistance develops. It has been suggested that adjuvant therapies, such as l-arginine and vitamin D could stimulate mycobactericidal and immunomodulatory actions against the infection, and thereby shorten the duration of therapy. It is of note that patients with tuberculosis are reported to have deficient vitamin D levels. Studies of the effects of vitamin D therapy in these patients have not yet been reported.

28.9
Nephrology

The kidneys and bones are both involved in calcium homeostasis; therefore, impaired renal function leads to defective calcium homeostasis and renal osteodystrophy, both in the young and the old. Chronic renal insufficiency induces osteoporosis, osteomalacia and secondary hyperparathyroidism by means of deficiencies in vitamin D metabolism. Observational studies have shown that the survival of patients with hyperparathyroidism may be improved by treatment with analogues of vitamin D, given while the patients are on dialysis. Chronic kidney disease (CKD) and end-stage kidney disease (ESKD), with the increased risk of fracture, are both the subjects of growing interna-

tional concern. The prevalence of both is expected to increase over the next decade together with the ageing of populations in many parts of the world. Many studies of these patients, both completed and ongoing, deal with the therapy and prevention of osteoporosis and fractures, including treatment with bisphosphonates. Another major consideration, also from an epidemiological point of view, is the close association of CKD with the risk of cardiovascular disorders, which of course are also increased in the older populations and may be associated with osteopenia/osteoporosis. The survival of patients with CKD has benefited from therapy with calcitriol and, in recent years, the more potent analogues have shown additional advantages. These beneficial effects are also due to improvements in the cardiovascular system. It is now hoped that early therapy will benefit the kidney, slow progression of disease and postpone the necessity for haemodialysis and transplantation.

During *haemodialysis* or following *kidney transplantation*, the osteopathy is somewhat improved or it may be "set" and remain static. Interesting observations had previously been made in the early years of this decade, on minimodelling in iliac bone in patients on dialysis, especially after parathyroidectomy. Recent studies also of bone biopsies of patients on dialysis included young, active, ambulatory patients, as well as postmenopausal women. A comprehensive approach is required for the management of patients after transplantation, due to the many possible factors involved: steroid usage, hypogonadism, persistent hyperparathyroidism, poor allograft function, age-related and other chronic co-morbidities, and nutritional factors. Nevertheless, studies have shown that vitamin D and calcium, bisphosphonates and calcitonin may be effective. Vitamin D-based therapies have already been shown to be effective for the prevention of graft rejection after renal transplantation; attention to lifestyle factors is also important. Various novel treatments are under investigation and results are awaited. Therapy-resistant osteoporosis is frequently encountered today as a consequence of chronic renal disease and haemodialysis. Patients with chronic renal insufficiency on long-term dialysis develop a complicated bone disorder called "renal osteodystrophy". The manifestations of this disorder are severe and greatly reduce patients' quality of life: severe bone pain, multiple fractures and extra-skeletal ossifications. Renal osteopathy is described in detail in Chap. 31.

28.10
Neurology and Psychiatry

Chronic disorders such as Parkinson's disease, transient ischaemic attacks, stroke, Alzheimer's, epilepsy, multiple sclerosis, amyotrophic lateral sclerosis and diabetic neuropathy increase the risk of falling and correlate with lower bone mass, caused by immobility and drugs. The same is true for depressive states in which physical activity is reduced and nutrition may be inadequate. Depression has also been associated with disorders of the cardiovascular and many other systems, osteoporosis, and increased serum levels of various cytokines, e.g. of the TNF-alpha system, which may even contribute to the development of the depressive disorder. There also appears to be a link between depression and cognitive function, which further complicates the condition. And, unfortunately, some studies have indicated that anti-depressive drugs such as the tricyclic antidepressants have an increased risk of falls and fractures.

Most patients with *Parkinson's disease* have an increased risk of osteoporosis and fractures. This applies particularly to elderly females. This risk is largely due to restrictions in physical mobility as a result of the disease itself. BMD should be monitored and appropriate measures taken, including specially adapted exercises for the individual patient. Individuals with intellectual and/or developmental disabilities are also prone to osteoporosis and fractures in the absence of preventive measures.

Many studies have found an increased risk of fractures in patients with *epilepsy* on therapy with anti-epileptic drugs (AEDs), for example carbamazepine. The increased risk is associated to some extent with length of exposure to the drug. Therefore, appropriate screening and monitoring of BMD is recommended, as is attention to nutrition and supplements of calcium and vitamin D as required.

Immobilization and impaired physical activity: simple and easily applicable counter-measures developed for astronauts to reduce bone loss before and during spaceflight have also been advocated for patients who are paralysed. Changes in BMD in patients with psychiatric disorders such as schizophrenia have been described, and the causes may be related to effects and lifestyle consequences of the condition itself, as well as those of the medications administered. Studies have shown that glucocorticoids represent a common factor in almost all psychiatric and somatic complex disorders, as well as in many of their therapies, and are involved in the pathophysiology of most of the organs and tissues in the body, including the skeleton. Consequently, they also play a part in the effects of psychiatric disorders on the bones. Mitochondrial changes and dysfunctions with age have been documented in the neurodegenerative disorders, including psychiatric conditions, which in turn affect the skeleton.

Adult and elderly patients with *multiple sclerosis* are liable to osteoporosis and injurious falls. Out of a total of 354 patients investigated, more than 50% reported injurious falls. Management of the accompanying osteoporosis and alleviation of the fear of falling are two of the most important components of therapy, alongside programs for the prevention of falls in these patients.

Charcot neuro-osteoarthropathy is considered to be of neurogenic origin. However, Charcot arthropathy occurs most frequently in patients with diabetes, and considering the relationship between diabetes and osteoporosis, the possibility has been put forward that Charcot arthropathy could be a late consequence of osteoporosis in diabetic patients – a most cogent reason for early diagnosis and therapy in these patients. Studies have also demonstrated that early diagnosis and conservative intervention, therapy and rehabilitation have good results and avoid surgery. In more advanced cases, surgery is necessary, for example to salvage tibiotalar arthrodesis in patients with very unstable ankles due to bimalleolar fractures complicated by the Charcot neuro-arthropathy. The results were better in patients who had received antiresorptive therapy beforehand in the acute phase. Patients with vascular complications, and possibly even osteonecrosis, required more extensive surgery. It has recently been shown that the level of C-reactive protein is a reliable indicator of the presence of infections in patients with Charcot's arthropathy. Increased levels were not found in patients with Charcot foot pathology, so that in these patients inflammatory cytokines were not involved in the condition.

28.11
Oncology

The diffuse metastatic spread of a solid tumour can mimic a primary osteoporosis, particularly in the absence of localized osteolytic and/or osteosclerotic lesions. Osteoporosis of uncertain aetiology accompanied by bone pain and pathologic fractures should always be thoroughly checked to rule out an underlying malignant condition, especially metastases of neoplasias of the breast, prostate and lungs, among others. The first induces mainly osteoporotic/osteolytic metastases, the second mainly osteosclerotic. Patients with brain tumours are particularly liable to develop osteopenia/osteoporosis due to a multiplicity of factors. These include: drugs, glucocorticoids, anti-epileptics, anti-coagulants, chemotherapy, radiotherapy, inadequate nutrition, partial immobilization and possible hemiplegia, and these must all be considered in the medical management. Localized osseous changes, such as vertebral compression fractures, may also occur and must be appropriately handled. Other malignant tumours, such as bronchial cancers, may also cause skeletal lesions, usually paraneoplastic, by means of secretion of parathormone-related proteins (PTHrP). Various localized changes in bone are also caused by bone tumours, such as the osteosarcomas. It has recently been demonstrated that metastatic breast cancer cells induce an inflammatory stress response in osteoblasts, with production of cytokines that attract osteoclasts and so establish an environment in which resorption is increased and formation is reduced.

It should be borne in mind that oncologic patients of all ages are subject to the development of osteoporosis due to the anti-neoplastic therapy, which frequently contains glucocorticoids, and the physical restrictions imposed by the cancers and their consequences. The use of bisphosphonates in early cancer has two main objectives:

- To prevent the adverse effects of the cancer treatments on the skeleton, and
- To counteract the effects of the cancer itself on the bones, as it has already been established that the bisphosphonates reduce the frequency and severity of skeletal complications in patients with osteotropic cancers.

It has already been demonstrated that patients with bone metastases from solid tumours together with increased resorption showed normalization of the bone resorption markers within 3 months of treatment with zoledronic acid. This is a major justification for early administration of bisphosphonates in patients with metastases of breast cancer, prostate cancer, lung cancer and other solid tumours. Moreover, postmenopausal women with early breast cancer who are on therapy with an aromatase inhibitor, such as Arimidex or letrozole, inevitably suffer extra bone loss which can effectively be prevented by immediate administration of a bisphosphonate such as alendronate or zoledronic acid, as shown in the results of the ZO-FAST Study (2008).

In addition, in patients who already have osseous complications, the bisphosphonates relieve bone pain, and in some cases they also improve survival of the patients. It is also pertinent to emphasize the probable part played by vitamin D, its receptors genetic variants and analogues in the prevention and the treatment of malignancies. This has been indicated by some prospective trials, for example in patients with renal cell carcinoma, and on-going investigations of vitamin D analogues for prostate cancer. The extraskeletal actions of vitamin D include pro-apoptotic, anti-metastatic, anti-angiogenic, anti-inflammatory, pro-differentiating and immunomodulating activities. Clearly, careful attention to vitamin D status is essential in both prevention and in treatment of malignancies.

28.12
Pulmonology

Patients with long-standing cortisone-dependent asthma bronchiale should be regularly monitored for prevention of osteoporosis. Patients with cystic fibrosis may have osteoporosis even before lung transplantation and this should be treated in advance. One of the systemic manifestations of chronic obstructive pulmonary disease (COPD) is skeletal muscle dysfunction, which is one factor in the development of osteopenia/osteoporosis in these patients. Moreover, the results of a population-based case control study (6763 cases) investigating the use of beta-2 agonists in patients with COPD, indicated that the severity of the underlying disease and not the therapy played a role in the increased risk of fractures in these patients.

28.13
Rheumatology and Immunology

Skeletal damage is a hallmark of many chronic rheumatic diseases such as rheumatoid arthritis (RA), ankylosing spondylitis (AS) and systemic lupus erythematosus (SLE) and is known as "inflammation-induced bone loss in the rheumatic diseases". Vitamin D exercises a regulatory function in the maintenance of immune-homeostasis and it has been demonstrated that the net effect of vitamin D is an enhancement of innate immunity. A role has been ascribed to vitamin D in autoimmune disorders such as multiple sclerosis and rheumatoid arthritis.

Additional bone loss in the rheumatic disorders due to long-term steroid therapy and immobilization aggravate the osteoporotic state. Various forms of skeletal destruction are recognized: local bone erosion, periarticular bone loss and generalized osteoporosis. Local bone erosion is the most typical example of inflammation-induced bone loss. The lesion affects the subchondral bone at the margins of the joints and it emerges at the interphase between articular cartilage and the underlying bone, first described as "caries of the joint ends". Generalized bone loss is another important and frequent feature of RA. About one third of RA patients are osteoporotic, and 10% suffer from vertebral fractures. These patients suffer a decrease of 2.5% in vertebral BMD and 5% in the BMD of the hip within the first year of disease, and bone loss is doubled a year later if the disease is not adequately treated. Severity of disease, as indicated by high inflammatory activity, is an independent risk factor for accelerated bone loss and increased fracture risk. In patients on long-term therapy with corticosteroids, this may be the determining factor, with a relatively minor effect of the corticosteroids on the BMD. Formation of osteoclasts is facilitated by the inflammation-induced expression of cytokines such as TNF, IL-6 and RANKL. Furthermore, monocytes and macrophages accumulate in the synovial inflammatory tissues and express receptors such as RANK in response to the cytokines, and these in turn stimulate the development of active osteoclasts. Studies have shown that the replicative capacity of osteoblasts decreases with ageing and contributes to periarticular

osteopenia in RA – more so than in patients with osteoarthritis.

To summarise: in the rheumatic disorders, the combination of joint pain, immobilization and glucocorticoid therapy inevitably leads to a further loss of bone. Early correction of vitamin D deficiency and initiation of bisphosphonate therapy is strongly advised. In patients with chronic polyarthritis, measurement of the density of the phalanges by ultrasound has proved a useful method to monitor the state of the bones.

To investigate the possibility that patients with *scleroderma* (systemic sclerosis, SSc) have an increased risk for developing osteoporosis, a survey was carried out with one group of patients suffering from non-inflammatory musculoskeletal disease, and another group with RA as controls. The results showed that the patients with SSc and those with RA had the same prevalence of osteoporosis, in addition to which the patients with SSc had a similar or lower BMD; this indicated that patients with SSc should be screened for BMD values and treated accordingly. It should be mentioned that many of the clinical manifestations of SSc often go unrecognized, indicating that greater awareness is needed. This is also true for the osseous complications, so that the possibility of preventive therapy may be missed. Moreover, the complications themselves, such as hepatic, thyroid and neurological disorders may include risk factors for osteoporosis.

Ankylosing spondylitis (AS) is a chronic rheumatic disorder primarily affecting the vertebral column and the sacroiliac joints. It induces extensive damage to the vertebral column conducive to fractures and spinal cord injury. Primary preventive measures are absolutely essential in order to prevent such injuries. Management of these patients once such an injury has occurred is complex and involves extensive rehabilitation. Any patient presenting with non-specific symptomatology should be carefully investigated for a possible specific aetiology before institution of therapy, with the possible exception of pain relief.

Osteoporosis and Drugs

29

A detailed drug history is of vital importance, since many medicines and substances can adversely affect the skeleton. A comprehensive list of drugs associated with increased risk for osteoporosis in adults has been outlined by the National Osteoporosis Foundation (Table 29.1).

29.1
Corticosteroid-Induced Osteoporosis

Steroid-induced osteoporosis is nearly always due to long-term therapy with one of the steroid hormones, only rarely to an endogenous Cushing syndrome. It should also be stressed that the underlying disorder itself often causes osteoporosis, which is then aggravated by the steroid therapy; examples include Crohn's disease, rheumatic disorders, collagenoses, organ transplants, bronchial asthma, malignant lymphomas, multiple myeloma and others.

The use of corticosteroids over a period of days or weeks, even in very high doses, will not result in clinically significant bone loss. But bone loss is evident within months of the start of steroid therapy. When treated over long periods of time – possibly years – about 50% of these patients will suffer from manifest osteoporosis (Fig. 29.1). Continuing bone loss is particularly likely in patients requiring more than 10 mg/day of prednisone. Children, young men and postmenopausal women are particularly vulnerable. A few patients may have an individual sensitivity to corticosteroids. Initial bone density measurement is recommended in all patients so that a baseline is established for later comparison.

Corticosteroid-induced osteoporoses have the following characteristics:
- They occur in 30–50% of patients on long-term steroid therapy.
- Osteoporosis affects the trabecular bone; therefore, fractures occur preferentially in vertebral bodies, ribs and femoral neck.
- The rate of bone loss is rapid – "fast losers", "very high turnover osteoporosis". A loss of up to 20% of the bone mass may occur in the first year of steroid therapy.
- Dramatic bone loss may result from even low doses of prednisone (7.5 mg or its equivalent).

Table 29.1. Drugs associated with an increased risk of generalized osteoporosis (alphabetical list)

Aluminium antacids
Antibiotics
Anticonvulsants
Antihypertensives
Aromatase inhibitors
Chemotherapeutics
Diuretics
Glucocorticosteroids
GnRH agonists
Heparin
Immunosuppressants
Isoniazid
Lithium
Loop diuretics (e.g. Lasix)
Tamoxifen
Thyroid hormone
Warfarin

R. Bartl, B. Frisch, *Osteoporosis*, DOI 10.1007/978-3-540-79527-8_29,
© Springer-Verlag Berlin Heidelberg 2009

29

Glucocorticoids have a multifaceted *effect on bone* (Fig. 29.2):

- Inhibition of osteoblast proliferation, differentiation and function
- Increased apoptosis of osteoblasts
- Stimulation of osteoclastic activity
- Decreased intestinal absorption of calcium
- Increased renal excretion of calcium
- Increased parathormone secretion
- Decreased secretion of calcitonin
- Decrease in number of bone remodelling units
- Occurrence of aseptic bone necroses
- Increased production of collagenases
- Decreased production of corticotropin and gonadotropin.

In addition, interactions of glucocorticosteroids with other factors also contribute to the pathogenesis of steroid-induced osteoporosis:

- Increased sensitivity of osteoblasts to parathyroid hormone (PTH) and to active vitamine D
- Decreased production of prostaglandin E
- Decreased local production of insulin-like growth factor (IGF)-1
- Effect on IGF binding proteins.

Various guidelines have been recommended for the therapy and prevention of corticosteroid-induced osteoporosis. The results of many reviews suggest that the risk of fracture appears shortly after the start of therapy and at relatively low daily doses above 5 mg/day. It is also likely that the bone mineral density (BMD) threshold for fractures in corticosteroid-induced osteoporosis differs from that in postmenopausal osteoporosis. Bone loss may be substantially reversible after stopping therapy and it is independent of underlying disease, age and sex. Patients with obstructive pulmonary disease showed increases in fracture risk comparable to those of the patients with arthropathies.

Users of *inhalation corticosteroid therapy* (ICS) also had higher risks of fracture, but this may be related to the underlying respiratory disease rather than to inhaled corticosteroid therapy. However, a quantitative systematic review has found deleterious effects of ICS on BMD. Budesonide appeared to be the ICS which had the least damaging effects on bone, followed by beclomethasone, dipropionate and triamcinolone.

As a general rule, one can assume that with oral therapy of more than 6 months duration, and at a dose

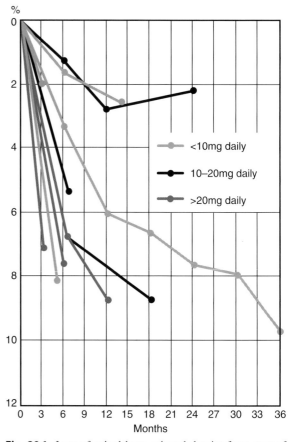

Fig. 29.1. Loss of spinal bone mineral density from start of corticosteroid therapy. Results of ten studies (modified from van Staa et al. [2002])

of more than the equivalent of 7.5 mg prednisone/day, a significant loss of bone will occur so that bisphosphonates are indicated for prevention. At higher doses the loss of bone may rise to 15% or more per annum so that when prescribing glucocorticoids the following *recommendations* should be followed:

- Check for the shortest possible duration of treatment to avoid adrenal cortical atrophy.
- Use glucocorticoids with the shortest half-life.
- Utilize local application whenever possible (creams, sprays etc.).
- Emphasize physical activity and muscle training.
- Prescribe vitamin D at 1000 IU daily.
- Make sure the patient ingests 1000–1500 mg calcium daily with food or supplements.

Therapy of corticosteroid-induced osteoporosis is the same as that of postmenopausal, but early use of preventive measures against corticosteroid-induced os-

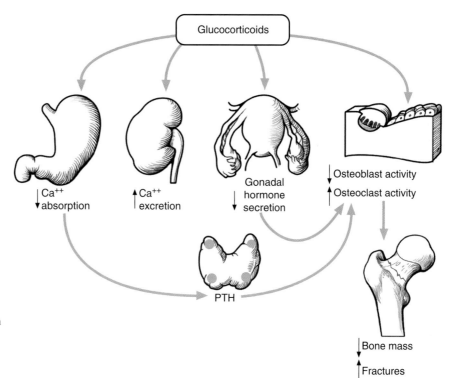

Fig. 29.2. Negative effects of glucocorticoids on calcium homeostasis, on the activity of bone cells and on bone mass. *PTH*, parathyroid hormone

teoporosis is highly recommended. In a recent trial, no difference was found between treatment with vitamin D or calcitriol; but alendronate was superior to either for treatment of glucocorticoid-induced bone loss. Therefore, the following recommendations for prevention and treatment are given:

- Physical activity and muscle training.
- Calcium and vitamin D supplements.
- Check and treat steroid-induced diabetes mellitus.
- Check for hypogonadism and treat as needed. Administration of testosterone to men whose testosterone levels are decreased by steroid therapy may increase BMD in the lumbar spine by 5% in 12 months.
- Start early with a modern nitrogen-containing bisphosphonate (e.g. alendronate once weekly 70 mg, or risedronate once weekly 35 mg).

Patients with problems of intestinal absorption, e.g. Crohn's disease or after a transplant, are preferably treated with infusions of a nitrogen-containing bisphosphonate (Zoledronate 5 mg annually). Before therapy is started, bone density should be measured at the lumbar spine and at the femoral neck. One of the following *treatment strategies* can then be applied according to the results:

- Normal bone density (T-score 2.0 to –1.0) and no additional risk factors: Calcium-rich diet, vitamin D and muscle training. Dual energy X-ray absorptiometry (DXA) control measurement at half-yearly intervals.
- Osteopenia and osteoporosis (T-score <–1.0): Strategy as above plus a modern bisphosphonate orally or by infusion.

29.2
Transplantation Osteoporosis

The number of transplants of solid organs such as kidney, liver, heart, lung and pancreas is rising steadily, together with an increase in the length of patients' survival times. For example, 98% of kidney, 87% of hepatic and 69% of heart transplant patients live longer than 1 year. Half of all transplant patients eventually develop osteoporosis with fractures and this substantially reduces their quality of life. Even now, as shown by a recent study, the fracture rates remain intolerably high at 20–40% of patients. The major cause of the fractures is the bone disease which could have preceded the transplant, and the subsequent conditions which follow it. In the absence of preventive measures, increased bone loss begins in the immediate postoperative period due to immobilization and immunosuppression, and continues thereafter due to many additional factors, such as possible neuropathy, reduced mobility and lack of exercise, nutritional factors and, above all, the immunosuppressive therapy which patients have to take. Patients who had diabetes before the transplant had significantly increased post-transplant fractures in the absence of prophylactic measures.

The *pathogenesis* of transplant osteoporosis is complex and only partly understood. General risk factors (inactivity, vitamin D deficiency, menopause, andropause, alcohol and nicotine) and some medications (diuretics, anticoagulants, corticosteroids and other immunosuppressive agents) are frequently involved. In addition, in many cases the diseased organ probably damaged the bone for long periods prior to transplantation. Biochemical markers of bone resorption are always elevated in the pre-transplantation phase. But the post-transplantation occurrence of fractures is due to immunosuppression with glucocorticoids, cyclosporin A and tacrolimus (FK506). Azathioprine increases the number of osteoclasts but not their resorptive activity. Loss of bone is especially prominent during the first year post-transplant. Put briefly, these recognized *pathogenic factors* are:

- Prior osteopenia/osteoporosis
- Immunosuppressive drugs
- Calcium and vitamin D deficiency
- Hypogonadism
- Poor mobility
- Poor nutrition.

During the first month after *cardiac transplantation*, the levels of testosterone decreased, but normalized during the second month. The levels of gonadotropins also decreased, suggesting an adverse effect of prednisone on the hypo-pituitary-gonadal axis. Subsequently, low testosterone levels are common. Therefore, these patients must be checked and treated also for BMD to avoid effects of hypogonadism and osteoporosis. Today, the situation is changing, especially if the patients have undergone assessment of bone density prior to transplant, and a program for preservation of the bones was initiated. This includes proper nutrition, calcium and vitamin supplements, early mobilization, targeted exercise therapy and antiresorptive treatment with one of the aminobisphosphonates. Studies on anabolic therapy, for example with PTH, have not been published to date.

It should be noted that *kidney transplant patients* require special attention: the presence of renal osteodystrophy, possibly with low bone turnover or even adynamic bone disease, is a contraindication for bisphosphonates. Vitamin D supplements are particularly important in kidney transplant patients as they may reduce post-transplant hyperparathyroidism. Results of a prospective trial of alfacalcidol alone, alendronate alone and the two together in renal transplant recipients showed that the combination was more effective in the improvement of bone mass than the separate use of either one alone. Pre-transplantation administration of vitamin D could also have a beneficial effect on the immune system and reduce the possibility of rejection. In addition, these patients are even at risk for cancer if the pre-transplant levels of vitamin D were low.

The presence of *pre-transplant diabetes* is also a significant risk factor for post-transplant fractures. Since the survival time of transplanted patients has now increased, it is important to stress that long-term preventive therapy must also be given!

Lifestyle, nutrition and risk factors: Previous experience has shown that long before a transplant, bone density should be measured and, if required, the appropriate therapy should be instituted well before transplantation: bisphosphonates, calcium, vitamin D or its active metabolites and muscle training. This should prevent bone loss before transplantation. In the post-transplantation period, up to 20% of the bone mass may be lost, particularly from the vertebral bodies and the femoral neck. Patients with liver, heart and lung transplants have a particularly high rate of loss. Aminobisphosphonates and calcitriol are the first choice for preventive therapy. Vitamin D-induced hypercalciuria must be avoided in patients with kidney transplants. In patients with hypogonadism, oestrogen or testosterone should be given. A calcium-rich diet and special exercises are also recommended for healthy bones. Calcitonin and fluoride, tested in clinical trials, were not found to be effective. Other factors such as sex and age may also impact on osteoporosis. For example, the early rapid loss of bone in men following renal transplantation can be prevented by bisphosphonates given i.v. at the time of transplantation and 1 month later.

29.3
Tumour Therapy-Induced Osteoporosis

Many treatment protocols in oncology lead to manifest osteoporosis. Irradiation causes local atrophy of bone and bone marrow due to the toxic effects on bone and bone marrow cells, while chemo- and hormone therapy induce systemic rarefaction of both trabecular and cortical bone. Moreover, these iatrogenic effects may even be increased by a direct effect on bone of the tumour itself, which could well have preceded the deleterious effects of the therapy.

Causes of osteoporosis during treatment of neoplasias include:
- Therapy-induced hypogonadism
- Glucocorticoids in chemotherapy protocols
- Toxic effects of chemotherapy
- Radiotherapy – also of the CNS in children because of brain tumours or acute leukaemias
- Immobilization
- Nutritional disturbances.

29.3.1
Tumour Therapy with Induction of Secondary Hypogonadism

Any chemotherapy with this effect will eventually also cause severe osteoporosis. Two groups of tumours are distinguished:
- Sex hormone-dependent neoplasias such as breast or prostatic cancer. Here the hypogonadism is part of the treatment strategy and substitution therapy cannot be given.
- Sex hormone independent-tumours such as Hodgkin's disease and other malignant lymphomas. In these cases hypogonadism is an unwanted side effect.

29.3.2
Hypogonadism with Breast Cancer

Premenopausal patients with breast cancer develop irreversible ovarian insufficiency within the first year of chemotherapy. BMD of the lumbar spine decreases by 8–10% and of the hips by 4–6% within 2 years of chemotherapy. However, if bisphosphonates are given at the same time as chemotherapy, this bone loss can largely be avoided. Moreover, therapy of ovarian insufficiency is integrated into the treatment schedule, especially that of patients with oestrogen receptor-positive tumours. This is achieved by means of gonadotropin-releasing hormone (GnRH) analogues, inhibitors of aromatase (especially those of the third generation) and oestrogen antagonists. Such antihormone therapy entails a considerable long-term risk of osteoporosis. *Tamoxifen*, a synthetic anti-oestrogen, has an antiresorptive effect on the bone but cannot make up for the lack of oestrogen stimulation of bone formation. In contrast, *aromatase inhibitors* markedly suppress plasma oestrogen levels by inhibiting aromatase, the enzyme responsible for the synthesis of oestrogens from androgenic substrates (Table 29.2; Fig. 29.3). Unlike tamoxifen, aromatase inhibitors have no stimulatory effect on bone. Consequently, non-steroidal aromatase inhibitors of the third generation have been shown to increase the risk of osteoporosis by a profound lowering of circulating oestrogen levels. Short-term use of letrozole (an aromatase inhibitor) has been shown to be associated with an increase in bone-resorption markers; and adjuvant therapy with anastrozole (also an aromatase inhibitor) is associated with a higher incidence of fractures than therapy with tamoxifen (ATAC Study). The steroidal aromatase inhibitor exemestane, however, significantly prevents bone loss and enhances bone mechanical strength. The steroidal action of exemestane's principal metabolite, 17-hydroexemestane, may account for the observed bone-preserving effects.

Development of osteoporosis under non-steroidal aromatase inhibitors or chemotherapy can be pre-

Table 29.2. Classification of aromatase inhibitors

Generation	Type 1 (Steroidal)	Type 2 (Non-steroidal)
First	None	Aminoglutethimide
Second	Formestane	Fadrozole
Third	Exemestane (Aromasin®)	Letrozole (Femara®)
		Anastrozole (Arimidex®)
		Vorozole

29

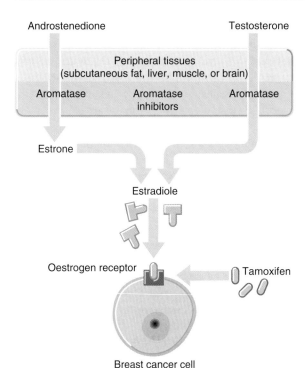

Fig. 29.3. Mechanism of action of aromatase inhibitors and tamoxifen (modified from Smith and Dowsett [2003])

vented or modified with concurrent use of bisphosphonates. Therefore, all patients with breast cancer should have a BMD (DXA of lumbar spine and hips) before commencing therapy. If osteopenic, *preventive therapy* with bisphosphonates should be instituted:

- Clodronate 1600 mg daily per os will increase the bone mass and most probably also decrease both skeletal and visceral metastases.
- Alendronate (10 mg) or risedronate (5 mg) daily orally can also be used as single therapy for prevention and treatment of osteoporosis.
- Alendronate (70 mg) or risedronate (35 mg) once weekly if authorized instead of the daily dose.
- Ibandronate (150 mg) once monthly.
- Alternatively ibandronate 3 mg i.v. at 3-monthly intervals according to the severity and type of osteoporosis.
- And last, but certainly not least, zoledronate 5 mg i.v. annually is recommended and has already been tested in clinical studies.

It is worth emphasizing that patients with osteoporosis and a history of breast cancer should not receive hormone substitution therapy, but only an aminobisphos-

phonate orally or intravenously. Raloxifene can also be given.

29.3.3
Hypogonadism and Prostatic Malignancy

Attainment of hypogonadism is one of the aims of therapy, particularly in all forms of metastatic cancer and a high postoperative PSA level. Possible modes of treatment are orchidectomy, GnRH analogues and anti-androgens. Patients who have received such treatments are at great risk of developing osteoporosis, and the appropriate diagnostic and therapeutic measures are indicated as for patients with mammary cancer.

29.3.4
Hypogonadism in Hodgkin's Disease and Other Malignant Lymphomas

Hypogonadism resulting from therapy of the malignant lymphomas is the most frequent in the group of the non-hormone-dependent neoplasias. Irreversible ovarian insufficiency and early menopause are induced in 30–60% of women after radio- and intensive chemotherapy. Because of the low proliferative index of Leydig cells, men are less likely to develop severe osteoporosis, though some degree of bone loss will be manifest later in life. BMD measurements at diagnosis should also be made in patients with lymphomas so that bisphosphonate therapy, if needed, can be given to prevent development of osteoporosis.

29.3.5
Anti-tumour Therapy with Direct Effect on Bone

Many protocols applied in oncology contain substances which, when given systematically, affect bones adversely and cause osteoporosis. However, the degree of damage and extent of bone loss depend on the frequency and/or duration of the cycles of chemotherapy. Measurement of BMD indicates when osteoporosis should be forestalled and/or treated.

29.3.6
Protocols Including Corticosteroids

Patients with malignant lymphomas and multiple myeloma receive chemotherapy protocols which include high doses of corticosteroids, but these are given intermittently, not continuously. In contrast to women with ovarian insufficiency, patients without hypogonadism did not suffer bone loss although high cumulative doses of prednisone were given. One possible explanation may be the relatively short exposure time, in addition to which the negative impact on bone of the bone marrow infiltration is reduced by the therapy, in the lymphomas and especially in multiple myeloma. It should also be remembered that the modern bisphosphonates have anti-tumour effects, for example on the myeloma cells, which contributes to their positive influence on remodelling of bone, osteoporosis and other osseous lesions.

29.3.7
Therapy Protocols Including Methotrexate and Doxorubicin

Many chemotherapeutic agents have not yet been investigated for their possibly harmful effects on bone. An exception is methotrexate given for rheumatoid arthritis: increased resorption of bone together with decreased formation have been reported with an ensuing high renal excretion of calcium, and reduction in BMD. One of the direct consequences of methotrexate appears to be a drop in the recruitment of osteoblast precursors. Children treated with methotrexate (e.g. in acute lymphatic leukaemia) are especially liable to considerable resorption of bone, although with cessation of methotrexate therapy the resultant osteopenia is reversible. Clinical studies of bone in patients with breast cancer treated with the protocols containing methotrexate (CMF protocol) have not yet been reported.

29.3.8
Therapy with Ifosfamide

This alkylating agent combined with cisplatin is used mainly for solid tumours. Depending on the amount given, it causes reversible or permanent damage of the proximal renal tubuli resulting in metabolic acidosis, loss of phosphate and hypercalciuria, which in turn lead to the clinical picture of osteoporomalacia. However, there is no information as yet, as to whether or not ifosfamide itself has a direct toxic effect on bone cells.

29.3.9
Treatment Strategy

The problem of osteoporosis in patients with malignancies is underestimated. Usually, an osteologist is only consulted when the patient has already sustained one or more fractures. This unsatisfactory situation could be avoided by timely "osteoprotection", which starts with a BMD measurement when the diagnosis is established and appropriate steps are taken depending on the results. These steps include the basic and specific measures outlined above.

The choice, dose, duration and intervals of bisphosphonate therapy are determined by the severity of bone loss and the patients' risk factors. When carefully chosen and correctly administered, the bone deficit can be eradicated and a positive bone balance with increases up to 10% in bone density obtained. A broad spectrum of bisphosphonates is available:

Oral administration:

- **Alendronate (Fosamax®)**
  10 mg daily
- **Alendronate (Fosamax®)**
  70 mg once weekly
- **Risedronate (Actonel®)**
  5 mg daily
- **Risedronate (Actonel®)**
  35 mg once weekly

Intravenous administration:

- **Ibandronate (Boniva®)**
  3 mg infusion/injection every 3 months
- **Pamidronate (Aredia®)**
  30 mg infusion every 3 months
- **Zoledronate (Aclasta®)**
  5 mg infusion annually
- **Clodronate (Ostac®)**
  600 mg infusion every 3 months

In summary, intravenous administration has some important advantages:

- Supportive treatment when i.v. chemotherapy is given at 4- to 6-week intervals
- Avoids gastrointestinal side effects
- Avoids problems of gastrointestinal absorption
- Avoids problems of compliance.

29.4
Drug-Induced Osteoporomalacia

Bone formation and mineralization require calcium and phosphate together with active metabolites of vitamin D. Drugs affecting the vitamin D system may cause both osteoporosis and osteomalacia by several mechanisms:

- *Blockers of vitamin D production*: Elderly and institutionalized individuals with limited nutrition and sunlight exposure are at particular risk.
- *Inhibitors of vitamin D absorption*: Vitamin D, a fat-soluble vitamin, is absorbed in the jejunum and ileum, in combination with bile acids. Therefore, bile acid binding resins such as cholestyramine and colestipol interfere with this process and inhibit vitamin D absorption.
- *Interference with vitamin D metabolism*: To be active, vitamin D must first be metabolized in the liver and then in the kidney. Drugs such as anticonvulsants or rifampicin induce drug-metabolizing enzymes in the liver which then accelerate the catabolism of vitamin D and its metabolites. Some reports have shown that 20–65% of patients with epilepsy receiving anticonvulsants such as phenytoin or phenobarbital developed osteoporosis and/or osteomalacia, especially if they were institutionalized. These patients were at an increased risk of fractures during their epileptic seizures. Patients taking these anticonvulsants require higher doses of vitamin D to achieve a positive calcium balance, with doses of up to 4000 IU per day. Anticonvulsants such as sodium valproate do not induce the hepatic drug-metabolizing enzymes and therefore have no impact on vitamin D metabolism.
- *Antagonists of vitamin D action*: Glucocorticoids interfere with intestinal calcium absorption, but they are not direct antagonists of vitamin D at the receptor level. There are no known drugs that directly interfere with the actions of active vitamin D at the target-tissue level.
- *Inhibitors of phosphate absorption*: Hypophosphatemia is a major cause of osteomalacia and the most important drug-induced form is caused by excessive ingestion of aluminium-containing antacids, which inhibit intestinal phosphate absorption.
- *Inhibitors of bone mineralization*: Aluminium-induced osteomalacia is mainly found in patients on haemodialysis and on total parenteral nutrition. Etidronate, the first bisphosphonate, also induced disturbances in mineralization when given in high doses. However, no reports have been published of osteomalacia caused by nitrogen-containing bisphosphonates. Bone biopsies of patients treated with alendronate for more than 7 years have shown no evidence of demineralization. Fluoride in high doses often showed evidence of abnormal mineralization, and this defect is aggravated by concomitant low calcium and vitamin D intake.

29.5
Antiepileptic Drug-Related Osteopathy, a Pressing Need for Better Understanding

It is well known (as described above) that anti-epileptic drugs (AEDs) have long-term effects on the state (health) of the bones, specifically with respect to bone density, vitamin D metabolism, as well as other risk factors for fractures. However, these aspects of AED therapy have not been adequately investigated in the studies published to date. It is therefore important to stress that patients with epilepsy on AEDs have an increased risk for bone loss, defects in mineralization and fractures. A patient on long-term therapy with an AED has a 2–3 times greater risk of fracture than the controls and, as demonstrated in the studies, 4–70% of patients, i.e. 50% on average, have demonstrable osteopathies. The type, dosage and duration of the anti-epileptic therapy determine the type of osteopathy and this is valid for enzyme-inducing as well as for non-enzyme-inducing medications.

The *pathogenesis* of AED-related bone disease remains controversial and multifactorial:

- Accelerated hepatic vitamin D metabolism by enzyme-inducing AEDs
- Altered vitamin K metabolism
- Lowered calcitonin levels in AED users
- Reduction of IGF-I and IGF-binding protein 3 (IGFBP-3)
- Direct inhibition of intestinal calcium absorption
- Reduced exercise levels, poor dietary calcium intake and reduced sunlight exposure
- Increased falls during seizure and at other times
- Lower levels of endogenous oestrogens
- Increased levels of sex hormone-binding globulin
- Inhibition of osteoblast-like cells.

The enzyme inducers such as phenytoin, primidone, phenobarbital and carbamazine have been particularly well investigated with regard to their effects on metabolism of vitamin D. However, loss of bone may occur in the absence of vitamin D deficiency. Moreover, combinations of osteoporosis and osteomalacia are frequently seen and must be taken into consideration when specific therapy is recommended. The question of what, if any, effect on bone is exerted by the modern AEDs such as lamotrigine, gabapentin and levetiracetam, is still under consideration.

Before administration of therapy, every patient should be thoroughly investigated, including bone density by DXA and lever of 25(OH) D in the serum to establish baseline values – similar to the approach to patients when long-term therapy with systemic corticosteroids is contemplated. Moreover, in addition to the clearly defined treatment of any osteopathy already present, patients with epilepsy should be advised on how to minimize epileptic attacks and falls.

In the light of all the above, the following therapeutic measures are recommended:

- Careful choice and dosage of the AED to reduce the frequency of epileptic attacks.
- Physical activity in particular for muscular development and maintenance and to improve co-ordination.
- Appropriate lifestyle to benefit the bones – no smoking!
- Nutrition – including a minimum of 1000 mg calcium daily.
- Vitamin D3 2000 IU daily, but more than 4000–5000 or even up to 15,000 IU daily if osteomalacia is already present at diagnosis. The patient's serum should be monitored. Patients on Phenytoin need higher doses of vitamin D. Alternatively, vitamin D may also be taken as weekly or monthly capsules of 20,000 IU, or given as intramuscular injections of 100,000 IU every 3 months.
- Active vitamin D metabolites e.g. Alphacalcidol or Calcitrol, should only be given in cases of marked osteomalacia, or if patients cannot accept the high doses of vitamin D3.
- Nutrition rich in vitamin K (such as dark green vegetables) or vitamin K supplements are given in rare cases for prevention of phenytoin-induced bone loss.
- When impending or manifest osteoporosis is diagnosed initially, nitrogen containing bisphosphonates or other medications can be given, as recommended by the FDA or other responsible authorities in individual countries.

AIDS Osteopathy

It is important to emphasize that today in 2008 there are well over 33 million people worldwide who are infected with the AIDS virus (acquired immune deficiency syndrome), and according to information given recently at an international televised meeting (Clinton Foundation), over 5 million more people are still infected annually. A high proportion of these are women and children. Many AIDS patients live in circumstances which do not enable them to receive the care and treatment outlined below, although greater international efforts in this direction are now being made. It has been estimated that currently there are about 1 million HIV-infected people in the US.

Put very briefly, the progression of HIV infection to the full-blown picture of AIDS is associated with loss of immunocompetence and its consequences, the occurrence of opportunistic infections and malignancies, while the immune dysregulation may lead to autoimmune phenomena such as vasculitis. Poor antibody responses have also been associated with premature exhaustion of B lymphocytes in HIV-infected patients. Fungal infections in particular increase the risk for disease progression. Co-infection with hepatitis C virus also has a deleterious effect and contributes to hepatic fibrosis. DNA microarray analysis has been used to predict hepatic fibrosis, thereby sparing the patients a liver biopsy. These patients also have reduced bone mineral density (BMD) and possibly osteopenia/osteoporosis.

Much knowledge has accumulated over the years from the work that has been done on the pathogenesis of AIDS (Table 30.1) and on the mechanisms of disease progression from infection with the virus to the full-blown clinical picture of AIDS. These insights are being used to assist in the development of a vaccine against AIDS that has widespread applicability. However, all attempts to accomplish this goal have so far not been successful, but concentrated efforts are on-going and results expected.

The introduction of HAART (highly active antiviral therapy) in 1995/1996 has changed the future and fate of people with AIDS; at least those who are able to receive and adhere to therapy with HAART. Since its introduction, some modifications and variations have been made and are available, and these contribute to the differences in both the beneficial effects and the adverse reactions reported during the past 10 years or so. Racial/ethnic differences, due to a variety of factors, have also been shown to play a part, as seen in the reactions of patients to therapies given for some of the disorders associated with AIDS, such as metabolic syndromes and malignancies, which in turn influence their consequences, such as osteopenia/ osteoporosis. Studies have shown that renal dysfunction, frequent in advanced HIV-AIDS, was improved after 2 years therapy with HAART. However, neurocognitive disturbances associated with HIV-AIDS were not affected by therapy with HAART. In contrast, therapy with HAART has resulted in a dramatic reduction in morbidity and mortality among HIV-AIDS patients.

It has been estimated that >40% of HIV-AIDS patients develop a malignancy during the course of their lives. Since the introduction of HAART and the increased survival, it is estimated that malignancies, mainly lymphomas and sarcomas, still occur in more than 40% of patients at some time in their lives. Possibly the incidence is so high due to the increased survival. The patients suffer from the so-called AIDS-related malignancies, but also from others such as lung

Table 30.1. Aetiology of AIDS osteopathy

Basic disorder
Haematopoietic cell defect?
T-cell activation
Bone marrow inflammation
Malnutrition
Gastrointestinal infections
Immobilization
Lipodystrophy
Testosterone deficiency
Vitamin D deficiency
Infections
Hyperparathyroidism
Glucocorticoids
Antibiotics
Protease inhibitors

cancer. The malignancies, their therapies and the consequences of both all have deleterious effects on the skeleton, which has greatly increased the prevalence of osteopenia/osteoporosis among patients with AIDS. The manifestations of rheumatic disorders in AIDS patients has changed with the introduction of HAART, but complications such as metabolic abnormalities, cardiovascular disorders and osteoporosis still occur. It should be clearly stated that rheumatic disease is also still prevalent even after therapy with HAART. Some studies have indicated that alendronate is the bisphosphonate of choice for the osteopenia/osteoporosis in patients on HAART therapy, although few comparative studies have been published. Since over 10 years have now passed since the introduction and use of HAART, reports of cases of resistance to therapy have increased and national authorities, as well as the WHO, have developed monitoring, assessment and prevention strategies to facilitate evidenced-based decision-making, concerning the various aspects of AIDS therapy.

30.1
Manifestations of AIDS Osteopathy

Many of the problems experienced by patients with AIDS require haematologic, immunologic and osteologic investigations. These problems include: cytopenias, lymphomas, infections, fever of unknown origin (FUO), haemorrhages, bone pain and pathologic

fractures. It is essential to emphasize that osteopathy in AIDS is an important, highly complex complication which has so far received too little attention. Haematologic disorders and neoplasias have been extensively described and are well recognized, but not osteological problems. Since the latest treatments for AIDS now achieve longer survival times, it is all the more important to pay attention to the quality of life for which mobility and therefore skeletal integrity are crucial, particularly for the millions of children involved, because many of the more than 40 million people with AIDS are young.

Drugs used to treat AIDS may also be harmful to the bones, as is the decreased physical activity of many patients. HIV therapy-induced changes in immune factors, which also participate in bone remodelling, have been implicated in the increased bone resorption in HIV-infected children and adolescents. In one study, evaluation of aspirates and bone marrow biopsies (n=120) frequently demonstrated dysplastic/aplastic changes in haematopoiesis, as well as inflammatory reactions in the stroma of the bone marrow. The bone itself also regularly exhibited changes designated as "AIDS Osteopathy" These changes are summarized as follows (Fig. 30.1a,b):

- Reduced bone density (osteopenia, osteoporosis)
- Increased osteoclastic activity [secondary hyperparathyroidism (HPT)]
- Disturbances in mineralization (osteomalacia).

Recent studies on the interaction of the AIDS infection and bone have postulated that the constant stimulation of T-cells leads to activation of osteoclasts and thereby increased resorption via osteoprotegerin. In adult men, the G–IGF-1 axis in the control mechanism of bone remodelling is apparently also involved. In addition to the direct viral and drug-induced damage to bone cells, marrow cells and stroma, as well as the anomalies of vitamin D metabolism, many other secondary risk factors are also involved (Table 30.1). Recent international studies of bone density by dual-energy X-ray absorptiometry (DXA) measurements in AIDS patients have now confirmed the frequent occurrence of osteopenia/osteoporosis and pathological fractures, and in some cases even of osteonecrosis, as shown in a large study of patients from 1999 to 2002. A recent study has demonstrated that pre- and postmenopausal women who are HIV+ are at increased risk for fragility fractures, compared with women in the general public, in many cases with the

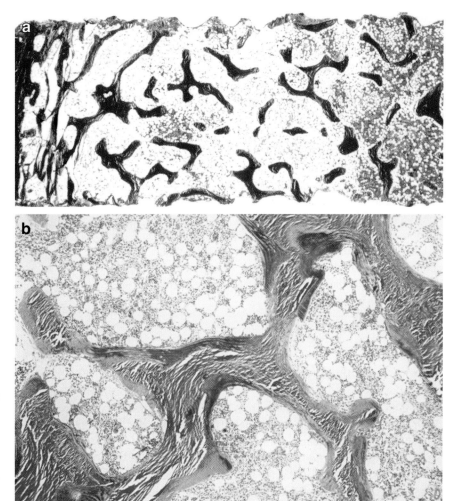

Fig. 30.1 a, b. (a) Iliac crest biopsy of a patients with AIDS: note marked marrow atrophy and osteoporosis, Gomori staining. (b) At higher magnification, signs of inadequate mineralization with increased amount of osteoid (*red*), Ladewig

same BMD as the controls. Should the patients undergo additional viral infections such as hepatitis C, they will be at risk for additional complications such as diabetes, steatohepatitis, subsequent advanced fibrosis and increased body mass index (BMI). The causes of the osteopathies in AIDS are very complex (as noted above) and are also influenced by the various therapies patients have received. These in turn affect the clinical, biochemical and radiological manifestations. Moreover, fractures in AIDS patients have a very strong adverse influence on quality of life, by the additional suffering and incapacity, the added requirements for care and nursing, the effect on morbidity and mortality, as well as contributing greatly to the cost of treatment, which is still a very important factor in many developing countries with a high prevalence of AIDS infection in the population. This also accounts for geographic differences in availability of HAART.

There are also differences in population-level as well as individual rates of adherence to antiviral therapy. Rates may vary according to age, sex, and educational levels, as well as social and economic environments. However, adherence has increased over time since HAART came into widespread use, and the greatly increased publicity, the participation of public figures and "celebrities" in the propagation of knowledge of the disease and its therapy have had a strong impact on the populations of countries most at risk for infection.

30.2 Diagnosis

Consequently, all AIDS patients should undergo an osteological evaluation at the time of diagnosis, including the following, if at all possible:

- X-ray of the lumbar spine in two planes
- DXA of lumbar spine and hip (annual monitoring)
- Examination of peripheral blood for calcium, phosphate, alkaline phosphatase, cross laps, PTH, vitamin D, TSH and testosterone/oestrogen
- Complete blood count (CBC).

Results of clinical trials published in 2005 have now been summarized and suggestions as to screening and treatment have been made. When appropriate indications are present (cytopenias, atypical cells in blood films etc.), and possibly (unclarified) osteopathies, a bone biopsy and aspirate should be obtained for clarification and diagnosis. It should be stressed that in AIDS the disorders of the bones of young people and adults begin in childhood – even in the neonatal and perinatal periods; therefore, appropriate management of the paediatric patient is crucial.

30.3
Treatment Strategies

All AIDS patients would benefit from implementation of the guidelines given under "Basic Therapy of Osteoporosis" which include physical activity (physiotherapy if possible), bone-preserving lifestyle, and adequate nutrition and supplements of calcium and vitamin D. However, should osteoporosis already be present at diagnosis (T<–2.5 SD), or if the density measurements decrease in spite of basic therapy (as above), then addition of an oral aminobisphosphonate is indicated. If difficulties arise with the oral route, then an aminobisphosphonate can be given i.v., which also forestalls problems of compliance and uncertainty as to whether or not the medication has been taken. The schedule is the same as previously noted:

- Alendronate 70 mg orally weekly
- Risedronate 35 mg orally weekly
- Ibandronate 3 mg i.v. every 3 months
- Zoledronate 5 mg i.v. annually

When osteomalacia and secondary HPT dominate the clinical picture, the daily supplement of vitamin D can be increased to 3000 IU; alternatively, an active metabolite of vitamin D can be substituted. Serum calcium must of course be monitored.

To *summarize*, every second AIDS patient develops some form of osteopathy during the course of the disease. This can be a combination of osteoporosis, osteomalacia and secondary HPT and frequently entails difficult clinical situations involving pathological fractures and bone pain. Studies are in progress to clarify to what extent the viral infection itself and/or the anti-viral therapy are/is responsible for the loss of bone mass. Secondary infections and lipodystrophy also add to the "osteoporomalacia". If the diagnostic investigations (as described above) are applied and the basic therapy implemented, then AIDS osteopathy can be diagnosed and prevented in its early stages and even successfully treated in the later ones. Studies have already been published on the efficacy of alendronate plus calcium and vitamin D on bone mineral density; however, most of the patients were male with an average length of 8 years HIV infection. Results of additional studies are pending.

Renal Osteopathy

31.1
Definition

Patients with chronic renal insufficiency and patients on long-term dialysis develop complicated bone disorders, also known as renal osteodystrophy or renal bone disease. This is often accompanied by severe bone pain, multiple fractures and extra-osseous calcifications, all of which considerably reduce the patient's quality of life. On a more optimistic note, it has recently been shown that therapy with statins inhibits or prevents decline in creatinine clearance and slows impairment of renal function. Moreover, statins also participate in the regulation of bone turnover. Renal osteodystrophy consists of a mixture of three subgroups – hyperparathyroidism (HPT), osteomalacia and osteoporosis – as seen in the three types of renal bone disease:

- High-turnover osteopathy with characteristics of primary HPT
- Osteomalacia with manifestations of severe inhibition of mineralization
- Low-turnover osteopathy with the picture of severe osteoporosis (adynamic bone disease).

31.2
Pathophysiology

Many factors influence both the type and extent of osteopathy:

- The renal disorder itself.
- Presence of associated diseases such as diabetes mellitus and amyloidosis.
- Severity of the renal insufficiency.
- Patient age – young patients are particularly severely affected, especially males up to 40 years. Subsequently, there are no differences between the sexes.
- Vitamin D deficiency.
- Dietary restrictions.
- Level of parathyroid hormones (PTH).
- Type of dialysis and length of time patient is on dialysis.
- Accumulation of toxic substances (e.g. aluminium, fluoride, iron).
- Glucocorticoid therapy.

Four of these factors play a decisive part in the pathogenesis of renal osteodystrophy:

- Anomalies of vitamin D metabolism.
- Extent of secondary HPT.
- Aluminium deposition on bone prevents mineralization.
- Immunosuppressive therapy with a negative bone balance.

The most significant of the above in the mechanism of renal bone disease are:

- Anomalies of vitamin D metabolism
- Degree of secondary HPT
- Deposition of aluminium on bone (prevents mineralization, is now infrequent)
- Immunosuppressive therapy inducing a negative bone balance.

R. Bartl, B. Frisch, *Osteoporosis,* DOI 10.1007/978-3-540-79527-8_31,
© Springer-Verlag Berlin Heidelberg 2009

31.3
Symptoms

The most important symptoms are *bone pain, skeletal deformities, muscle weakness and anomalies of growth in young patients.*

31.4
Biochemical Investigation

The following parameters of bone metabolism should be measured: calcium and phosphate, alkaline phosphatase and osseous alkaline phosphatase, PTH, metabolites of vitamin D 25 and 1.25, aluminium and the Desferal test.

Radiologic signs: These may demonstrate characteristic changes seen in osteomalacia (Looser's zones) or in secondary HPT (e.g. subperiosteal bone resorption of the phalanges) such as subcutaneous and arterial calcifications, subperiosteal erosions and "rugger jersey" spinal column. Three components of renal osteodystrophy can be identified and classified in histology of bone:

- Alterations of remodelling: osteitis fibrosa cystica or adynamic bone
- Disturbance of mineralization: osteomalacia, previously associated with aluminium
- Reduction in bone mass: osteopenia, osteoporosis, partly due to glucocorticoids.

31.5
Radiological Investigation

All the characteristic signs of osteomalacia (Looser's zones) (Fig. 31.1) and of secondary HPT may be present (e.g. subcutaneous and arterial calcifications, subperiosteal erosions, osteolytic lesions in the phalanges) (Fig. 31.2). The "rugger jersey" sign (three layers) in the cancellous bone of the vertebral bodies is found in 60–80% of patients (Fig. 31.3). However, in daily practice, the diagnosis may not be straightforward because biochemical and radiological findings do not always match or accurately reflect the extent of damage to the bones.

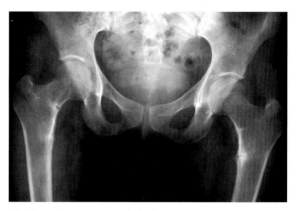

Fig. 31.1. Looser zones of the femoral neck

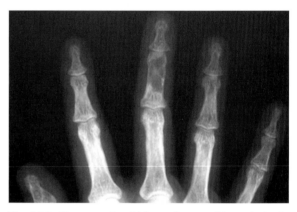

Fig. 31.2. Hyperparathyroid bone disease with marked subperiosteal bone resorption involving the phalanges

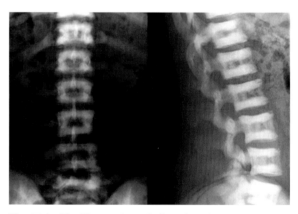

Fig. 31.3. The "Rugger jersey" sign (three layers) in the cancellous bone of the vertebral bodies

A *bone biopsy* may be essential in situations in which definitive identification of the type of renal osteodystrophy is required for therapeutic decisions, as when parathyroidectomy is considered. Renal bone disease is classified according to three histological features best evaluated in a bone biopsy:

- *Disturbances of mineralization* (osteomalacia, previously also associated with aluminium) (Fig. 31.4)
- *Anomalies of bone remodelling* (osteitis fibrosa cystica; or adynamic bone disease) (Figs. 31.5 and 31.6)
- *Reduction in bone mass* (osteopenia/osteoporosis, possibly partly glucocorticoid-induced) (Fig. 31.5).

Various histomorphometric parameters of bone remodelling, such as the formation period (FP) and the quiescent period (QP), may permit a clearer identification of osteomalacia and low-turnover conditions. Moreover, detailed studies of bone biopsies have led to the recognition of a variant of adynamic bone disease (ABD) with PTH-independent osteoclastic resorption, implicating other factors conducive to osteoclast activation in these cases.

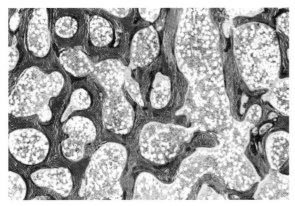

Fig. 31.4. Iliac crest biopsy of a patient with renal osteopathy: characteristics of osteomalacia (*red*, osteoid) and secondary hyperparathyroidism ("dissection osteoclasia"), Ladewig

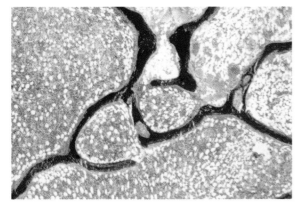

Fig. 31.5. Small trabeculae showing dissecting bone resorption

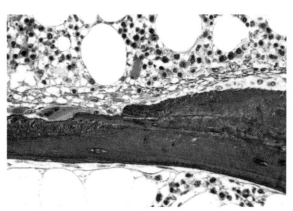

Fig. 31.6. At higher magnification, increased osteoclastic activity (*left*) and seam of osteoblasts (*right*) with endosteal fibrosis, Gomori staining

31.6
Treatment Strategies

Advances in dialysis techniques and the use of active metabolites of vitamin D have radically changed the manifestations and *therapy* of renal osteodystrophy over the last 20 years. Previously, osteomalacia and secondary and tertiary HPT were major hurdles, but today severe and therapy-resistant osteoporosis is a major problem. It is characterized by markedly reduced osseous remodelling – ABD – previously due to aluminium deposition on bone. With early institution of bisphosphonate therapy together with active metabolites of vitamin D, the emphasis is on prevention, since the early management of secondary HPT will decrease the number of patients requiring surgery. Inhibition of bone resorption in high-turnover renal osteodystrophy is especially beneficial. In resistant cases with high levels of PTH and enlargement of the parathyroid glands, excision is indicated.

A recent study compared the survival benefit of oral vitamin D in 7203 haemodialysis patients with the survival of 8801 haemodialysis patients who had not received vitamin D, as part of the CORES study carried out in six Latin American countries. The study was carried out for a period of 16 months. The results showed that the haemodialysis patients who received the oral active vitamin D daily in low doses, i.e. 1 µg, had the highest survival advantage. The patients who were on active vitamin D showed significant reductions in mortality related to cardiovascular, infectious and neoplastic co-morbidities

31

compared to the controls. The results of this study confirmed earlier reports on some of the putative actions of vitamin D. However, according to recent studies, the question as to whether all patients with chronic renal disease should receive calcitriol has not yet been definitively answered and randomized trials are awaited.

Today the situation has changed due to the increasing application of bisphosphonates. The aim of therapy is prevention by means of early intervention with bisphosphonates and active metabolites of vitamin D. Since patients on dialysis require protection of the gastrointestinal tract, intravenous bisphosphonate therapy is the method of choice. The following *protocol* is recommended:

- **Ibandronate (Bon(v)iva®)**
  3 mg injection every 3 months.
- **Zoledronate (Aclasta®)**
  5 mg infusion annually.

Because of its half-life in the serum of up to 16 h, patients should receive the bisphosphonate on completion of dialysis. When resistance to bisphosphonates occurs in patients with high PTH levels and demonstrable enlargement of the parathyroid glands, parathyroidectomy is indicated. Children with renal osteodystrophy require special evaluation and individual therapy for which European Guidelines have been published (Klaus et al. 2006).

32.1
Complex Regional Pain Syndrome (CRPS)

32.1.1
Definition

Also known as *algodystrophy*, *Sudeck's disease* or *sympathetic reflex dystrophy*, this disorder is a highly unpleasant, unpredictable and painful complication of injuries and trauma, especially fractures. The cause, development and effective treatment of CRPS are largely unknown. It has not been observed in children. Putative *causes* range from disorders of vegetative innervation to endocrine and psychosomatic disorders. Triggers of CRPS include fractures, operations, infections and nerve injuries. The severity of the underlying injury bears no apparent relationship to the severity of the symptoms of Sudeck's disease, which can be triggered even by trivial trauma. Most frequently affected are joints of the hand (90%), followed by the ankle and knee joints. Two types are recognized: *Type 1* develops after a trauma, while *Type 2* is triggered by a peripheral nerve injury.

32.1.2
Clinical Findings

These consist of a triad of sympathetic, motoric and sensory manifestations with five characteristic symptoms:

In collaboration with Christoph Bartl MD, Department of Orthopaedic and Trauma Surgery, University of Ulm, Germany

- Disproportionately strong pain (Fig. 32.1)
- Swelling and unusual warmth of the affected area
- Skin discoloration of the affected area
- Increased hair growth on the area involved
- Stiffness of the joints involved.

32.1.3
Diagnosis

The results of the following investigations contribute to the *diagnosis*:
- Thermography (area of overheating)
- Bone scan (area of increased uptake)
- X-ray (patchy rarefaction of bone)
- MRI (oedematous areas around the joints involved)
- Alleviation of pain by sympathetic blockade – designated as "sympathetically maintained pain" (SMP) confirms the diagnosis.

32.1.4
Course of Disease

This can be divided into *three main stages* (though questioned by some experts):
- *Inflammation* stage (up to 3 months): Typical symptoms include localized pain, blue discoloration and overheating of the skin, dough-like oedema and functional limitations of the joint. MRI shows presence of bone marrow oedema.
- *Dystrophy* stage (3–6 months): The dermatologic symptoms regress, leaving a trophic disorder of the

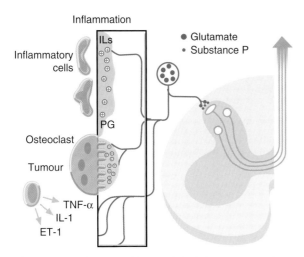

Fig. 32.1. Mechanisms of bone pain in inflammatory and on-cologic disorders

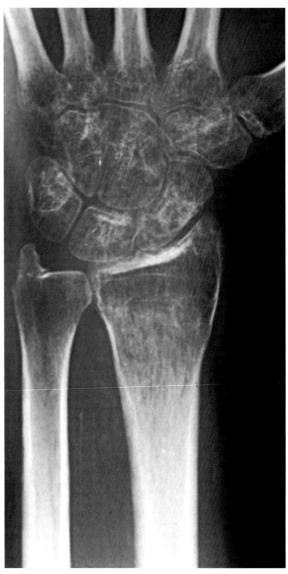

Fig. 32.2. Massive spotty decalcification of the hand in complex regional pain syndrome, Stage III

skin. There is an increase in restriction of joint movement and spotty areas of demineralization are seen on X-rays.

- *Atrophy* stage (6–12 months): This end stage is characterized by generalized atrophy of skin, muscles and bone (Fig. 32.2). Stiffness of the joint is further increased as massive rarefaction of bone occurs.

32.1.5
Treatment Strategies

A relationship of confidence and trust must be established between patient and doctor to ease the fear, tension and anxiety which always accompany this chronic condition. First, it is essential to break the vicious circle of pain and dystrophy by rest and physiotherapy. Surgery is only indicated for stabilization of a fracture or later for correction of a deformity. However, it should be noted that early surgical intervention carries the risk of aggravating the condition.

Immobilization, analgesics, anti-inflammatory drugs and cold dressings to counteract overheating are useful measures in stage I. Blockade of the sympathetic nerve supply (stellate) and calcitonin therapy have also been successful at this stage. Physiotherapy and exercises are strongly recommended in stages II and III.

32.1.6
Bisphosphonates

Since 1988, four international trials performed with pamidronate showed alleviation of pain in most cases and cure in some. This constitutes genuine progress in the treatment of M. Sudeck. Clodronate and alendronate were equally effective. Similar results were also achieved in patients treated with one of the following aminobisphosphonates given for 4–6 months:

- **Ibandronate (Bondronat®)**
  Infusion of 6 mg monthly, 4 times, the first
  infusion only 2 mg in 100 ml NaCl solution
  over 15 min
- **Pamidronate (Aredia®)**
  Infusion of 60 mg monthly, 4–6 times, the first
  infusion only 30 mg in 500 ml NaCl solution
  over 30–60 min
- **Zoledronate (Aclasta®)**
  5 mg infusion over 30 min given once only

The initial low doses of 3 mg ibandronate or 30 mg
pamidronate were used to avoid the possible acute-phase
reactions (previously described), which could be much
more pronounced in patients with Sudeck's disease than
in other patients. Occasionally, acute-phase reactions
occurred after the second infusion, but were milder.
Many patients – some already morphine-dependent
– have been cured by this therapy. In others, the pain
was alleviated to such a degree that analgesics were no
longer required. Since the bisphosphonates have not yet
been authorized for treatment of Sudeck's disease, the
patient's informed consent must be obtained and documented. A systemic review, published in April 2008,
confirmed the potential of bisphosphonates to reduce
pain, but evidence-based trials are still awaited.

32.2
Transient Osteoporosis and the Bone Marrow Oedema Syndrome (BMOS)

This section deals with transient (or transitory) osteoporosis and the bone marrow oedema syndrome
(BMOS) separately. However, it should be stressed at
the outset that bone marrow oedema and transitory
osteoporosis occur sequentially and both are manifestations which may be due to any of a long list of
possible causative factors. Up-to-date studies found
that these conditions are more frequent in men than
in women, and often more than one site is affected,
either in the same or in another joint. Shifting BMO,
in all the cases investigated, was transient. Though
frequently unilateral, bilateral transient osteoporosis
of the hip in male patients has also been observed.
Other studies have indicated that progression to ar-

ticular collapse and fracture may occur. Moreover,
the conditions are preceded by and associated with
changes in vascularity (ischaemia) which in turn can
lead to osteonecrosis. Hence the urgency for early
diagnosis and therapy to avoid these complications
and the surgery which may well be required.

The question as to whether BMOS and transient
osteoporosis should (or should not) be regarded as
separate entities has not yet been completely resolved.
Recent studies have pointed out that BMOS and transient osteoporosis should not be regarded as separate
entities, but rather as signs of an ongoing process involving the knee, hip joint or femoral head. Moreover,
as mentioned above, both may occur in many different
conditions, separately or in combination. Examples of
such conditions are inflammatory and septic arthritis,
synovial disorders, stress fractures, neoplasias, reflex
sympathetic dystrophy, complex regional pain syndrome and others. There is also a link with vitamin
C deficiency. These correlations are relevant both for
the determination of the exact diagnosis and for the
therapy of patients presenting with musculoskeletal
pain, and they emphasize the need for early recognition both for treatment and as a preventive measure.

32.2.1
Transient Osteoporosis

Transient osteoporosis has been defined as a rapidly
developing painful osteopenia/osteoporosis of benign
nature and of various possible aetiologies. Neural and
circulatory mechanisms have been implicated as causative factors. This disease is more frequent in men, although women may also be affected, sometimes even
bilaterally in the third trimester of pregnancy, or in
the post-partum period. Spontaneous remissions frequently occur. Clinically two groups are recognized:
- Regional transient osteoporosis of the hip
- Regional migratory osteoporosis with involvement
  of various joints.

32.2.1.1
Diagnosis

The patients complain of severe pain and limitation
of movement in the affected joints. In the later stages,
X-ray films show local bone loss. Initially, MRI is

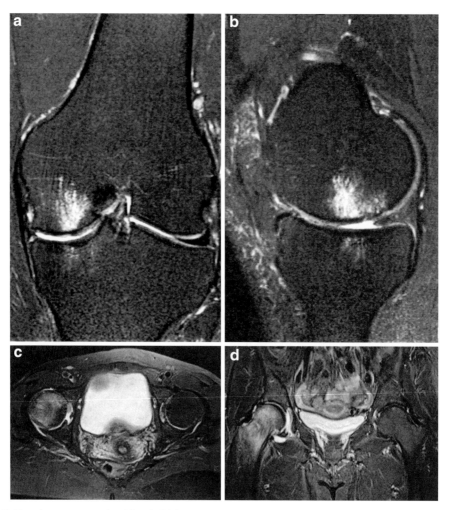

Fig. 32.3. (**a**, **b**) Transient osteoporosis with painful bone marrow oedema in the region of the distal femur. (**c**, **d**) Transient osteoporosis with painful bone marrow oedema in the femoral head and neck, MRI

needed to demonstrate bone marrow oedema near the affected joints (Fig. 32.3a–d) and this is required in order to establish the diagnosis, which should be made in the earliest possible stages as occasionally bone marrow atrophy and oedema may precede osteonecrosis (Fig. 32.4). This can also be demonstrated by MRI, should it develop. In some cases, areas of demineralization around the hip joint may be seen in X-rays of that region. Occasionally, healing of the transitory osteoporosis takes place in 4–6 months, even without therapy. In cases with severe pain not relieved by medication, surgical intervention may be required to lessen the intraosseous pressure. To establish the diagnosis, various conditions such as localized immobilization osteoporosis, osteonecrosis,

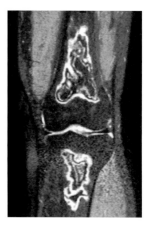

Fig. 32.4. Widespread osteonecrosis of the femur and tibia after chronic and progressive "transient osteoporosis" and nicotine abuse

osteochondrosis dissecans and Sudeck's disease must be ruled out by MRI.

32.2.1.2
Treatment Strategies

An important therapeutic measure is to relieve the joint of any stress and weight-bearing, which may be difficult in cases with bilateral transient osteoporosis, especially of the hip. Frequently this is followed by spontaneous regression of the symptoms, which appears to indicate that overloading of the joint may have contributed to the cause.

Bisphosphonates are recommended for rapid relief of pain and reduction of the bone marrow oedema. A bisphosphonate is given intravenously monthly for 4–6 months according to the following schedule:

- **Ibandronate (Bondronat®)**
  6 mg infusion monthly, the first infusion only 2 mg
- **Pamidronate (Aredia®)**
  60 mg infusion monthly, the first infusion only 30 mg
- **Zoledronate (Aclasta®)**
  5 mg as a single infusion

After the final infusion, an MRI should be made to monitor the affects of therapy and to check for residual oedema or osteonecrosis as mentioned above.

32.2.2
Bone Marrow Oedema Syndrome

BMOS is now recognized as a common cause of pain in the musculoskeletal system in general and in joints of the extremities in particular: hips, knees, feet, shoulders, elbows and hands as well as joints of the spinal column. Moreover, some patients may present with bilateral involvement, and a migratory transient BMOS has already been characterized. In addition to the pain felt during movement and exercise, the patients also experience pain at rest, which is caused by the increased intraosseous pressure. BMOS, possibly preceding aseptic or avascular osteonecrosis (Fig. 32.4), also occurs in paediatric oncology patients, sports men and women as well as in highly-trained

athletes, for example tennis players with an upper limb syndrome, or in young soccer players at the pubic symphysis. Patients with osteoporosis and in particular patients with rheumatic disorders such as osteoarthritis of various joints are also prone to develop BMOS in the affected joints. It stands to reason, therefore, that any patient with musculoskeletal pain should be carefully checked for BMOS by MRI in addition to other clinically indicated investigations. Various *classifications of BMOS* have been proposed; the following is practical and widely used:

- **Ischemic BMOS**
  - Osteonecrosis
  - Transient osteoporosis
  - Osteochondrosis dissecans
  - Complex regional pain syndrome (CRPS)
- **Mechanical BMOS**
  - Bone contusion ("bone bruise")
  - Stress fractures
  - Microfractures
- **Reactive BMOS**
  - Osteoarthritis
  - Rheumatoid arthritis
  - Postoperative BMOS
  - Neoplasias

32.2.2.1
Diagnosis

MRI, with or without various refinements, is indicated for the diagnosis of BMOS. Other clinical and laboratory examinations including X-rays of the affected joints and bones are required to identify the specific pathology and this may vary in each patient, considering the many possible causes (see above).

During the past decade, MRI proved to be the imaging method of choice for the evaluation of patients with painful bones and/or joints. The most important constituents of the joint, in particular the cartilage, the subchondral bone, the capsular-ligament system and the surrounding soft tissues, can be evaluated with MRI. The correct interpretation of the MRI findings is of decisive importance for therapeutic decisions. Bone marrow oedema, with its typical signal pattern in the MRI, is a common but non-specific finding in painful local bone and joint lesions (Figs. 32.5a,b and 32.6a–c). Because only marrow structures are involved in the initial stages of BMOS, X-ray, CT or even bone

32

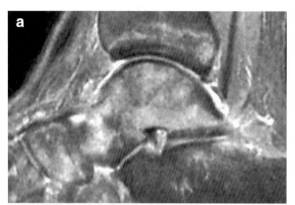

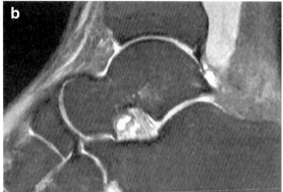

Fig. 32.5. (a) Widespread traumatic bone marrow oedema syndrome of the talus, distal tibia and foot following an ankle supination trauma. The 19-year-old patient had complex regional pain syndrome-like symptoms for more than 6 months. **(b)** At 3 months following treatment with an intravenous bisphosphonate (3 infusions of 6 mg ibandronate) the patient is pain-free with full restoration of his sports activities (MRI)

scan are not useful for initial diagnosis. BMOS is also not visualized on arthroscopy. It is characterized by low signal intensity compared with unaffected cellular bone marrow on T1-weighted images. On T2-weighted images, especially when fat-suppression techniques are used, high signal intensities in the low-signal areas of the T1-weighted images are typical for BMOS.

A bone marrow biopsy in BMOS shows increased extracellular fluid together with inflammatory vascular reactions and decreased haematopoiesis. The *main histologic findings* are (Fig. 32.7a–c):

- Hypocellular marrow with oedema in the marrow spaces.
- Dilatation of sinusoidal lumina and disruption of their walls.
- Spatial disorganization of the haematopoietic cell lines.
- Reactive plasmacytosis and fine fibrosis.
- Production of woven bone in the subchondral osseous region in cases of "bone bruise".
- Increased osseous reaction with hyperactive osteoclasts, osteoblasts and osteocytes.
- Increased osteoid volumes and seams (see Bartl & Frisch 1993, Biopsy of Bone in Internal Medicine).

The characteristic symptom of BMOS is pain during mechanical loading, but the severity of pain does not always correlate with the intensity and extent of BMOS seen on MRI. Nevertheless, a final control by MRI is useful to document the efficacy of therapy.

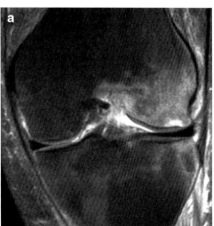
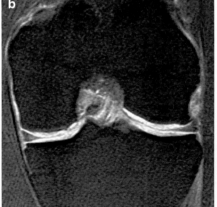
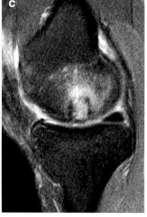

Fig. 32.6. (a) Traumatic bone marrow oedema syndrome (BMOS) ("bone bruise") of the medial femoral condyle in a 58-year-old patient who had no sign of osteonecrosis or osteoarthritis and no abnormalities visible on X-ray. **(b)** Complete regression of the BMOS after one infusion of 5 mg zoledro-nate. At 3 months later the patient is completely free of pain (MRI). **(c)** Reactive BMOS of the femoral condyle following osteochondral transplantation. Complete restoration of the painful BMOS after treatment with zoledronate 5 mg i.v.

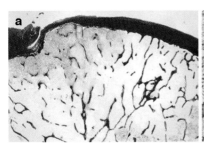 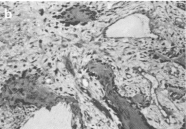 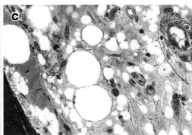

Fig. 32.7. Histology in the area of a "bone bruise" lesion. (**a**) Low magnification of a section of a "bone bruise" lesion with marked oedema (*light brown*) in the subchondral region. (**b**) Mi-crofracture with production of new woven bone in the subchondral region (Giemsa staining). (**c**) Massive bone marrow oedema in the surrounding bone marrow area (Gomori staining)

32.2.2.2
Treatment Strategies

Therapy ranges from operative, i.e. core decompression to conservative with drugs such as *iloprost*, a prostacyclin analogue and the *bisphosphonates*, in addition to measures such as *limited weight-bearing* and activity of the joint(s) involved, and physical therapy. Therapeutic management of BMOS also depends on the basic disease. Pain is mainly caused by the increased intraosseous pressure (normal pressure 20–30 mmHg). Therefore, mechanical unloading by partial weight bearing or by *drilling the oedematous lesion* may lead to pain relief. *Non-steroidal anti-inflammatory drugs* (NSAIDs) and medications for pain are only of limited value.

32.2.3
Bisphosphonates

According to our experience, however, *bisphosphonate* treatment proved to be the first choice for effective therapy. With respect to side effects, about 10% of the cases experienced an "*acute phase reaction*" with fever and flu-like symptoms 1 day after the first infusion. Symptomatic therapy can be given for this, but is rarely required. An acute phase reaction occurs only after the first infusion, rarely after the second and then is very mild. In the past 4 years we have treated 355 patients with BMOS of the talus (see Fig. 32.5a,b), knee (see Fig. 32.6a,b) and/or femoral head.

We used intravenous bisphosphonates of the third generation (see Chap. 3), and a complete, rapid regression of the bone marrow oedema was found in 78% of the cases, documented by MRI and clinical controls (Figs. 32.5 and 32.6). Relapse within 2 years occurred

in only 10 patients, but again there was a good response to bisphosphonate therapy.

In all cases of BMOS and independent of the basic disorders, we start with one of the following two bisphosphonate protocols:

> • **Ibandronate (Bondronat®)**
>   6 mg infusion (15-min duration) monthly, MRI control after the 3rd or 4th infusion, the number of infusions depending on the degree of pain relief
> • **Zoledronate (Aclasta®)**
>   A single 5 mg infusion (30 min duration), MRI control 3 months later

32.3
Vanishing Bone Disease
(Gorham-Stout Syndrome)

32.3.1
Definition

This syndrome is also known as *"massive osteolysis"*, *"disappearing bone disease"* and *"phantom bone"*.

Gorham's vanishing bone disease is the ultimate osteoporosis showing complete disassociation of the normal coupling mechanism. The cause is unknown, though over-activity of cytokines, especially Il-6, has been implicated. Gorham's disease is occasionally fatal. This disorder was first described by Jackson in 1938 as "a boneless arm" (Fig. 32.8). In 1953, Gorham and Stout published 24 cases and emphasized the angiogenic component of the disease. Subsequent

32

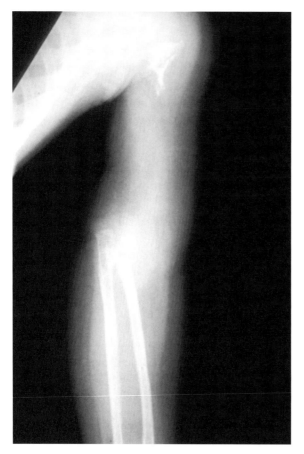

Fig. 32.8. Almost complete disappearance of the left humerus in a 14-year-old patient with Gorham-Stout syndrome

surveys of the literature revealed nearly 150 documented cases (Devlin et al. 1996); more have been reported since then, up to 175 cases as of February 2008. Occasionally, the disease has also been identified in children, as in a recent case in the humerus of a 14-year-old boy.

32.3.2
Aetiology and Pathophysiology

The cause has not yet been elucidated. Hemangiomatosis and lymphangiomatosis have been implicated, possibly due to an endothelial defect, with production of abnormally high levels of cytokines which stimulate osteoclasts. Some studies have reported the presence of numerous leaky lymphatic vessels near the osteolytic lesions as well as chylous ascites. Investigations have now revealed several lymphangiogenic

pathways that could be relevant in Gorham's disease. Many investigators have described prominent osteoclasts, particularly in the lytic front of the lesions. However, no reactive osteoblastic activity has ever been documented indicating that the physiological "coupling" between bone resorption and bone formation has been completely abrogated. This clearly demonstrates a communication defect between osteoclasts and osteoblasts resulting in the absence of stimulation of osteoblasts, i.e. no reaction to the osteoclastic activity. In one patient, initially high levels of interleukin (IL)-6 – a cytokine that stimulates osteoclasts and is produced by various cell types including endothelial cells, either directly or by way of VEGF, was implicated – dropped after therapy with bisphosphonates and radiation.

32.3.3
Clinical Findings

A review of the recent literature based on findings in 46 patients revealed the following features):
- It affects young adults without preference for male or female.
- Genetic, endocrinologic and metabolic disturbances have not been found.
- It starts in a single bone and spreads to adjacent bones.
- In 38 of 46 cases the condition was already polyostotic at diagnosis.
- Pelvis, vertebrae, ribs, proximal bones of the extremities and cranial bones are frequently involved.
- Progression and spread of the disease are unpredictable.
- When the ribs are affected, pulmonary insufficiency is frequently a lethal consequence.
- Chylothorax is a common complication.

32.3.4
Diagnosis

The diagnosis of Gorham-Stout syndrome is established by X-rays which demonstrate the absence of bone in the affected areas. Occasionally, vertebral compression fractures in severe osteoporosis must be considered in the differential diagnosis. When localized to the mandible, it must be differentiated from osteonecrosis due to other causes (Mignona et al. 2005) (see also Chap. 34). In early phases of the disorder, osteolytic lesions due to a malignancy must be ruled out. Bone biopsies taken from an involved area show increased osteoclastic resorption by morphologically normal osteoclasts. The absence of osteoblasts is particularly striking. This indicates complete abrogation of the "coupling" mechanism. The resorption lacunae are filled with fibroblasts, blood vessels and oedematous connective tissue. Infiltration of the involved areas by plasma cells, lymphocytes and mast cells suggests an immunologic component.

32.3.5
Treatment Strategies

Before the introduction of bisphosphonates, progression of Gorham-Stout syndrome was inexorable. All previous attempts to treat this condition have failed. But, as in all other states of skeletal destruction: immediate initiation of bisphosphonate therapy proved to be highly effective. Case reports have demonstrated rapid disappearance of local symptoms and pain after i.v. administration of bisphosphonates; moreover, follow-up over the subsequent 24 months revealed a stable condition with no evidence of progression (Hammer et al. 2005).

32.3.6
Bisphosphonates

Focal osteolysis – the unbalanced hyperactive osteoclastic resorption – can be halted immediately by intravenous bisphosphonates, which stop progression of the disease. The following are recommended:

- **Ibandronate (Bondronat®)**
  6 mg infusion monthly for 4–6 months
- **Zoledronate (Aclasta®)**
  5 mg single infusion

X-rays should be taken every 4–6 months for follow-up. Restitution of the vanished bone has not been observed, even under therapy with bisphospho-

nates. Trials with anabolic agents have not yet been reported.

32.4
Fibrous Dysplasia

Fibrous dysplasia is a local developmental fibro-osseous aberration of the skeleton. The aetiology is not clear, but it does not appear to be hereditary. Increased production of Il-6 has been implicated as a causative factor. The disease occurs mainly in the first two decades of life, and both sexes are affected (Fig. 32.9). When there are polyostotic fibrous dysplasias of bone together with *café au lait* skin pigmentation and endocrine disorders, the condition is known as Albright's syndrome, or McCune Albright syndrome (MAS). The underlying pathologic process is substitution of

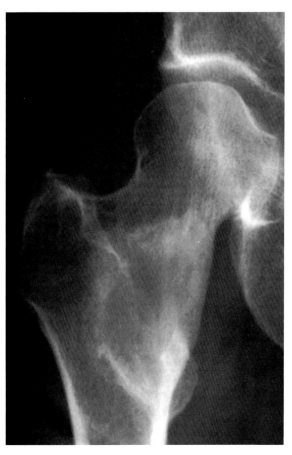

Fig. 32.9. Fibrous dysplasia of the right proximal femur

fibrous tissue for both bone marrow and bone with activation of osteoclasts. The aim of therapy is normalization of the increased osteoclastic activity by administration of bisphosphonates.

The main clinical symptoms and signs are:
● Bone pain
● Osteolysis or local osteopenia
● Deformity of bone
● Spontaneous fractures.

The pelvis, long bones and skull are particularly prone to this disorder. Malignant transformation occurs in less than 1% of cases. Both mono- and polyostotic variants are recognized.

Surgical correction was the only treatment available until recently. Early administration of bisphosphonates can curtail secondary osteoclastic bone destruction and thereby prevent deformity of bone. Successful treatment with bisphosphonates has already been reported, although the patient groups were small. The studies underscored the alleviation of pain, improvement in function, decrease of fracture risk and prevention of deformity. In practice, intravenous bisphosphonate therapy is recommended, but should be administered at an osteological clinic, after informed consent has been obtained and documented.

● **Ibandronate (Bondronat®)**
   6 mg infusion monthly
● **Pamidronate (Aredia®)**
   60 mg infusion monthly
● **Zoledronate (Aclasta®)**
   5 mg infusion annually

X-rays, CT and/or bone scans can be used for monitoring.

32.5
Paget's Disease of Bone

Paget's disease or Morbus Paget (named after Sir James Paget who first accurately described the disease in 1877) is also called *osteodystrophia deformans* or *osteitis deformans*. It is a localized non-inflammatory disease of bone caused by uncontrolled, increased bone resorption, by pathological large multinucleated osteoclasts, which in turn induces disorganized bone formation. This disease illustrates graphically what happens when there is complete local deregulation of osteoclasts together with partial abrogation of "coupling" in the osteological meaning of the term. Osteoblasts are stimulated to replace the resorbed bone, but the osteoid is randomly produced and not laid down as lamellae, so that the resulting bone is dense but mechanically inadequate. The focally greatly increased bone turnover is accompanied by hypervascularization and increased blood flow. Deformities of the effected bones are the rule. Mono- and polyostotic forms of Paget's disease are recognized.

About 1–3% of people over 40 years of age have Paget's disease of bone (more men than women, 3:2), but initially only 5% are symptomatic or require therapy. More recent estimates put the number of affected people (55 years or older) at 2–7% in the US and Western Europe. The cause of Paget's disease is presumed to be a viral infection of osteoclasts and/or an abnormality on chromosome 18, resulting in multinucleated, hyperactive and unregulated giant osteoclasts. Mutations in SQSTMI have been associated in up to 40% of familial and sporadic cases. Other genetic anomalies have been found, but the aetiology of Paget's disease has not yet been determined. Moreover, why all osteoclasts are not involved is still a complete mystery!

The following *symptoms* are indicative of Paget's disease: the variability of the symptoms that characterize Paget' disease is caused by the variability of the locations.
● Pain and warmth of the affected area (pelvis, spine, extremities, skull).
● Bone pain that is stabbing and deep and often stronger at night. Pain could also be due to compression of nerves or associated arthrosis.
● Bending and deformities of the effected bones with risk of spontaneous fractures ("sabre tibia", "hat that became too small" appearance).
● When the base of the skull is involved, hearing loss and damage to the cranial nerves can occur.
● Compression fractures may result if the vertebrae are involved.
● Secondary arthrosis can occur due to incorrect weight-bearing.
● When large areas of the skeleton are affected, the accompanying hypercirculation may cause cardiac insufficiency.

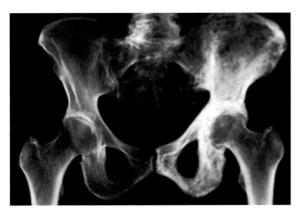

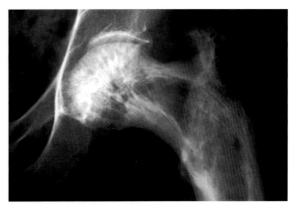

Fig. 32.10. Paget's disease of bone with widespread painful involvement of the left pelvis, sclerotic stage

Fig. 32.11. Paget's disease of bone in the left femur with deformation and thickening of the shaft and an especially large Ward's triangle

- Inner ear involvement can cause deafness. It has been assumed that Beethoven's deafness was caused by Paget's disease of bone.

The *course* of the disease can be divided into three stages which are identified locally:
- *Lytic stage*: The osteolytic process spreads at the rate of 1 cm annually.
- *Repair stage*: also called "mixed stage": After the period of rapid resorption osteoblasts fill the cavities with bone, thereby producing cement lines with the mosaic patterns characteristic of Paget's disease.
- *Sclerotic stage*: When the disease has progressed for several years, relatively large areas consist of dense bone, but this is not capable of weight-bearing or stress (Fig. 32.10).

Transition from mono- to polyostotic forms of Paget's disease must be excluded by periodic X-ray examinations and bone scans.

32.5.1
Diagnosis

Imaging techniques highlight a focal increase in bone remodelling, and depict the extent of skeletal involvement (mono- or polyostotic). In addition, characteristic X-rays plus increased alkaline phosphatase levels, as well as other markers of bone remodelling in the serum confirm the diagnosis. Conventional X-ray and/or CT demonstrate typical changes and the following points are considered:
- Alterations in contours of the bone
- Careful evaluation is required when the vertebrae are effected
- Thickening of the cortical bone
- Coarsened trabecular structure with alternating lytic and sclerotic regions (Fig. 32.11)
- Narrowing of the foramina of the spinal column (Fig. 32.12)

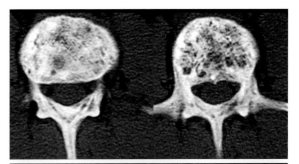

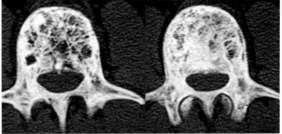

Fig. 32.12. Paget's disease of bone in the area of the lumbar spine (CT). Note the altered structure of the trabecular bone. Significant narrowing of the vertebral canal is evident (*bottom right*)

32

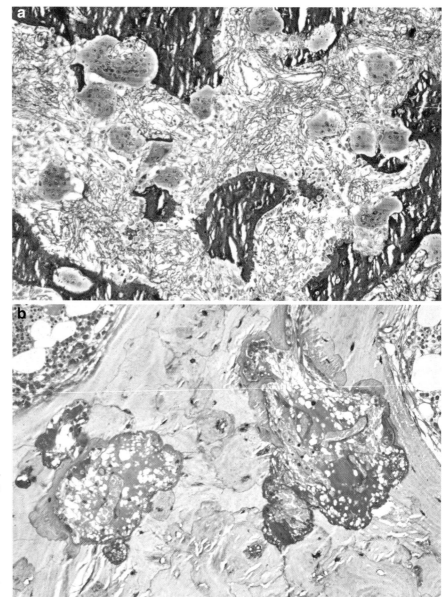

Fig. 32.13a,b. Typical histology of bone in Paget's disease. (**a**) Multiple multinucleated and active osteoclasts in deep resorption lacunae. Note the marked fibrosis in the marrow spaces, Gomori staining. (**b**) Marked remodelling with dissecting osteoclasia and mosaic structures in the adjacent bone, Giemsa staining

- Thickening of the skull
- Fibrosis and hypervascularization of the bone marrow surrounding the foci of involved bone.

Bone biopsy can be useful in the initial stages of Paget's disease for differential diagnosis and to rule out metastasis or arthrosis. The most important features (Fig. 32.13a,b) are:

- Cement lines forming mosaic structures, and woven bone

- Multinucleated osteoclasts containing nucleoli and showing signs of activity: localization in resorption bays, presence of pronounced ruffled membranes
- Striking reactive osteoblastic bone formation
- Fibrosis and hypervascularization of the surrounding bone marrow
- Two histologically unmistakable features characterize Paget's disease: the giant, multinucleated osteoclasts and the mosaic structure of the newly formed bone.

Biochemical markers of disease activity are *alkaline phosphatase* in blood and pyridinoline crosslinks in urine. The level of osteocalcin in the serum is used for monitoring. Osteocalcin production by osteoblasts is dependent on vitamin K; the level reflects the degree of bone remodelling.

For *differential diagnosis* the following must be excluded:
- Skeletal metastasis
- Primary bone tumour
- Malignant lymphoma
- Severe arthrosis
- Primary hyperparathyroidism and renal osteopathy.

The danger of later transformation to sarcoma is minimal (<1%), particularly in the present era of bisphosphonate therapy. Tumour-associated Paget-like lesions seen on X-rays, CT or scans must be investigated by bone biopsy, but are rare.

32.5.2
Treatment Strategies

Treatment is indicated if there are local changes, pain, and risk of complications that may require neurosurgical or orthopaedic intervention, and if there are high alkaline phosphatase levels (more than 5 U/l). Skeletal deformities and fractures require orthopaedic interventions. Two separate indications for therapy are derived from the clinical course of the disease:
- *Alleviation of symptoms*: severe headaches, backaches and radicular nerve pain
- *Prevention of complications*: fractures, deafness, paralyses, skeletal deformities, sarcomatous transformation

Bisphosphonates are the treatment of choice, and many have been authorized for use in Paget's disease of bone (see below). The latest is zoledronate, and now that this is authorized, therapy of Paget's disease is simplicity itself. For patients with extensive and/or active disease (as indicated by high levels of alkaline phosphatase in serum), intravenous administration is the method of choice. Analgesics or NSAIDs are now rarely required. The following protocols for infusion can be used:

- **Pamidronate (Aredia®)**
  30 mg infusion to begin with, then 60 mg in 500 ml NaCl given slowly for 30–60 min monthly until the pain has been alleviated and the alkaline phosphatase level has returned to normal. Thereafter only regular clinical and biochemical monitoring is required
- **Ibandronate (Bondronat®)**
  Given in 250 ml NaCl infusion for 15 min monthly, 2 mg for the first and 6 mg for subsequent infusions till normalization as above
- **Zoledronate (Aclasta®)**
  5 mg infusion for 15 min. Usually one infusion is enough to normalize the bone markers. Thereafter monitoring as above

Alternatively, oral therapy can be given, preferably one of the potent aminobisphosphonates:

- **Tiludronate (Skelid®)**
  400 mg daily for 3 months
- **Clodronate (Ostac®)**
  800 mg daily for 3 months
- **Alendronate (Fosamax®)**
  40 mg daily for 3 months (authorized in the US)
- **Risedronate (Actonel®)**
  30 mg daily for 2–3 months

Bisphosphonates halt progression and may even induce regression of Paget's disease. This is usually accomplished within 2–6 months depending on the intensity of therapy. Histologically, therapeutic success is indicated by decrease in osteoclast number and formation of lamellar bone. The effects of therapy can last for several years. Should symptoms such as bone pain and/or a rise in markers of bone resorption recur, administration of a bisphosphonate should be repeated. The following markers are generally involved: alkaline phosphatase, osteocalcin and ß-CrossLaps. Therapy with a different bisphosphonate is given if resistance is suspected. Bone scans and X-rays are used to check for spread and/or malignant transformation and should be carried out annually (or semi-annually as required) as part of monitoring of the disease and the efficacy of therapy. Current reviews of Paget's disease have confirmed the long-term safety and efficacy of zoledronic acid 5 mg for attainment of long-lasting remissions.

Periprosthetic Osteoporosis and Aseptic Loosening of Prostheses

33

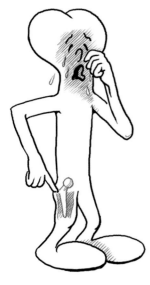

Total joint arthroplasty of the hip and knee has become one of the most frequent and rewarding operations in orthopaedic surgery. Worldwide more than one million such prostheses are implanted annually. With the steady rise in life expectancy, long-term complications related to implant loosening and periprosthetic fractures are on the rise. Efforts to sustain and improve the clinical survival of total joint implants have thus generated great interest.

33.1
Pathogenesis

Stability of the prosthesis within the surrounding bone is the decisive factor for flawless functioning and longevity of the implants. Osteolysis is a multifactorial process stemming from host, prosthesis and surgical factors. Billions of wear particles are generated at material interfaces and are dispersed along the ef-

In collaboration with Christoph Bartl, MD, Department of Orthopaedic and Trauma Surgery, University of Ulm, Germany

fective joint space, into bone and the adjacent soft tissue, inducing an inflammatory reaction that leads to osteoclast activation and finally causing osteolysis. Over time, without proper treatment, osteolysis may progress to aseptic loosening and failure of the implant (Fig. 33.1). Initially most patients may have no clinical symptoms despite radiographic evidence of osteolysis or bone loss. Usually patients only become symptomatic when implant loosening, implant failure or periprosthetic fractures occur.

The main factors involved in periprosthetic osteolysis and aseptic loosening following total joint arthroplasty are (Figs. 33.2 and 33.3):

- *Wear debris-induced osteolysis*: Integration of the implant into the surrounding bone can be hindered by an inflammatory reaction ("foreign body reaction") induced by macrophages absorbing small particles, mainly polyethylene and metallic wear debris, leading to activation of RANKL and OPG which then trigger osteoclastic activity. Another important factor is the inhibition of osteoblast function mediated by wear particles. Finally, osteolysis and bone loss around the implant occur.

- *Micromovement between surfaces*: Implants that do not achieve adequate initial fixation will exhibit micromotion in response to load. The greater the area of friction the more osteoclasts are activated, causing osteolysis around the implant which leads to *fatigue failure at interfaces*. When the distance between bone and implant exceeds 150 μm, connective tissue membranes are formed between implant and bone as well as between implant and cement. These membranes hinder the osteo-integration of the prosthesis. Many biochemical mediators are

R. Bartl, B. Frisch, *Osteoporosis*, DOI 10.1007/978-3-540-79527-8_33,
© Springer-Verlag Berlin Heidelberg 2009

247

33

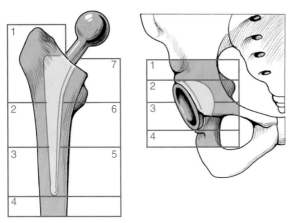

Fig. 33.1. Zones of prosthesis loosening according to Gruen

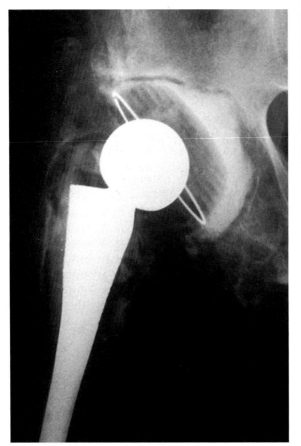

Fig. 33.2. Peri-implant bone resorption ("linear osteolysis") at the interface of the acetabular component, "radiolucent lines"

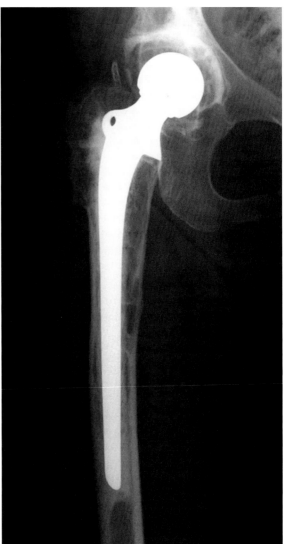

Fig. 33.3. Peri-implant bone resorption at the interface of the femoral ("geographic osteolysis") and acetabular component ("linear osteolysis")

involved: cytokines, prostaglandins, metalloproteases and collagenases.

• *Inappropriate mechanical load and stress shielding*: Insertion of an implant leads to new biome-

chanical relationships between various regions of the surrounding bone and implant. Bone regions around the implant receiving high loads of stress result in bone apposition and higher bone density, whereas bone regions receiving lower stress loading react with bone loss ("*stress shielding*" according to *Wolffs' law*). Appropriate load transmission is an essential factor in maintaining bone volume. Optimal load transfer is influenced by implant design and stiffness of the implant. Bone loss around the implant due to stress shielding can account for up to 50% of the former bone stock in underloaded regions, which has been demonstrated by dual-energy X-ray absorptiometry (DXA) measurements. Finally periprosthetic fractures can occur.

- *Surgical trauma*: Thermic and mechanical necrosis caused by the surgical procedure and cementing techniques alter bone quality.
- *Postoperative immobilization*: The postoperative decrease in weight-bearing results in local immobilization osteoporosis. Overall, postoperative bone loss mainly occurs in the first 6 months and can reach up to 50% of the former bone stock.

33.2
Diagnosis

Slight loosening of the implant remains symptomless for long periods. Significant loosening causes considerable pain on weight-bearing and sudden movements, eventually resulting in a feeling of complete instability. Pain on rotation of the leg in a patient with a hip implant indicates loosening of the shaft and pain on axial compression may indicate loosening of the cup. Radiolucent lines more than 2 mm wide indicate loosening, but localized and limited osteolysis, while incomplete radiolucent lines per se do not constitute evidence of loosening of the implant. Migration of the prosthesis over time is diagnostic: migration of >5 mm indicates loosening. Implant migration indicates local bone loss which is a significant problem in revision surgery. Besides standard radiographs, bone scans are also useful for the detection of regions of high bone turnover around implants, while computed tomography can be used to quantify the amount of bone lost.

33.3
Treatment Strategies

Causative therapy consists of replacing the prosthesis. Indications for this are pain, functional limitations and migration of the implant. Accompanying osteoporosis and loss of bone stock around the implant can turn this operation into a more dangerous and difficult one than the index operation. However, recent advances in technology and materials for cementing may improve long-term results in the future. Intensive research is underway to improve the survival of the implants, including local application of bisphosphonates and implant coating with osteoinductive factors. Implantation of cementless implants is recommended for younger patients with bone of good quality, as less bone is removed, which ensures a more favourable situation if a revision procedure has to be undertaken later.

Various *modifications to improve osteointegration of implants* are under investigation:

- Optimization of prosthetic design with optimal load transfer to the bone
- Better cementing techniques
- Local application of growth factors (hydroxylapatite, TGF-β, BMP-2) as well as parathyroid hormone to improve osteo-integration of the implant.

33.4
Bisphosphonates

Early administration of nitrogen-containing bisphosphonates inhibits peri-implant osteoclastic resorption. This has been demonstrated in numerous animal experiments which showed a decrease in bone loss around the implant. Current clinical studies are hampered by short follow-ups. A recently published meta-analysis of six randomized controlled studies showed that bisphosphonates given in the immediate postoperative period prevented periprosthetic bone loss and resulted in a higher periprosthetic bone mineral density (BMD) at the end of the study period compared to controls.

In cases where total joint arthroplasty is planned, *therapy with bisphosphonates can be given in the following situations*:

- *Underlying systemic or local osteoporosis*: a higher bone density in the perioperative period may reduce the postoperative bone loss and extent of periprosthetic osteolysis.
- *Underlying chronic inflammatory joint disorder*: Inhibition of osteoclasts and suppression of osteoclast activating mediators, as well as an increase in bone density can help to reduce postoperative bone loss and increase the time of implant survival.

33

The following *treatment protocols* are recommended. Dosages and time intervals depend on the type and severity of the underlying condition:

> • **Alendronate (Fosamax®)**
>   70 mg orally once weekly
> • **Risedronate (Actonel®)**
>   35 mg orally once weekly
> • **Pamidronate (Aredia®)**
>   30–60 mg intravenously every 3 months
> • **Ibandronate (Bonviva®)**
>   3 mg intravenously every 3 months
> • **Ibandronate (Bonviva®)**
>   150 mg orally monthly
> • **Zoledronate (Aclasta®)**
>   5 mg intravenously annually

The following *parameters are used to monitor therapy*:

- Clinical examination
- Control radiographs
- DXA (bone densitometry) (Fig. 33.4)
- Markers of bone.

To establish the efficacy of bisphosphonates in preventing bone loss after total joint arthroplasty, more randomized clinical trials with large numbers of patients, long-term follow-up and clinically relevant endpoints (functional outcomes, revision rates) have to be conducted. However, the current results for prevention of periprosthetic bone loss with bisphosphonates are very promising.

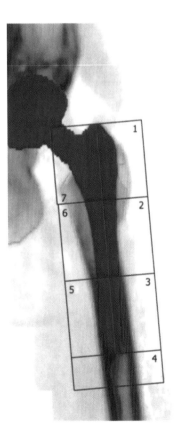

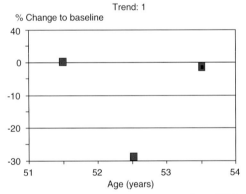

Region	BMD (g/m^2)	BMC (g)	Surface area (cm^2)
1	0.741	1.01	1.37
2	0.946	1.23	1.30
3	1.343	4.10	3.06
4	1.270	5.86	4.61
5	1.414	2.81	1.99
6	1.002	4.21	4.20
7	0.679	1.15	1.70

Trend: 1

Date measure	Age (years)	BMD (g/cm^2)	Change to Baseline (%)	Change to Baseline (%/year)
18.06.2008	53.5	0.741	-1.5	-0.8
20.06.2007	52.5	0.534	-29.0	-28.7
14.06.2006	51.5	0.752	Baseline	Baseline

Fig. 33.4. Dual-energy X-ray absorptiometry monitoring of bone mineral density in periprosthetic region (using Lunar Prodigy): Decrease of bone mineral density (*BMD*) in the first year without bisphosphonate therapy and increase of BMD in the second year under treatment with the bisphosphonate zoledronate 5 mg i.v. annually. *BMC*, bone mineral content

Bone loss in the oral cavity occurs due to many conditions which may be grouped into diseases of bacterial aetiology and oral bone loss associated with systemic disease (e.g. osteoporosis). Periodontitis (parodontitis, paradontosis) is an inflammation of the tissues (the gums) surrounding the teeth, which leads to resorption of the alveolar bone and can progress to abscess formation with loosening and shedding of teeth. Inflammation of the gums with loosening of the teeth is a clear indication for an immediate dual-energy X-ray absorptiometry (DXA), dental investigation and appropriate treatment.

34.1
Oral Bone Loss and Systemic Osteoporosis

It has long been postulated that oral bone loss may be related to systemic conditions which predispose the patient to osteoporosis. Indeed, some of the same risk factors are present. In postmenopausal women, an association between results of systemic measures of osteoporosis (DXA of hip and spine) and oral bone mineral density was demonstrated in several studies. There is also evidence that loss of teeth may be related to systemic bone mass. Some studies also reported a relationship between systemic bone loss and residual ridge resorption.

34.2
Pathogenesis of Periodontitis

Periodontal inflammation is due to bacteria in the plaques on the teeth causing inflammatory reactions and resorption of the alveolar bone of the jaws. Matrix metalloproteinases participate in the destruction of the periodontal tissues by splitting extracellular molecules. Mediators of inflammatory reactions such as prostaglandin (PGE_2), interleukin 1 (IL-1) and tumour necrosis factor (TNF) are also involved in the resorption of the alveolar bone. Other participants in the process are collagenases, macrophages and osteoclasts. The diagnosis is usually not in doubt. Rarely, however, a specific cause may be found, such as for example a patient with Gorham's disease presenting with an osteolytic lesion confined to the mandible. The patient was successfully treated with the bisphosphonate zoledronate.

34.3
Clinical Findings

Examination of the inside of the mouth reveals inflammation, possibly even purulent, of the gums leading to resorption of the alveolar bone surrounding the teeth, which are loosened and may fall out on pressure.

34.4
Treatment Strategies

Elimination of the dental plaque harbouring the bacteria is an essential prerequisite for successful treatment. This is accomplished by mechanical removal, cleansing and topical application of antibiotics such as tetracycline or metronidazole. Non-steroidal anti-inflammatory drugs decrease the level of prostaglandin in the area of the inflamed gums, and thereby reduce the loss of alveolar bone.

34.5
Bisphosphonates

Bisphosphonates minimize resorption and loss of alveolar bone in the inflamed areas. They inhibit both osteoclastic activity and collagenases (metalloproteinases). This has been demonstrated in many studies using oral alendronate preparations.

Local application of bisphosphonates in toothpaste has also been tested. Topical application of etidronate decreases plaque formation and thereby also bacterial infections. Many clinical studies have examined a possible connection between systemic osteoporosis and buccal bone loss leading to loosening and loss of teeth. Presumptive mechanisms include the following: all the bones of the skeleton are affected in generalized osteoporosis, including those of the jaws; therefore, a systemic low bone mass in the skeleton includes the jaw bones so that there is a propensity for the teeth to fall out. Systemic factors which influence systemic bone loss also modify the local tissue reactions to a periodontal infection.

Cases of *osteonecrosis of the jaw* have been reported following treatment with high-dose bisphosphonates, almost exclusively in cancer patients treated intravenously and in the presence of additional risk factors, such as immunosuppression, chemotherapy, corticosteroids and poor oral hygiene (Fig. 34.1a,b). Bisphosphonate-associated osteonecroses of the jaws have been observed mainly in patients receiving high-

dose, long-term i.v. bisphosphonate therapy, rarely in patients on oral therapy. In a study of 335 patients, treatment with alendronate was not associated with a higher incidence of complications secondary to dental procedures, and no cases of osteonecrosis of the jaw were observed. The incidence of tooth loss was decreased by more than 40% in the patients treated with oral alendronate. Therefore, given the large number of women (millions) routinely taking, or who have taken, oral bisphosphonates, the very small risk of developing osteonecrosis should be considered with due regard to the benefit in retarding alveolar bone loss and treating systemic osteoporosis.

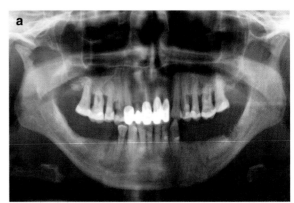

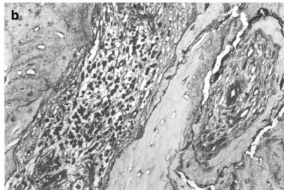

Fig. 34.1a, b. Osteonecrosis of the jaw in a patient with metastatic breast cancer under long-term treatment with i.v. bisphosphonate. (**a**) X-ray showing necrotic area in the left side of the mandible. (**b**) Histology from this area demonstrating necrotic bone tissue with empty osteocytic lacunae and inflammatory reaction in the surrounding marrow, Giemsa staining

35.1
Links Between Osteoporosis and Cancer

Recent studies have raised the question of a possible link between osteoporosis and cancer, as demonstrated by a report on a cohort of 23,935 men and women with osteoporosis who were investigated for risk of cancer. The patients were divided into two groups: up to 70 years of age, who appeared to be at increased risk of cancer; and a second group: older than 70 years who appeared to be at decreased risk of cancer. The results suggested that the risk factors associated with earlier or later onset of osteoporosis were also related to an increased or decreased risk of cancer, respectively.

35.2
Tumour-Induced Hypercalcaemia (TIH)

Hypercalcaemia is found in about 1% of all hospitalized patients, caused by malignancy in 46% of all cases, and by primary hyperparathyroidism (pHPT) in 35%. In the remaining 19%, other conditions are responsible. These include sarcoidosis, immobilization and medications such as thiazides or active metabolites of vitamin D.

Patients with mild hypercalcaemia have no symptoms. The term hypercalcaemic syndrome refers to a constellation of symptoms independent of the aetiology including renal, gastrointestinal and neuro-psychiatric changes. This syndrome has a wide clinical spectrum from asymptomatic to lethal. It is charac-terized by severe dehydration which is caused by the following sequence of events: hypercalcaemia – hypercalciuria – polyuria – polydipsia – polyuria. Nausea and vomiting further increase the fluid and electrolyte loss. The result is hypopotassemia together with disturbances of cardiac rhythm. Moreover, fatigue, depression and a general deceleration of cognitive function indicate additional neuropsychiatric involvement. In severe cases, the condition may progress to a hypercalcaemic crisis with somnolence and coma.

All patients with cancer are subject to hypercalcaemia in the advanced stages of malignancy, in particular patients with breast cancer or with multiple myeloma, less frequently with neoplasms of the lung or prostate. Hypercalcaemic episodes occur in 30% of patients with metastatic tumours and in 50% of patients with multiple myeloma.

Hypercalcaemia of malignancy is characterized by elevation of serum calcium with suppression of normal parathyroid secretion. The increase in serum calcium is due to aggressive local osteolyses, increased renal excretion and increased tubular re-absorption of calcium. *Two types of TIH are recognized*:

- *Osteolytic hypercalcaemia*: Tumour cells in the bone marrow secrete osteoclast-stimulating factors (IL-6, TGF), which stimulate massive osteoclastic resorption with release of calcium from the bone.
- *Humoral hypercalcaemia*: Many tumours produce parathyroid hormone-like substances (PTHrP) which bind to PTH receptors in bone and kidney and trigger the normal physiological effects of PTH (para-neoplastic syndromes). In addition, granulomas, e.g. in tuberculosis, sarcoidosis and sarcomas

R. Bartl, B. Frisch, *Osteoporosis*, DOI 10.1007/978-3-540-79527-8_35,
© Springer-Verlag Berlin Heidelberg 2009

and tumour-induced production of active vitamin D metabolites (e.g. in lymphomas) can lead to hypercalcaemia.

35.2.1
Treatment Strategies in TIH

Bisphosphonates have greatly simplified the treatment of hypercalcaemia. A single 2-h infusion of one of the following is generally effective, especially those with high potency, e.g. ibandronate and zoledronate:

- Clodronate (Ostac®) 1500 mg
- Pamidronate (Aredia®) 90–120 mg
- Ibandronate (Bondronat®) 6 mg
- Zoledronate (Zometa®) 4 mg

After rehydration, the bisphosphonate is infused slowly (1–4 h) in plenty of fluid (e.g. 500 ml of physiological saline), in order to avoid renal damage. The therapeutic activity comes into effect after a delay of 2–4 days (longer with Pamidronate), and normal levels of calcium are obtained within 4–7 days and maintained for a period of several weeks, depending on the aggressivity of the tumour and which of the bisphosphonates was used (zoledronate 88%, ibandronate 78%, pamidronate 70%). Generally, the period of normalization ranges from 2 to 4 weeks, with a success rate of 70–95%. If a satisfactory result is obtained with zoledronate, then the second infusion should be given 7 days later. Treatment is repeated if and when elevation of serum calcium recurs. A dose of 4 mg zoledronate via 15-min infusion is recommended for initial treatment of hypercalcaemia of malignancy (HCM) and 8 mg for relapsed or refractory hypercalcaemia. The median durations of complete responses were 32 (4 mg) and 43 (8 mg) days respectively.

Patients with renal failure should receive 30–50% lower doses, and longer infusion times are recommended (e.g. pamidronate 0.5 mg/min). Disturbances of renal function and/or local side effects at the site of infusion have not been reported for ibandronate. Moreover, as the hypercalcaemia is normalized, an improvement in renal function is also achieved. Bisphosphonate therapy is less effective and of shorter duration

when there is a high level of PTHrP. The extraskeletal effects of PTHrP are not influenced by bisphosphonate therapy. In life-threatening situations, when the level of calcium must be lowered rapidly, the combination of a bisphosphonate with calcitonin is recommended, because this reduces the serum calcium level within a matter of hours by increasing the renal excretion of calcium. The calcitonin acts rapidly and bridges the gap till the bisphosphonate begins to exert its effect.

35.3
Tumour-Induced Bone Pain (TIBP)

Bone pain is the most frequent symptom in patients with osseous metastases. More than 50% of these patients experience bone pain before or at the time of diagnosis of skeletal metastases. The pain is constantly present and may increase in intensity. Multiple myeloma and osteomyelosclerosis are also often accompanied by severe bone pain. Bone pain has a complex, incompletely understood aetiology. Mechanical factors include:
- Increased pressure in the bone marrow
- Bending or distortion of bone
- Stretching of the periosteum and/or endosteum
- Destruction of bone.

Inflammatory, humoral and neural factors also play a role (Fig. 35.1). Prostaglandins, histamine, serotonin, bradykinin and other cytokines can all act as triggers

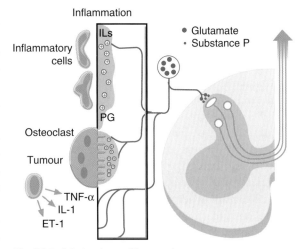

Fig. 35.1. Mechanisms of bone pain

or as modulators. Bone pain is mediated primarily by stimulation of nociceptors (pain receptors) in the periosteal and endosteal sheaths of the bones. It can also be caused by irritation and lesions of the afferent nerve fibres within the bone marrow. These fibres regulate blood flow through bone, bone marrow and sinusoids. Sensory nerve fibres are also present, as demonstrated for example by the pain induced when bone marrow is aspirated. Results of recent studies have implicated the RANKL/OPG system as a major factor in triggering bone pain. Moreover, tumour cells themselves secrete cytokines which stimulate T-lymphocytes and osteoclasts, which leads to further release of inflammatory mediators as bone is resorbed. Generalized bone pain is also caused by the increased pressure resulting from bone marrow infiltration (metastatic, leukaemic) or by oedema of the bone marrow. Paraneoplastic bone pain is mediated indirectly by the tumour by way of the hormone-like substances it secretes.

The *treatment of bone pain* in patients with malignancies should be an integral part of the overall management. Bone pain in cancer patients may have various causes:

- Due to the tumour itself (85%)
- Due to therapy (17%)
- Associated with the tumour (9%)
- Independent of the above (9%).

35.3.1
Treatment Strategies in TIBP

The first aim is elimination of the cause of the bone pain by specific therapy of the condition diagnosed if possible, for example:

- Vitamin D for osteomalacia
- Antibiotics for osteomyelitis
- Radiotherapy for focal neoplastic lesions.

Treatment of tumour-induced bone pain also includes:

- Physical therapy (exercises, physiotherapy)
- Central and peripheral analgesics
- Additional medications (antidepressants, tranquilizers, muscle relaxants)
- Invasive therapy (peridural or intrathecal opioids)
- Antineoplastic therapy (chemo- and radiotherapy)
- Antiresorptive therapy (bisphosphonates, calcitonin).

The alleviation of TIBP by bisphosphonates has been demonstrated in several placebo-controlled clinical trials. The effect is often felt within a day and may last for weeks or months, depending on the dose administered. However, not all physicians, even experts in the field, are aware of the alleviation of bone pain by bisphosphonates. Markers of bone resorption correlate closely with the analgesic effect. Success of bisphosphonate therapy is indicated by:

- Reduction of pain intensity
- Reduction in use of analgesics
- Reduction in need for radiotherapy
- Reduction in surgical interventions.

The following **protocols** are recommended for tumour-induced bone pain:

- **Clodronate (Ostac®)**
  600 mg infusion every 3–4 weeks
- **Clodronate (Ostac®)**
  1600 mg orally daily
- **Pamidronate (Aredia®)**
  60–120 mg infusion every 3–4 weeks
- **Zoledronate (Zometa®)**
  4 mg i.v. infusion every 3–4 weeks
- **Ibandronate (Bondronat®)**
  2–6 mg infusion every 3–4 weeks
- **Ibandronate (Bondronat®)**
  50 mg orally daily

Until recently, bisphosphonates were given when bone pain was presumably caused by osteolytic lesions. Pain induced by osteoblastic metastases, osteomyelosclerosis or systemic mastocytosis also responds rapidly and for long periods to bisphosphonate therapy. In practice, all large studies of metastatic carcinoma and multiple myeloma have confirmed the analgesic effects of bisphosphonates on pain due to osteolytic as well as osteoblastic and mixed metastases. This indicates that relief of bone pain by bisphosphonates is not due exclusively to inhibition of osteoclasts, but that the bisphosphonates also act on other cells such as T-lymphocytes and stromal cells and thereby exert an effect on the RANKL/OPG system.

35.4
Skeletal Manifestations in Multiple Myeloma (MM)

Multiple myeloma is not only a malignant disease of the bone marrow, but it is also a generalized disorder of bone characterized by skeletal destruction (Fig. 35.2). The skeleton must therefore be carefully examined together with investigation of haematopoiesis and the myeloma itself. These investigations should ideally be completed before organ complications have developed so that early preventive and supportive measures can be undertaken. Bone specific findings and symptoms at the time of diagnosis include:

- Bone pain 55%
- Osteolyses 45%
- Osteoporosis 40%
- Spontaneous fractures 18%
- Hypercalcaemia 16%.

A systematic X-ray examination of the axial skeleton is essential for initial diagnosis and monitoring. Bones most frequently affected are those of the skull (Fig. 35.3), thoracic and lumbar vertebrae, followed by other bones which enclose haematopoietic bone marrow. The structure of the osseous lesions is determined by the basic growth pattern of the MM within the bone marrow: osteolyses with the nodular type and osteoporosis with the interstitial type. Osteosclerosis has been found in less than 3% of myeloma patients.

When the histologic *growth pattern of the myeloma* is correlated with osteoclastic bone remodelling, two groups can be distinguished:

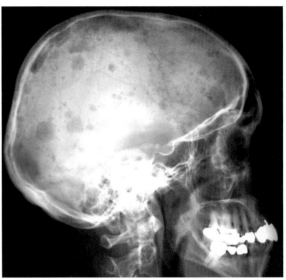

Fig. 35.3. X-ray of skull illustrating typical punched-out lesions in a patient with multiple myeloma

- *Paratrabecular* (Fig. 35.4a,b) and/or nodular growth patterns with high-grade osteoclastic resorption
- *Interstitial* loose infiltration without apparent increased osteoclastic resorption

The first is associated with a distinctly less favourable prognosis, and therapy with bisphosphonates is clearly indicated. Change to an interstitial type under bisphosphonate therapy carries a more favourable prognosis with it.

35.4.1
Treatment Strategies in Skeletal Manifestations of MM

Though chemotherapy reduces the tumour mass considerably, it does little to repair osteolytic bone lesions or to prevent further loss of bone. First-generation bisphosphonates also showed little effect. On the other hand, modern bisphosphonates such as clodronate or pamidronate given intravenously in placebo-controlled trials were effective in the treatment of *skeletal-related events* (SREs). The broad range of indications for therapy with bisphosphonates in myeloma should be taken into account when planning the management of each patient. The effect of ibandronate on osteoclastic bone remodelling and on myeloma cells is impressively demonstrated in Fig. 24.3a,b. Results of previous clinical experience as well as of clinical trials have highlighted the follow-

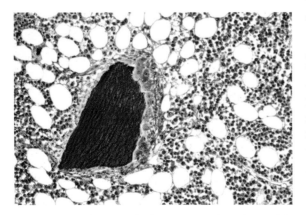

Fig. 35.2. Massive osteoclastic bone resorption of an ossicle with myeloma cells in the vicinity, Gomori staining

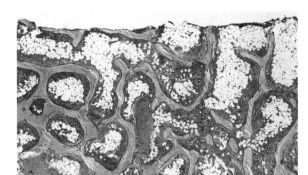

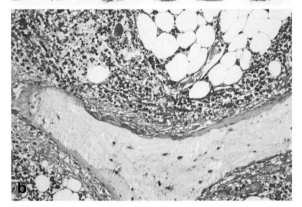

Fig. 35.4. (**a**) Example of paratrabecular infiltration in multiple myeloma and the effect on bone, Giemsa staining. (**b**) Higher magnification showing that the paratrabecular layer of cells consists almost entirely of myeloma cells activating the osteoclastic resorption, Giemsa staining

ing indications for bisphosphonate therapy in multiple myeloma:

- Hypercalcaemia
- Bone pain
- Osteoporoses
- Osteolyses
- After radiotherapy for osteolyses.

The protocols used for therapy of SREs are given below:

- **Pamidronate (Aredia®)**
  60–120 mg infusion every 3–4 months
- **Clodronate (Ostac®, Bonefos®)**
  600–900 mg infusion every 3–4 months
- **Ibandronate (Bondronat®)**
  6 mg infusion every 3–4 months or 50 mg orally daily
- **Zoledronate (Zometa®)**
  4 mg infusion every 3–4 months

In the case of dehydration and/or hypercalcaemia, infusion of a bisphosphonate should be carried out after rehydration and slowly to avoid renal damage, which is almost the rule in myeloma. Therefore, it is always best to choose bisphosphonates with the longest half-life in the serum to minimize the possible renal damage. The significance of bisphosphonate therapy in multiple myeloma lies in *prevention of skeletal complications*. Institution of bisphosphonate therapy at the time of diagnosis will lead to significant abrogation or at least to a clearly delayed appearance of skeletal complications, such as osteolysis, osteoporosis, fractures, hypercalcaemia and bone pain. Furthermore, it has been demonstrated conclusively that the aminobisphosphonates exert an *antiproliferative effect on tumour cells*, i.e. they inhibit growth of myeloma cells both directly and indirectly as described below. Therapy with zoledronate or ibandronate triggered a number of activities which were even enhanced when dexamethasone or chemotherapy with paclitaxel was added:

- Increased apoptosis of myeloma cells
- Reduction of osteoclastic and stromal cell production of IL-6
- Anti-angiogenic effect on blood vessels and stromal cells (changes similar to those seen after therapy with thalidomide)
- Cytotoxic effect on myeloma cells through activation of T-lymphocytes
- Interference with cellular interactions such as:
  - Inhibition of matrix metalloproteinase-1 secretion (stimulated by IL-1).

35.5
Skeletal Metastases –
The Fundamental Problem
in Clinical Oncology

Metastasis is a fundamental problem in clinical oncology. Once established in the skeleton or elsewhere, the malignancy is systemic and can no longer be cured by surgery alone. This is the reason that tumours are regarded as systemic from the moment osseous or other metastases are detected. Some even consider all malignant tumours as systemic from the moment they are established and certainly as soon as they have attained a clinically detectable size.

Skeletal metastases can remain dormant and symptomless for many years. But when they begin to spread, metastases cause a drastic reduction of the patient's quality of life due to complications such as pain, immobility, fractures, spinal cord compression, hypercalcaemia and haematopoietic insufficiency. The situation is made even worse by the fear, depression and hopelessness which inevitably accompany the physical condition. Prevention of metastatic spread is as yet unattainable simply because it has already occurred in many patients before the tumour itself was diagnosed. Studies have shown that over 10% of patients with breast cancer have metastases which have been dormant for over 10 years. Cases of recurrence of metastatic spread after more than 20 years (or even longer) have also been reported. What intrinsic and/or extrinsic factors enable malignant cells to survive in a state of "hibernation" or dormancy, and what events/circumstances trigger their subsequent awakening and renewed growth have not yet been completely elucidated.

The lungs, liver and bone marrow act as filters for disseminated circulating malignant cells and are the most frequent sites for hematogenic spread. Of these, the bone/bone marrow environment offers ideal conditions for establishment of metastases. However, the frequency of metastatic involvement of the skeleton at autopsy varies from 25 to 85%, probably due to differences in the method and thoroughness of search. Skeletal metastases are found at autopsy in 70%–85% of patients with tumours of the breast, prostate and lung, but fewer than half of these had been recognized clinically during the patients' lifetime. The overall impression from previous studies is that up to 90% of all patients who die of malignant tumours had skeletal metastases. Certain tumours exhibit *osteotropism*, that is, a particular affinity to metastasize to the bones. These include tumours of the breast, prostate, lung, kidney and thyroid, and they are responsible for over 80% of all metastases in bone.

Metastases "home" to bones which house red haematopoietic marrow (Fig. 35.5a,b). Several factors are responsible for this proclivity: the extensive vascular system, the thin vascular walls, often without a basal membrane, and the slow blood flow through the sinusoids in the bone marrow. These are ideal conditions for intravascular tumour cells to migrate into the surrounding tissues and to implant, i.e. establish themselves ("seed and soil" hypothesis). A greater understanding of the molecular mechanisms of skel-

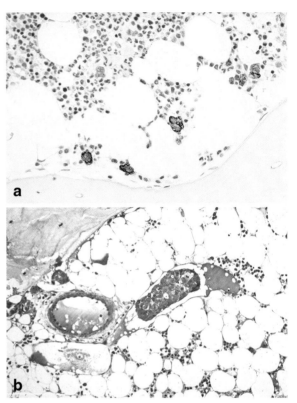

Fig. 35.5 a,b. Initial stages in the process of establishment of metastases in the bone marrow. (**a**) Dissemination of tumour cells in the bone marrow and incipient adhesion to the surface of the bone (immunohistology). (**b**) Large intravascular tumour embolus and small interstitial clusters of tumour cells in hypocellular bone marrow, Giemsa staining

etal metastases is expected to lead to the development of more targeted therapy. Some progress has already been made with respect to factors released by the tumour cells, the bone cells and the environmental mesenchymal cells. Tumour cells produce predominantly growth factors and cytokines that stimulate either osteoclasts or osteoblasts. Growth factors re-

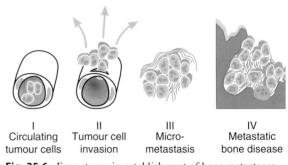

I	II	III	IV
Circulating tumour cells	Tumour cell invasion	Micro-metastasis	Metastatic bone disease

Fig. 35.6. Four stages in establishment of bone metastases

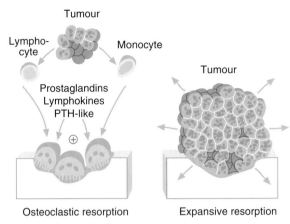

Fig. 35.7. Cells and factors involved in metastatic osteolysis and bone loss: two types of mechanisms

Table 35.1. Histologic bone reactions in various primary tumours (% of cases with metastatic bone disease)

	Breast	Prostate	Bronchus
Normal	5	0	28
Osteoporosis/lysis	20	7	18
Mixed form	41	38	27
Trabecular sclerosis	22	0	26
Woven bone	12	55	0

approach – to inhibit tumour growth by targeting the bone marrow microenvironment.

As outlined above, an *osseous reaction* with markedly increased remodelling, particularly resorption, occurs in 93% of patients with skeletal metastases, and bone turnover markers are used for diagnosis, prognosis and as predictors of skeletal complications in many solid tumours. Two types of bone resorption in metastatic bone disease are known: osteoclastic and expansive by the tumour cells themselves (Figs. 35.7 and 35.8a,b). The type of osseous reactions to the metastases depends on the primary tumour. Usually osteoclastic resorption is accompanied by osteoblastic formation. Metastases of breast cancer exhibit this mixed osteoclastic/osteoblastic reaction, while the metastases of prostatic carcinomas evoke an almost exclusively osteoblastic reaction with production of woven bone (Table 35.1).

leased from the bone matrix support and maintain the tumour cells themselves – a kind of vicious cycle is established whereby the environment and the metastases support each other (Fig. 35.6). The elucidation of this process has suggested new therapeutic avenues of

35.6
Skeletal Metastases of Breast and Prostate Cancer

35.6.1
Bone Reactions in Breast Cancer

Mammary carcinoma is the most frequent malignant tumour in women. It effects one out of ten women, is fatal in 30% of cases and over 75% of patients will have osseous metastases with progression of the disease. The average survival after the appearance of osseous metastases is approximately 2–3 years. The prognosis is much worse (only a few months) when visceral metastases have occurred.

Destruction of bone and replacement of haematopoietic tissue by the tumour or by the cytotoxic effects of chemotherapy, or both, lead to the following complications:

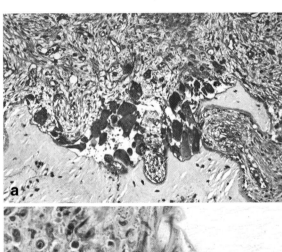

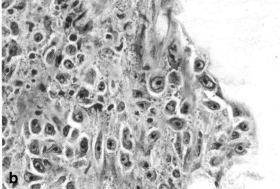

Fig. 35.8a,b. Iliac crest biopsies illustrating (**a**) osteoclastic and (**b**) direct tumour cell osteolyses in metastatic bone disease, all Giemsa staining

35

- Bone pain 60–80%
- Osteoporosis 40–50%
- Pathologic fractures 10–30%
- Hypercalcaemia 10–30%
- Bone marrow failure 20%
- Spinal cord compression 10%.

35.6.2
Treatment Strategies in Metastatic Breast Cancer

Before beginning therapy for breast cancer, certain goals are set:

- Prevention of development of metastasis by tumour cells already dispersed in the body.
- Treatment of micrometastases and prevention of skeletal destruction once bone marrow involvement has been detected, for example, by MRI, bone scan or bone biopsy. The efficacy of bisphosphonates in this setting has already established.
- Prevention and treatment of osteoporosis: It should be noted that bone loss may be due to the patient's age, to the disease itself and to therapy, any or all of which can cause osteoporosis resulting in pathologic fractures. Recent studies have indicated that this bone loss can be prevented by bisphosphonates, and skeletal integrity maintained.
- Treatment of pre-existing skeletal complications, as in patients with advanced breast cancer or complications associated with radiotherapy or other procedures (palliative treatment). Administration of

bisphosphonates after radiotherapy can accelerate the re-calcification of osteolytic lesions after radiation.
- Prophylaxis with bisphosphonates is becoming ever more significant, also in view of the minimal side effects of these drugs.
- On completion of radio- and chemotherapy, after surgery, treatment with aromatase inhibitors, anastrazole or letrozole, is initiated. Bisphosphonate therapy is continued as long as this treatment is continued, for up to 5 years. Results of a study with zoledronic acid 4 mg given bi-annually by i.v. infusion for 5 years have documented the prevention of bone loss in these postmenopausal patients on therapy with letrozole after the first year of therapy.

35.6.3
Bisphosphonates for the Prevention of Metastasis

Bisphosphonates form an integral part of the management of breast cancer (Fig. 35.9). Clinical studies of patients treated with clodronate over a 3-year period have shown a 50% reduction in skeletal metastases. The survival time of patients on long-term therapy with clodronate or ibandronate was significantly increased. However, these studies did not produce uniform results with respect to visceral metastases and survival. It is clear that patients who had circulating tumour cells or high levels of bone sialoprotein (BSP) benefit most from this type of adjuvant therapy. BSPs are produced by osteoclasts and tumour cells and play

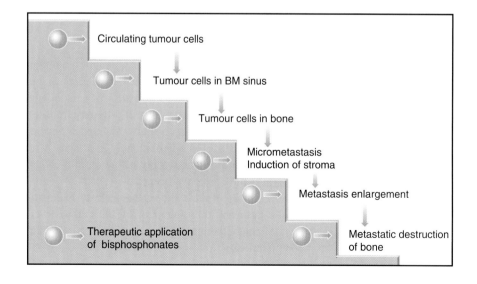

Fig. 35.9. Cascade of reactions in the development of skeletal metastases and the inhibitory effects of bisphosphonates. *BM*, bone marrow

an important part in cell–matrix interactions in bone, e.g. adhesion of osteoclasts to collagen type I.

35.6.4
Bisphosphonates for the Prevention of Skeletal Complications

Micrometastases – as well as larger established metastases – are demonstrable on MRI, tumour markers in blood and by bone biopsy. At this point, these metastases have not evoked any osseous reactions demonstrable by bone scan or X-ray, and administration of bisphosphonates can prevent their establishment and development on and in the bones.

35.6.5
Bisphosphonates for the Treatment of Skeletal Complications

Bisphosphonates have strong antiresorptive effects and also some degree of osteoreparative (recalcification) effect (Fig. 35.10). They can prevent unwanted bone loss following radiotherapy. Administration of bisphosphonates leads to increased formation of callus which accelerates healing of bone defects. A dose of 1000 IU vitamin D daily (after exclusion of hypercalcaemia!) promotes mineralization of the newly formed bone. However, since complete restoration of normal bone structure in large osteolytic lesions can take years, it is all the more important to prevent them. Previous studies have shown that bisphosphonates can prevent SREs: new osteolytic lesions, pathologic fractures, hypercalcaemia, spinal cord compression and bone pain, thereby reducing the need for surgery and radiotherapy. Clinical studies on the renal safety and the efficacy of bisphosphonates in patients treated for over 10 years have now been published. A modest increase in survival of premenopausal patients was also observed. Administration of a bisphosphonate such as clodronate together with irradiation of an osteolytic lesion is thought to have an additive effect. The presence of visceral metastases, though probably predictive of a shorter survival, is no justification for not giving bisphosphonates. In addition, numerous articles from many countries have now confirmed the efficacy of bisphosphonates for skeletal protection in patients with breast cancer. Many have emphasized the efficacy of early administration of bisphospho-

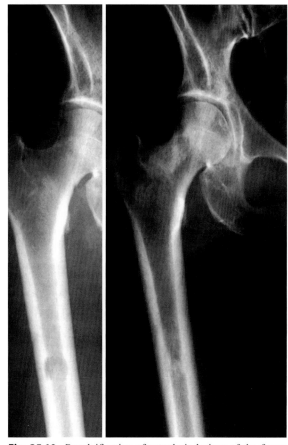

Fig. 35.10. Recalcification of osteolytic lesions of the femur under bisphosphonate and chemotherapy in a patient with metastatic breast cancer

nates, for example immediately following neoadjuvant chemotherapy, to evaluate effects on cellular apoptosis, proliferation and on angiogenesis, in addition to the effects on the actions of the bone cells for prevention of the osteoblastic and/or osteolytic effects stimulated by the tumour cells.

Treatment of skeletal complications is best achieved by monthly intravenous or daily oral administration of bisphosphonates:

- **Pamidronate (Aredia®)**
  90 mg infusion monthly
- **Ibandronate (Bondronat®)**
  6 mg infusion monthly
- **Ibandronate (Bondronat®)**
  50 mg orally daily
- **Zoledronate (Zometa®)**
  4 mg infusion monthly

These protocols automatically include both treatment and prevention of osteoporosis; note that both oral and i.v. administration are now available. The optimal duration of bisphosphonate therapy in this clinical setting has not yet been established. A diet rich in calcium and a vitamin D supplement should also be prescribed after exclusion of hypercalcaemia.

35.6.6
Bone Reactions in Prostatic Cancer

A total of 10–20% of patients with prostatic cancer have bone metastases at the time of diagnosis; some may be small. Consequently, whole-body MRI has been advocated for complete as possible detection of skeletal metastases of prostate cancer. Moreover, the simultaneous demonstration of associated skeletal complications is an advantage. Whereas osteolytic lesions predominate in multiple myeloma and breast cancer, metastases of prostatic cancer are characterized by their osteoblastic reactions evoked by a number of mediators (Fig. 35.11).

In spite of the preponderance of bone formation, bisphosphonates are also indicated both as a preventive and a palliative measure due to the significant role played by the osteoclasts because of the "coupling" of processes involved in bone remodelling even in these metastases. Moreover, experimental studies have shown that the tumour cells can produce the receptor activator of RANKL, which activates osteoclasts.

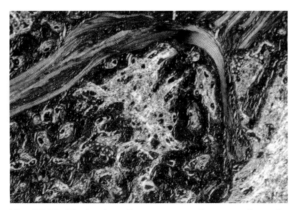

Fig. 35.11. Diminution of marrow space by woven bone deposited on the lamellar trabecula, as well as in the marrow space in a patient with skeletal metastases of prostate carcinoma, Gomori staining polarization

Matrix metalloproteinases, which degrade bone matrix, are also secreted by the prostatic tumour cells. Moreover, after therapy with bisphosphonates, a rapid and prolonged alleviation of pain, together with a reduction in requirements of analgesics, has been reported by patients with prostatic skeletal metastases. The improvement in the pain score also coincides with a decrease in resorption products in blood and urine. The considerable risk of osteoporosis due to therapeutic hypogonadism constitutes another justification for the early initiation of bisphosphonate therapy. The effects of androgen deprivation therapy are far reaching including changes in body composition: lean mass, fat mass and muscle mass, as well as reduction in BMD. Encouraging results have already been obtained with high doses of parenteral clodronate, alendronate, pamidronate and ibandronate. Bisphosphonate treatment of painful osseous metastases due to hormone refractory prostate cancer resulted in a significant decrease in pain and a corresponding significant reduction in the daily consumption of analgetics in 75% of patients. Each parameter correlated with an increase in the Karnofsky index, mainly due to better mobility. Therefore, bisphosphonates have a definite role in the palliative management of symptomatic hormone refractory prostate cancer. It has already been established that therapy with bisphosphonates decreases the risk of skeletal complications in men with androgen independent prostate cancer and bone metastases. Moreover, preliminary trials of chemotherapy (taxane) together with a bisphosphonate (zoledronate) have shown good results, as have preliminary results of therapy with denosumab, a human monoclonal antibody to RANKL.

Consensus Guidelines have recently been published for the introduction of bisphosphonates into the management of metastasizing cancers (Berensen 2005). Studies on the benefits of zoledronate in the prevention of skeletal complications have already been published. In addition, studies aimed at the prevention of skeletal metastases are currently under way with ibandronate. A retrospective analysis of patients with non-small cell lung cancer treated with zoledronate for 21 months showed a statistically significant correlation between the therapy and increased survival. It should also be mentioned that zoledronate is the only bisphosphonate that has demonstrated statistically significant long-term benefits in patients with renal cell carcinoma. New Consensus Guidelines on the use of bisphosphonates in solid tumours have just been published.

Finally, a word of caution: the possibility of bisphosphonate-induced *necrosis of the jaws* (ONJ) must not be forgotten when giving potent bisphosphonates, especially intravenously. The patient must be fully informed, consultation with the dentist is strongly recommended, and a consent form must be signed before therapy is started, particularly if used for indications not yet completely authorized. Therefore, it is advisable to check whether administration of bisphosphonates for the prevention of metastases in patients with the tumours mentioned above has already been authorized, as for example zoledronate for treatment of patients with bone metastases in the US. The efficacy of bisphosphonates for prevention of skeletal metastases is now being investigated in many clinical trials and results are awaited. Treatment-induced bone loss can also occur in cancers other than those mentioned above, for example certain sarcomas.

One last important group comprises the *long-term cancer survivors*, who should be regularly monitored for the state of the skeleton, so that timely preventive therapy can be given if and when required. This applies to children as well as to adults. Finally, in certain specific cases, tumour-induced skeletal destruction may require a completely different approach, for example in the case of malignant vertebral compression fractures: radionuclide therapy for the malignant cells and injection of polymethyl methacrylate to support the vertebral body. Studies for the optimal treatment of such fractures are underway.

The first systematic review of cardiovascular risk factors, with insulin resistance as a common denominator, was published in 1988 by G. Reaven under the title of "Syndrome X". Since then, recognition and identification of Syndrome X, known today as the *metabolic syndrome* (MetSyn) has been steadily increasing, especially during the first decade of the 21st century. It should be emphasized that this steady increase parallels the increase in obesity almost the world over, in the developed countries, but also in the so-called underdeveloped countries. It is important to stress that all ages may be affected by obesity from the youngest of the young to the oldest of the old. Therefore, all ages are also vulnerable to the consequences of obesity including the MetSyn and the risk factors for cardiovascular disease, as well as metabolic bone disorders including osteoporosis that it represents. The MetSyn is also a representative of the up-to-date disease classification now being applied as more comprehensive information on the basic underlying physio-pathological pathways leading to disorders and diseases has become available, and is still being revealed by the ongoing investigations.

Recent (2008) estimates of the *prevalence of obesity* in the populations of some countries include the following:

USA	24–33% of both genders
Netherlands	23–37%
Spain	19% male and 6% female
Germany	42%
European Union in general	25% of both genders
Arabian oil-rich countries	30% male and 40% female
Taiwan	4–22% of both genders

Even though these values depend on different criteria, they demonstrate unequivocally the high numbers of obese people in many parts of the world today.

Varying *definitions of the MetSyn* have been proposed, of which the following three are widely used internationally, though many countries have published their own versions:
● World Health Organization (WHO).
● National Cholesterol Education Program Adult Treatment Panel 111 (NCEP-ATP-111).
● 3rd International Diabetes Federation (IDF).

Some investigators in the US have also utilized the US National Health and Nutrition Evaluation Survey (NHANES) to define the MetSyn. However, it should be clearly stated that each of these definitions has its own values for the criteria used: for example differences in the cut-off values of waist circumference, an indication of visceral obesity. Therefore, there may be significant differences in the results of investigations depending on which definitions and criteria were applied, even to the same participants. For example, a lower waist cut-off value would include significantly more participants with MetSyn than a higher cut-off value! In the latest edition of the *Merck Manual*, the MetSyn is described as follows:

"The Metabolic Syndrome is characterized by excess abdominal fat causing at least two of the following: insulin resistance, dyslipidemia, and hypertension. Causes, complications, diagnosis and treatments are similar to those of obesity." Dyslipidemia itself is also a risk factor for osteoporosis. In addition, the *Merck*

Manual lists the following *criteria* for diagnosis of the Meta Syn:

- Waist circumference, cut-off values (cm) 102 cm for men, 88 cm for women
- Fasting glucose (mg/dl) >110 mg/dl
- 2-h postprandial glucose >140 mg/dl
- Blood pressure mmHg >139/85
- Triglycerides, fasting >150 mg/dl
- Low density lipoprotein (LDL) cholesterol >100 mg/dl
- High density lipoprotein (HDL) cholesterol <40 mg/dl for men, <50 mg/dl for women
- Increases in bone mass index (BMI) >35, and body fat distribution (Fig. 36.1a–c)

It has been suggested that the simple measurements of BMI, waist circumference and blood pressure will identify most young adults with MetSyn and therefore at risk for type 2 diabetes and cardiovascular disease, as well as the consequences of both. Additional criteria can then be evaluated in the positive patients so that preventive strategies can immediately be initiated. The *Merck Manual* also states that the syndrome is very common and, as an example, that possibly almost half of people over 50 years of age in the US are affected.

The excess abdominal fat (Fig. 36.1a–c) in obese patients eventually leads to hepatic and muscular insulin resistance, to hyperglycaemia, to hyperinsulinemia, to dyslipidaemias and to hypertension, resulting in diabetes mellitus and cardiovascular diseases – the latter two both being risk factors for osteoporosis. Additionally, uric acid levels in the serum are elevated and a prothrombotic state may develop, thereby indicating involvement of the renal and haematopoietic systems, which in turn are interwoven with the metabolism of the bones as witnessed by renal osteodystrophy, osteopenia and osteoporosis. The immune system is also involved in the MetSyn, with increases in inflammatory cytokines, and clearly this also affects the metabolism of the bones, resulting in osteopenia/osteoporosis, among other osteodystrophies.

It has been suggested that the peroxisome proliferator-activated receptors (PPARS) play an important part in the pathogenesis of the MetSyn. The PPARS are a sub-group of the nuclear hormone receptor family of ligand-activated transcription factors. The PPARS have been implicated in diabetic nephropathy, glomerulosclerosis and progression of renal disease with its accompanying osteodystrophy. Cystatin C is

also associated with the MetSyn in dyslipidaemic patients as a significant marker for risk of cardiovascular and renal disease. The MetSyn itself has been implicated in the pathogenesis of chronic hepatitis C (CHC) as well as non-alcoholic liver disease.

The bone mineral density (BMD) and fracture risk in patients with the MetSyn is determined by the balance between the "beneficial" effects of obesity and the detrimental effects of hyperglycaemia, and when the latter prevails osteoporosis results. Many other factors, conditions and disorders are associated with the MetSyn, but only some can be mentioned in this brief review: calcium homeostasis, levels of vitamin D and parathyroid hormone, neuro-endocrine factors, androgen deprivation therapy, endothelial cell dysfunction as an initial step in atherosclerosis, bi-polar disorders, polycystic ovary syndrome and psoriasis in the adolescent population. The bones may be affected in all of them.

Increases in BMI and the waist circumference in any patient are frequently regarded as signs that the patient should be screened for the MetSyn, utilizing one of the recognized definitions, so that appropriate preventive measures can immediately be initiated if the results are positive.

According to some authorities, the MetSyn is currently considered the most important public health threat of the 21st century.

It has been estimated that in patients with the MetSyn the risk of cardiovascular disease and diabetes is increased 1.5- to 2-fold. Nevertheless, many questions still remain unresolved in spite of the astronomical amount of work already published. There are concerns about the criteria applied, for which there is no consensus as yet, and there are some investigators (a minority), who even question whether the diagnosis of MetSyn has any additional value in clinical practice today. However, taking into account the high estimated percentages of obese people in many populations, the recognition of the MetSyn as a direct consequence of obesity provides an unparalleled and highly significant opportunity for dissemination of widespread information and knowledge, for early diagnosis and application of effective preventive measures to decrease the incidence of cardiovascular morbidities – the number one killer (medically speaking) in the world today!

Moreover, as pointed out in numerous investigations, there are many diseases associated with

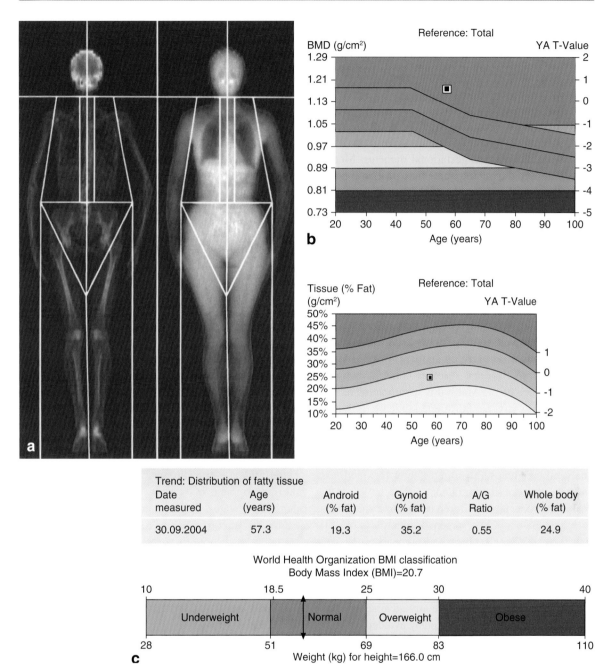

Fig. 36.1. (a) Dual-energy X-ray absorptiometry measurement (Lunar Prodigy Advance) of the total body used for measuring bone density and body composition. (b) Measurement of BMD of total hip (c) Measurement of the body mass index and the percentages of body fat in the different areas (gynoid versus android), important cardiovascular risk factors in the metabolic syndrome

increased body weight and increased BMI: life span is shortened and the risk of sudden death is increased. In addition to all the varieties of cardiovascular disorders, as well as diabetes and its accompanying co-morbidities including osteoporosis, studies have demonstrated that osteoarthritis, sleep apnoea and certain forms of cancer are also increased. In the human body many metabolic and immune response pathways are highly integrated and the proper function of the one is dependent on that of the other.

These interwoven pathways can be viewed as central homeostatic mechanisms, the dysfunctions of which lead to chronic metabolic disorders such as the MetSyn and its consequences, hence the current threat to global human health.

It is of interest that there is a relationship between *gestational diabetes* and the MetSyn, as demonstrated by the results of a case control study of 58 women with and 58 women without gestational diabetes. MetSyn was diagnosed during the immediate postnatal period using the criteria of the National Cholesterol Education Program (NCEP-ATP111) only in the study group but not in the controls.

As mentioned previously, the MetSyn also occurs even in *very young children*. A Chinese study of the MetSyn in obese children born large for gestational age showed that in this group the prevalence was 65%, significantly lower than the 45% for children born with size appropriate for gestational age. Moreover, hypertension and hypertriglyceridaemia with its risk of osteoporosis were components of the MetSyn in these obese children. Another study investigated the prevalence of the MetSyn in a sample of racially and ethnically diverse 8th grade students in the US: 9.5% of the youths were positive using the IDF criteria. The parameters evaluated included: height, weight and waist circumference; fasting blood samples were analyzed for glucose, insulin, a factor for insulin resistance, and for lipids. Other reports have emphasized that overweight children belong to a special risk category and should be screened, regardless of other risk factors. These reports also emphasize the need for early prevention by means of adherence to dietary guidelines, physical activity and other lifestyle factors. This is particularly important in children who are still growing and therefore any adverse effect on the skeleton should be scrupulously avoided. Initiated early enough, these simple measures have already proven to be highly effective. However, as in practically everything else, there are exceptions. A cohort of Australian Aboriginal children age 9–14 years was studied: 14% had MetSyn, 6.4% were overweight, 4.9% were obese and 26.2% had an elevated waist circumference. However, >50% of the children with MetSyn were neither overweight nor obese, although a tendency for central obesity was already evident in these children, indicating that measurement of waist circumference would help to identify children at high risk of MetSyn and therefore of deleterious effects on

the bones. Results of other investigations have shown that changes in plasma lipids and lipid fractions also appear to be early markers of the MetSyn with risk of osteoporosis in obese prepubertal children. If left untreated, these children might not attain an adequate peak bone mass.

Quite a number of investigations have been carried out on the *genetics* of MetSyn. However, to date, no single gene or cluster of genes has been consistently replicated for the MetSyn among different populations, possibly due to the complex interplay between genes and environment which occurs for expression of the MetSyn, and possibly also due to the lack of agreement on the definition of the phenotype. Moreover, some authors have advocated investigation of the various components of the MetSyn separately. New experimental approaches, such as combination of gene expression profiling with linkage and correlation analyses, among others, are expected to yield positive results. Additional studies have already demonstrated a potential involvement of the Il-15 pathway with muscle and bone phenotypes and with predictors of the MetSyn. A single gene defect in Wnt signalling has also been linked to coronary artery disease and multiple cardiovascular risk factors.

Many *associations of the MetSyn with other disease* entities have also been described in specific racial and/or ethnic groups. To mention but a few: the development of chronic kidney disease (CKD), depressive states, inflammatory conditions, risk of cataract extraction and severe periodontitis, which in turn may predispose to osteonecrosis of the jaw bones in patients with other contributory factors, such as a malignancy under treatment with intravenous chemotherapy.

Finally, a practical approach to the MetSyn (Blaha et. al. 2008): After studying numerous publications from January 1988 to December 2007, the authors have outlined a comprehensive management plan: the ABCDE approach. The motive and goals were and are to increase awareness of the inherent dangers in obesity and to aid the general public, and particularly doctors, to recognize the risks of obesity and to stimulate early diagnosis and immediate initiation of preventive measures and of management strategies according to the ancient proverb: *Prevention is better than cure!*

The *ABCDE approach*:

"A" for assessment of cardiovascular risk and aspirin therapy

"B" for blood pressure control

"C" for cholesterol management

"D" for diabetes prevention and dietary advice and recommendations

"E" for exercise therapy: turn fat into muscles and energy!

The authors regard this alphabetical approach as a practical framework for recognition, diagnosis and implementation of a comprehensive evidence-based management plan for the reduction of cardiovascular risk and its consequences on a large scale.

To end on an optimistic note: recent studies have demonstrated multiple beneficial effects of moderate wine consumption in the protection against development of the MetSyn and its related medical complications, including osteoporosis.

So let's raise a glass and drink to everybody's good health!

Bibliography

Introduction

The most relevant and useful books and articles are given at the end of the text. The 42 books listed contain comprehensive summaries and reviews of the different aspects of osteoporosis published over the past 10 years or so. They also contain extensive and exhaustive reference lists.

In addition to the other books recently published (not listed here), an astronomical number of articles on all aspects of osteoporosis has appeared in the international literature. These are readily available over the internet. For example, the key words "disorders of bone" yielded over 144,936 citations and of these more than 3600 for 2008 alone! Consequently, it is clearly impossible to cite all or even most of the very recent and up-to-date articles, with the result that only a few could be listed. An attempt has been made to include articles which made specific points appearing in the text.

Books on Osteoporosis

1. Arden N (2006) Osteoporosis. Remedica, London
2. Avioli L (2000) The osteoporotic syndrome. Academic Press, San Diego
3. Avioli L, Krane S (1997) Metabolic bone disease and clinically related disorders. Academic Press, San Diego
4. Barlow D, Francis R, Miles A (2001) The effective management of osteoporosis. Aesculapius Medical Press, London San Francisco Sydney
5. Bartl R (2008) Osteoporose – Prävention, Diagnostik, Therapie. 3. Auflage, Thieme, Stuttgart New York
6. Bartl R (2006) Antiosteoporotika. Wissenschaftliche Verlagsgesellschaft, Stuttgart
7. Bartl R, Frisch B (1993) Biopsy of bone in internal medicine – an atlas and sourcebook. Kluwer Academic Publishers, Dordrecht Boston London
8. Bartl R, Frisch B (2002) Bisphosphonates for bones: guidelines for treatment in all medical disciplines. Blackwell, Berlin
9. Bartl R, Frisch B (2004) Osteoporosis, prevention, diagnosis, therapy. Springer, Berlin Heidelberg New York
10. Bartl R, Frisch B, von Tresckow E, Bartl C (2007) Bisphosphonates in medical practice. Springer, Berlin Heidelberg New York
11. Bilezikian J, Raisz L, Martin J (2008) Principles of bone biology, 3rd edn. Academic Press, San Diego
12. Cooper C, Woolf A (2006) Osteoporosis. Elsevier, Edinburgh
13. Cummings S, Cosman F, Jamal S (2002) Osteoporosis: an evidence-based guide to prevention and therapy. American College of Physicians, Philadelphia
14. Duque G, Kiel D (2008) Osteoporosis in older persons. Springer, London
15. Eastell R, Baumann M, Hoyle N, Wieczorek L (eds) (2001) Bone markers, biochemical and clinical perspectives. Martin Dunitz, London

16. Favus MJ (Ed) (1999) Primer on the metabolic bone diseases and disorders of mineral metabolism. Lippincott, Philadelphia

17. Fleisch H (2000): Bisphosphonates in bone disease, 4th edn, Academic Press, San Diego

18. Frisch B, Bartl R (1998) Biopsy interpretation of bone and bone marrow. Arnold, London

19. Geusens P, Sambrook P, Lindsay R (eds) (2005) Osteoporosis in clinical practice. Springer, Berlin Heidelberg New York

20. Grampp S (2003) Radiology of osteoporosis. Springer, Berlin Heidelberg New York

21. Gueldner S, Grabo T, Newman E, Cooper D (2008) Osteoporosis, clinical guidelines for prevention, diagnosis, and management. Springer, Berlin Heidelberg New York

22. Henderson JE, Goltzman D (eds) (2000) The osteoporosis primer. Cambridge University Press, Cambridge

23. Hosking D, Ringe J (2000) Treatment of metabolic bone disease – management strategy and drug therapy. Martin Dunitz, London

24. Kanis J (1998) Pathophysiology and treatment of Paget's disease of bone, 2nd edn. Martin Dunitz, London

25. Kleerekoper M (2005) Drug therapy for osteoporosis. Taylor & Francis, London

26. Kleerekoper M, Siris E, McClung M (eds) (1999) The bone and mineral manual. Academic Press, London

27. Lanham-New S, O´Neill T, Morris R et al. (2007) Managing osteoporosis. Clinical Publishing, Oxford

28. Marcus R (2008) Osteoporosis. Academic Press, San Diego

29. Marcus R, Feldman D, Kelsey J (eds) (1996) Osteoporosis. Academic Press, San Diego

30. Martin B, Burr D, Sharkey N (1998) Skeletal tissue mechanics. Springer, Berlin Heidelberg New York

31. McDermott M, Zapalowski C, Miller P (eds) (2004) Osteoporosis. Hanley & Belfus, St. Louis

32. McIlwain H, Bruce D (1999) The osteoporosis cure. Avon Books, New York

33. Meunier PJ (1998) Osteoporosis: diagnosis and management. Martin Dunitz, London

34. Mundy G (1999) Bone remodelling and its disorders, 2nd edn. Martin Dunitz, London

35. Notelovitz M (1999) Osteoporosis: prevention, diagnosis and management. Professional Communications, Caddo

36. Orwoll E (Ed) (1999) Osteoporosis in men. Academic Press, San Diego

37. Riggs B, Melton L (1995) Osteoporosis etiology, diagnosis and management, 2nd edn. Lippincott-Raven, Philadelphia

38. Ringe J, Meunier P (1996) Osteoporotic fractures in the elderly. Thieme, Stuttgart

39. Rosen C, Glowacki J, Bilzikian J (eds) (1999) The aging skeleton. Academic Press, San Diego

40. Rubens R, Mundy G (Eds) (2000) Cancer and the skeleton. Martin Dunitz, London

41. Wolff J (1986) The law of bone remodelling. Springer, Berlin Heidelberg New York

42. Woolf A (1994) Osteoporosis. Martin Dunitz, London

Chapter 1 Epidemiology of Osteoporosis

1. Boonen S, Singer A (2008) Osteoporosis management: impact of fracture type on cost and quality of life in patients at risk for fracture I. Curr Med Res Opin 24:1781–1788

2. Borgstrom F, Johnell O, Kanis JA, Jonnson B, Rehnberg C (2006) At what hip fracture risk is it cost-effective to treat? International intervention thresholds for the treatment of osteoporosis. Osteoporos Int 17:1459–1471

3. Burge R, Dawson-Hughes B, Solomon D et al. (2007) Incidence and economic burden of osteoporotic-related fractures in the United States. 2005–2025. J Bone Miner Res 22:465–475

4. Cohen M Jr (2006) The new bone biology: pathologic, molecular, and clinical correlates. Am J Med Genet A 140:2646–2706

5. Cole Z, Dennison E, Cooper C (2008) Osteoporosis epidemiology update. Curr Rheumatol Rep 10:92–96

6. Cooper C, Atkinson EJ, Jacobsen SJ, O'Fallon WM, Melton LJ (1993) A population based study of survival after osteoporotic fractures. Am J Epidemiol 137:1001–1005

7. Cooper C, Campion G, Melton L 3rd (1992) Hip fractures in the elderly: a world-wide projection. Osteoporos Int 2:285–289

8. Cooper C, Jakob F, Martin-Mola E et al. (2008) Fracture incidence and changes in quality of life in women with an inadequate clinical outcome from osteoporosis therapy: the Observational Study of Severe Osteoporosis (OSSO). Osteoporos Int 19:493–501

9. Cree M, Juby A, Carriere K (2003) Mortality and morbidity associated with osteoporosis drug treatment following hip fracture. Osteoporos Int 14:722–727

10. Cummings S, Xu L, Chen X et al. (1994) Bone mass, rates of osteoporotic fractures, and prevention of fractures: are there differences between China and Western countries? Chin Med Sci J 9:197–200

11. Delmas P, Rizzoli R, Cooper C (2005) Treatment of patients with postmenopausal osteoporosis is worthwhile. The position of the International Osteoporosis Foundation. Osteoporos Int 16:1–5

12. Delmas PD, Siris E (2008) NICE recommendations for the prevention of osteoporotic fractures in postmenopausal women. Bone 42:16–18

13. Eichler H, Kong S, Gerth W et al. (2004) Use of cost-effectiveness analysis in health-care resource allocation decision making: how are cost-effectiveness thresholds expected to emerge? Value Health 7:518–528

14. El Maghraoui A, Koumba B, Jroundi I et al. (2005) Epidemiology of hip fractures in 2002 in Rabat, Morocco. Osteoporos Int 16:597–602

15. Fleurence RL, Iglesias CP, Torgerson DJ (2006) Economic evaluations of interventions for the prevention and treatment of osteoporosis: a structured review of the literature. Osteoporos Int 17:29–40

16. Fogarty P, O'Beirne B, Casey C (2005) Epidemiology of the most frequent diseases in the European a-symptomatic post-menopausal women. Is there any difference between Ireland and the rest of Europe? Maturitas 52(Suppl 1):S3–S6

17. Gemalmaz A, Oge A (2008) Knowledge and awareness about osteoporosis and its related factors among rural Turkish women. Clin Rheumatol 27:723–728

18. Hasserius R, Karlsson M, Nilsson B et al. (2002) Non-participants differ from participants as regards risk factors for vertebral deformities: a source of misinterpretation in the European Vertebral Osteoporosis Study. Acta Orthop Scand 73:451–454

19. Hasserius R, Karlsson M, Nilsson B et al. (2003) Prevalent vertebral deformities predict increased mortality and increased fracture rate in both men and women: a 10-year population-based study of 598 individuals from the Swedish cohort in the European Vertebral Osteoporosis Study. Osteoporos Int 14:61–68

20. Häussler B, Gothe H, Göl D et al. (2007) Epidemiology, treatment and costs of osteoporosis in Germany – the Bone EVA Study. Osteoporos Int 18:77–84

21. Johannesson M, Jonsson B (1993) Economic evaluation of osteoporosis prevention. Health Policy 24:103–124

22. Johnell O, Kanis JA (2006) An estimate of the worldwide prevalence and disability associated with osteoporotic fractures. Osteoporos Int 17:1726–1733

23. Kanis J, Johnell O, Oden A et al. (2000) Long-term risk of osteoporotic fracture in Malmo. Osteoporos Int 11:669–674

24. Kanis J, Adams J, Borgström F, Cooper C, Jönsson B, Preedy D et al. (2008) The cost-effectiveness of alendronate in the management of osteoporosis. Bone 42:4–15

25. Kanis J, Borgstrom F, Johnell O, Oden A, Sykes D, Jonsson B (2005) Cost-effectiveness of raloxifene in the UK. An economic evaluation based on the MORE study. Osteoporosis Int 16:15–25

26. Kanis J, Borgstrom F, Zethraeus N et al. (2005) Intervention thresholds for osteoporosis in the UK. Bone 36:22–32

27. Kanis J, Burlet N, Cooper C et al. (2008) European guidance for the diagnosis and management of osteoporosis in postmenopausal osteoporosis. Osteoporos Int 19:399–428

28. Kanis J, Johnell O, De Laet C et al. (2002) International variations in hip fracture probability: implications for risk assessment. J Bone Miner Res 17:1237–1244

29. Kanis J, Johnell O, Oden A et al. (2000) Risk of hip fracture according to the World Health Organization criteria for osteopenia and osteoporosis. Bone 27:585–590

30. Kanis J, Johnell O, Oden A et al. (2005) Intervention threshholds for osteoporosis in men and women: a study based on data from Sweden. Osteoporos Int 16:6–14

31. Kanis J, Jonsson B (2002) Economic evaluation of interventions for osteoporosis. Osteoporos Int 13:765–767

32. Kanis J, Oden A, Johnell O et al. (2003) The components of excess mortality after hip fracture. Bone 32:468–473

33. Kanis J, Stevenson M, McCloskey E et al. (2007) Glucocorticoid-induced osteoporosis: a systematic review and cost-utility analysis. Health Technol Assess 11:1–256

34. Levy P, Levy E, Audran M et al. (2002) The cost of osteoporosis in men: the French situation. Bone 30:631–636

35. Lippuner K, von Overbeck J, Perrelet R et al. (1997) Incidence and direct medical costs of hospitalisations due to osteoporotic fractures in Switzerland. Osteoporosis Int 7:414–425

36. Maalouf G, Gannagé-Yared M, Ezzedine J et al. (2007) Middle East and North Africa consensus on osteoporosis. J Musculoskelet Neuronal Interact 7:131–143

37. Martin A, Sornay-Rendu E, Chandler J et al. (2002) The impact of osteoporosis on quality-of-life: the OFELY cohort. Bone 31:32–36

38. Murray CJL, Lopez AD (eds) (1996) The global burden of disease and injury series, vol II. Global health statistics: a compendium of incidence, prevalence and mortality estimates for over 200 conditions. Harvard School of Public Health on behalf of the World Health Organization and the World Bank, Harvard University Press, Cambridge, MA

39. Nadrash T, Plushner S, Delate T (2008) Clinical pharmacists' role in improving osteoporosis treatment rates among elderly patients with untreated atraumatic fractures. Ann Pharmacother 42:334–340

40. Nielsen D, Ryg J, Nissen N et al. (2008) Multidisciplinary patient education in groups increases knowledge on osteoporosis: a randomized controlled trial. Scand J Public Health 36:346–352

41. Pérez Castrillón J, de Luis D, Duenas-Laita A (2008) Atherosclerosis and osteoporosis. Minerva Med 99:45–54

42. Philips S, Fox N, Jacobs J, Wright E (1988) The direct medical costs of osteoporosis of American women aged 45 and older. Bone 9:217–219

43. Richmond J, Aharonoff G, Zuckerman J, Koval K (2003) Mortality risk after hip fracture. J Orthop Trauma 17:S2–S5

44. Saw S-M, Hong C-Y, Lee J et al. (2003) Awareness and health beliefs of women towards osteoporosis. Osteoporos Int 14:595–601

45. Schürch MA, Rizzoli R, Mermillod B et al. (1996) A prospective study on socioeconomic aspects of fracture of the proximal femur. J Bone Miner Res 11:1935–1942

46. Shatrugna V, Kulkarni B, Kumar P et al. (2008) Relationship between women's occupational work and bone health: a study from India. Br J Nutr 99:1310–1315

47. Shichikawa K (2003) Establishment of the International Assessment Committee of Bone and Joint Diseases. J Rheumatol Suppl 67:66–68

48. Sidibe E (2005) Menopause in Africa. Ann Endocr (Paris) 66:105–107

49. Strom O, Borgstrom F, Sen SS, Boonen S, Haentjens P, Johnell O et al. (2007) Cost-effectiveness of alendronate in the treatment of postmenopausal women in 9 European countries – an economic evaluation based on the fracture intervention trial. Osteoporos Int 18:1047–1061

50. Tosteson A, Melton III L, Dawson-Hughes B et al. (2008) Cost effective osteoporosis treatment thresholds: the United States perspective. Osteoporos Int 19:437–447

51. World Health Organization (1994) Assessment of fracture risk and its application to screening for postmenopausal osteoporosis. Technical Report Series 843. WHO, Geneva

52. World Health Organization (2001) Macroeconomics and health: investing in health for economic development: report of the Commission on Macroeconomics and Health. World Health Organization, Geneva

53. World Health Organization (2007) Assessment of osteoporosis at the primary health care level. Summary Report of a WHO Scientific Group. WHO, Geneva

54. Zethraeus N, Ben Sedrine W, Caulin F, Corcaud S, Gathon HJ, Haim M (2002) Models for assessing the cost-effectiveness of the treatment and prevention of osteoporosis. Osteoporos Int 13:841–857

55. Zethraeus N, Borgström F, Ström O, Kanis J, Jönsson B, on behalf of the Committee of Scientific Advisors of the International Osteoporosis Foundation (2007) Cost-effectiveness of the treatment and prevention of osteoporosis – a review of the literature and a reference model. Osteoporos Int 18:9–23

56. Zethraeus N, Ström O, Borgström F et al. (2007) The cost-effectiveness of the treatment of osteoporosis, hypertension and hyperlipidaemia in Sweden. Osteoporos Int 18:9–23

57. Zethraeus N, Ström O, Borgström F et al. (2008) The cost-effectiveness of the treatment of high risk women with osteoporosis, hypertension and hyperlipidaemia in Sweden. Osteoporos Int 19:819–827

Chapter 2 Biology of Bone

1. Abu-Amer Y, Darwech I, Otero J (2008) Role of the NF-kappaB axis in immune modulation of osteoclasts and bone loss. Autoimmunity 41:204–211

2. Ahlborg H, Johnell O, Turner C et al. (2003) Bone loss and bone size after menopause. N Engl J Med 349:327–334

3. Ammann P, Rizzoli R (2003) Bone strength and its determinants. Osteoporos Int (Suppl 3):S13–S18

4. Atkinson H, Rosano C, Simonsick E et al. (2007) Cognitive function, gait speed decline, and comorbidities: the health, aging and body composition study. J Gerontol A Biol Sci Med Sci 62:844–850

5. Bar-Shavit Z (2008) Taking a toll on the bones: regulation of bone metabolism by innate immune regulators. Autoimmunity 41:195–203

6. Boivin G, Meunier P (2003) The mineralisation of bone tissue: a forgotten dimension in osteoporosis research. Osteoporos Int 14(Suppl 3): S19–S24

7. Bonewald L (2003) Osteocyte biology. Curr Opin Orthop 14:311–316

8. Bouxsein M (2003) Bone quality: where do we go from here? Osteoporos Int 14:S118–S127

9.   Boyce B, Xing L (2008) Functions of RANKL/ RANK/OPG in bone modeling and remodeling. Arch Biochem Biophys 473:139–146

10. Boyde A (2003) The real response of bone to exercise. J Anat 203:173–189

11. Boyle W, Simonet W, Lacey D (2003) Osteoclast differentiation and activation. Nature 423:337–341

12. Briana D, Gourgiotis D, Boutsikou M et al. (2008) Perinatal bone turnover in term pregnancies: the influence of intrauterine growth restriction. Bone 42:307–313

13. Browner W, Lui L, Cummings S (2001) Associations of serum osteoprotegerin levels with diabetes, stroke, bone density, fractures, and mortality in elderly women. J Clin Endocr Metab 86:631–637

14. Buckwalter J, Glimcher M, Cooper R, Recker R (1995) Bone biology: part I: structure, blood supply, cells, matrix and mineralisation. J Bone Joint Surg 77A:1256–1275

15. Burr D (1993) Remodeling and the repair of fatigue damage. Calcif Tissue Int 53(Suppl 1): S75–S80

16. Burr D (2002) The contribution of the organic matrix to bone's material properties. Bone 31:8–11

17. Cherian P, Siller-Jackson A, Gu S et al. (2005) Mechanical strain opens connexin 43 hemichannels in osteocytes: a novel mechanism for the release of prostaglandin. Mol Biol Cell 16:3100–3106

18. Civitelli R (2008) Cell-cell communication in the osteoblast/osteocyte lineage. Arch Biochem Biophys 473:188–192

19. Clarkin C, Emery R, Pitsillides A et al. (2008) Evaluation of VEGF-mediated signaling in primary human cells reveals a paracrine action for VEGF in osteoblast-mediated crosstalk to endothelial cells. J Cell Physiol 214:537–544

20. Colopy S, Benz-Dean J, Barrett J et al. (2004) Response of the osteocyte syncytium adjacent to and distant from linear microcracks during adaptation to cyclic fatigue loading. Bone 35:881–891

21. Corvalán C, Gregory C, Ramirez-Zea M et al. (2007) Size at birth, infant, early and later childhood growth and adult body composition: a prospective study in a stunted population. Int J Epidemiol 36:550–557

22. Currey J (2003) Perspective: how well are bones designed to resist fracture. J Bone Miner Res 18:591–598

23. Da Costa Gómez T, Barrett J, Sample S et al. (2005) Up-regulation of site-specific remodeling without accumulation of microcracking and loss of osteocytes. Bone 37:16–24

24. Dai J, Rabie A (2007) VEGF: an essential mediator of both angiogenesis and endochondral ossification. J Dent Res 86:937–950

25. Danova N, Colopy S, Radtke C et al. (2003) Degradation of bone structural properties by accumulation and coalescence of microcracks. Bone 33:197–205

26. Datta H, Ng W, Walker J et al. (2008) The cell biology of bone metabolism. J Clin Pathol 61:577–587

27. Donahue H (2000) Gap junctions and biophysical regulation of bone cell differentiation. Bone 26:417–422

28. Duque G, Troen B (2008) Understanding the mechanisms of senile osteoporosis: new facts for a major geriatric syndrome. J Am Geriatr Soc 56:935–941

29. Ettinger M (2003) Aging bone and osteoporosis: strategies for preventing fractures in the elderly. Arch Intern Med 163:2237–2246

30. Flier J (2002) Is brain sympathetic to bone? Nature 420:619–622

31. Frank G (2003) Role of estrogen and androgen in pubertal skeletal physiology. Med Pediatr Oncol 41:217–221

32. Frost H (2000) The Utah paradigm of skeletal physiology: an overview of its insights for bone, cartilage and collagenous tissue organs. J Bone Miner Metab 18:305–316

33. Frost H (2001) From Wolff's law to the Utah paradigm: insights about bone physiology and its clinical applications. Anat Rec 262:398–419

34. Frost H (2001) Why should many skeletal scientists and clinicians learn the Utah paradigm of skeletal physiology? J Musculoskelet Neuronal Interact 2:121–130

35. Frost H (2003) Bone's mechanostat: a 2003 update. Anat Rec A Discov Mol Cell Evol Biol 275:1081–1101

36. Genetos D, Kephart C, Zhang Y et al. (2007) Oscillating fluid flow activation of gap junction hemichannels induces ATP release from MLO-Y4 osteocytes. J Cell Physiol 212:207–214

37. Hadjidakis D, Androulakis I (2006) Bone remodeling. Ann N Y Acad Sci 1092:385–396

38. Hamrick M, Ferrari S (2008) Leptin and the sympathetic connection of fat to bone. Osteoporos Int 19:905–912

39. Harada S, Rodan G (2003) Control of osteoclast function and regulation of bone mass. Nature 423:349–355

40. Hayer S, Steiner G, Görtz B et al. (2005) CD44 is a determinant of inflammatory bone loss. J Exp Med 201:903–914

41. Hayman A (2008) Tartrate-resistant acid phosphatase (TRAP) and the osteoclast/immune cell dichotomy. Autoimmunity 41:218–223

42. Hikiji H, Takato T, Shimizu T et al. (2008) The roles of prostanoids, leukotrienes, and platelet-activating factor in bone metabolism and disease. Prog Lipid Res 47:107–126

43. Hofbauer L, Brueck C, Shanahan C et al. (2007) Vascular calcification and osteoporosis – from clinical observation towards molecular understanding. Osteoporos Int 18:251–259

44. Hofbauer L, Khosla S, Dunstan C et al. (2000) The roles of osteoprotegerin and osteoprotegerin ligand in the paracrine regulation of bone resorption. J Bone Miner Res 15:2–12

45. Hofbauer L, Kühne C, Viereck V (2004) The OPG/RANKL/RANK system in metabolic bone disease. J Musculoskelet Neuronal Interact 4:268–275

46. Hofbauer L, Schoppet M (2004) Clinical implications of the osteoprotegerin/RANKL/RANK system for bone and vascular diseases. JAMA 292:490–495

47. Jee W, Tian X (2005) The benefit of combining non-mechanical agents with mechanical loading: a perspective based on the Utah Paradigm of Skeletal Physiology. J Musculoskelet Neuronal Interact 5:110–118

48. Jee W, Tian X, Setterberg R (2007) Cancellous bone minimodeling-based formation: a Frost, Takahashi legacy. J Musculoskelet Neuronal Interact 7:232–239

49. Jiang J, Siller-Jackson A, Burra S (2007) Roles of gap junctions and hemichannels in bone cell functions and in signal transmission of mechanical stress. Front Biosci 12:1450–1462

50. Karsenty G, Wagner E (2002) Reaching a genetic and molecular understanding of skeletal development. Dev Cell 2:389–406

51. Kennedy O, Brennan O, Mauer P et al. (2008) The behaviour of fatigue-induced microdamage in compact bone samples from control and ovariectomised sheep. Stud Health Technol Inform 133:148–155

52. Khosla S (2001) Minireview: the OPG/RANKL/RANK system. Endocrinology 142:5050–5055

53. Ko K, McCulloch C (2001) Intercellular mechanotransduction: cellular circuits that coordinate tissue responses to mechanical loading. Biochem Biophys Res Commun 285:1077–1083

54. Kobayashi S, Takahashi H, Ito A et al. (2003) Trabecular minimodeling in human iliac bone. Bone 32:163–169

55. Kollet O, Dar A, Shivtiel S et al. (2006) Osteoclasts degrade endosteal components and promote mobilization of hematopoietic progenitor cells. Nat Med 12:657–664

56. Kuro-o M (2008) Klotho as a regulator of oxidative stress and senescence. Biol Chem 389:233–241

57. Lanham S, Roberts C, Cooper C et al. (2008) Intrauterine programming of bone. Part 1: alteration of the osteogenic environment. Osteoporos Int 19:147–156

58. Lanham S, Roberts C, Perry M et al. (2008) Intrauterine programming of bone. Part 2: alteration of skeletal structure. Osteoporos Int 19:157–167

59. Larciprete G, Valensise H, Di Perro G et al. (2005) Intrauterine growth restriction and fetal body composition. Ultrasound Obstet Gynecol 26:258–262

60. Lee N, Sowa H, Hinoi E et al. (2007) Endocrine regulation of energy metabolism by the skeleton. Cell 130:456–469

61. Lee T, Staines A, Taylor D (2002) Bone adaptation to load: microdamage as a stimulus for bone remodelling. J Anat 201:437–446

62. Litmanovitz I, Dolfin T, Arnon S et al. (2007) Assisted exercised and bone strength in preterm infants. Calcif Tissue Int 80:39–43

63. Liu D, Jiang L, Dai L (2007) Substance P and its receptors in bone metabolism. Neuropeptides 41:271–283

64. Liu X, Sajda P, Saha P et al. (2008) Complete volumetric decomposition of individual trabecular plates and rods and its morphological correlations with anisotropic elastic moduli in human trabecular bone. J Bone Miner Res 23:223–235

65. Manolagas S (2000) Birth and death of bone cells: basic regulatory mechanisms and implications for the pathogenesis and treatment of osteoporosis. Endocr Rev 21:115–137
66. Marakoglu I, Gursoy U, Marakoglu K et al. (2008) Periodontitis as a risk factor for preterm low birth weight. Yonsei Med J 49:200–203
67. Mittendorfer-Rutz E, Wasserman D, Rasmussen F (2008) Fetal and childhood growth and the risk of violent and non-violent suicide attempts: a cohort study of 31,953 men. J Epidemiol Community Health 62:168–173
68. Mödder U, Khosla S (2008) Skeletal stem/osteoprogenitor cells: current concepts, alternate hypotheses, and relationship to the bone remodeling compartment. J Cell Biochem 103:393–400
69. Muir P, Sample S, Barrett J et al. (2007) Effect of fatigue loading and associated matrix microdamage on bone blood flow and interstitial fluid flow. Bone 40:948–956
70. Naaraja S, Lin A, Guldberg R (2007) Age-related changes in trabecular bone microdamage initiation. Bone 40:973–980
71. Noble B (2008) The osteocyte lineage. Arch Biochem Biophys 473:106–111
72. Nuttall M, Gimble J (2000) Is there a therapeutic opportunity of either prevent or treat osteopenic disorders by inhibiting marrow adipogenesis? Bone 27:177–184
73. O'Brien F, Hardiman D, Hazenberg J et al. (2005) The behavior of microcracks in compact bone. Eur J Morphol 42:71–79
74. Onley R (2003) Regulation of bone mass by growth hormone. Med Pediatr Oncol 41:228–234
75. Orwell E (2003) Men, bone and estrogen: unresolved issues. Osteoporos Int 14:93–98
76. Osmond C, Barker D (2000) Fetal, infant and childhood growth are predictors of coronary hart disease, diabetes, and hypertension in adult men and women. Environ Health Perspect 108(Suppl 3):545–553
77. Phan T, Xu J, Zheng M (2004) Interaction between osteoblast and osteoclast: impact in bone disease. Histol Histopathol 19:1325–1344
78. Pignolo R, Suda R, McMillan E et al. (2008) Defects in telomere maintenance molecules impair osteoblast differentiation and promote osteoporosis. Aging Cell 7:23–31
79. Rauner M, Sipos W, Pietschmann P (2007) Osteoimmunology. Int Arch Allergy Immunol 143:31–48
80. Reid I (2008) Relationships between fat and bone. Osteoporos Int 19:595–606
81. Reilly G (2000) Observations of microdamage around osteocyte lacunae in bone. J Biomech 33:1131–1134
82. Riggs L (2000) The mechanisms of estrogen regulation of bone resorption. J Clin Invest 106:1203
83. Robinson J, Moore V, Owens J et al. (2000) Origins of fetal growth restriction. Eur J Obstet Gynecol Reprod Biol 92:13–19
84. Roord J, Ramaekers L, van Engelshoven J (1978) Intra-uterine malnutrition and skeletal retardation. Biol Neonate 34:167–169
85. Sato K, Takayanagi H (2006) Osteoclasts, rheumatoid arthritis, and osteoimmunology. Curr Opin Rheumatol 18:419–426
86. Sayer A, Cooper C (2005) Fetal programming of body composition and musculoskeletal development. Early Hum Dev 81:735–744
87. Schett G (2007) Joint remodelling in inflammatory disease. Ann Rheum Dis 66(Suppl 3): iii42–iii44
88. Seaman E (2003b) Periosteal bone formation – a neglected determinant of bone strength. N Engl J Med 349:320–323
89. Shun-ichi H, Rondan G (2003) Control of osteoblast function and regulation of bone mass. Nature 423:349–355
90. Suematsu A, Takayanagi H (2007) Interplay between the immune and skeletal cells in the regulation of inflammatory bone destruction. Nihon Rinsho Meneki Gakkai Kaishi 30:22–28
91. Takayanagi H (2002) Cross-talk between immune and skeletal systems. Nippon Rinsho 60:2287–2295
92. Takayanagi H (2005) Introduction to osteoimmunology. Nippon Rinsho 63:1505–1509
93. Takayanagi H (2005) Mechanistic insight into osteoclast differentiation in osteoimmunology. J Mol Med 83:170–179
94. Takayanagi H (2007) Osteoclast differentiation and activation. Clin Calcium 17:484–492
95. Takeda S (2008) Genomic approaches to bone and joint diseases. Control of bone remodeling by hormones and neuronal pathways. Clin Calcium 18:216–221

96. Takeda S, Elefteriou F, Levasseur R et al. (2002) Leptin regulates bone formation via the sympathetic nervous system. Cell 111:305–317

97. Taketa S, Karsenty G (2008) Molecular bases of the sympathetic regulation of bone mass. Bone 42:837–840

98. Taylor D, Hazenberg J, Lee T (2007) Living with cracks: damage and repair in human bone. Nat Mater 6:263–268

99. Teitelbaum S (2000) Bone resorption by osteoclasts. Science 289:1504–1508

100. Tilg H, Moschen A, Kaser A et al. (2008) Gut, inflammation and osteoporosis: basic and clinical concepts. Gut 57:684–694

101. Tung S, Iqbal J (2007) Evolution, aging, and osteoporosis. Ann N Y Acad Sci 1116:499–506

102. Turner C (2002a) Biomechanics of bone: determinants of skeletal fragility and bone quality. Osteoporos Int 13:97–104

103. Turner C (2002b) Mechanotransduction in skeletal cells. Curr Opin Orthop 13:363–367

104. van Oers R, Ruimerman R, Tanck E et al. (2008) A unified theory for osteonal and hemi-osteonal remodeling. Bone 42:250–259

105. Waldorff E, Goldstein S, McCreadie B (2007) Age-dependent microdamage removal following mechanically induced microdamage in trabecular bone in vivo. Bone 40:425–432

106. Wells J, Chomtho S, Fewtrell M (2007) Programming of body composition by early growth and nutrition. Proc Nutr Soc 66:423–434

107. Whitfield J (2003) Primary cilium – is it an osteocyte's strain-sensing flowmeter? J Cell Biochem 89:233–237

108. Wolf G (2008) Energy regulation by the skeleton. Nutr Rev 66:229–233

109. You L, Temiyasathit S, Lee P et al. (2008) Osteocytes as mechanosensors in the inhibition of bone resorption due to mechanical loading. Bone 42:172–179

110. Young M (2003) Bone matrix proteins: their function, regulation, and relationship to osteoporosis. Osteoporos Int 14(Suppl 3):S35–S42

111. Zaidi M, Blair H, Moonga B et al. (2003) Osteoclastogenesis, bone resorption, and osteoclast-based therapeutics. J Bone Miner Res 18:599–609

112. Zaidi M, Moonga B, Sun l et al. (2003) Understanding osteoclast formation and function: implications for future therapies for osteoporosis. Curr Opin Orthop 14:341–350

Chapter 3 Pathogenesis of Osteoporosis

1. Ackert-Bicknell C, Salisbury J, Horowitz M et al. (2007) A chromosomal inversion within a quantitative trait locus has a major effect on adipogenesis and osteoblastogenesis. Ann N Y Acad Sci 1116:291–305

2. Akune T, Ohba S, Kamekura S et al. (2004) PPARgamma insufficiency enhances osteogenesis through osteoblast formation from bone marrow progenitors. J Clin Invest 113:846–855

3. Bone C, Einhorn T (2003) Overview of osteoporosis: pathophysiology and determinants of bone strength. Eur Spine J 12:90–96

4. Czerwiński E, Badurski J, Marcinowska-Suchowierska E et al. (2007) Current understanding of osteoporosis according to the position of the World Health Organization (WHO) and International Osteoporosis Foundation. Ortop Traumatol Rehabil 9:337–356

5. Duque G, Troen B (2008) Understanding the mechanisms of senile osteoporosis: new facts for a major geriatric syndrome. J Am Geriatr Soc 56:935–941

6. Epstein S, Inzerillo A, Caminis J, Zaidi M (2003) Review: disorders associated with acute rapid and severe bone loss. J Bone Miner Res 18:2083–2094

7. Hazenberg J, Taylor D, Lee T (2007) The role of osteocytes and bone microstructure in preventing osteoporotic fractures. Osteoporos Int 18:1–8

8. Justesen J, Stenderup K, Ebbesen E et al. (2001) Adipocyte tissue volume in bone marrow is increased with aging and in patients with osteoporosis. Biogerontology 2:165–171

9. Kang S, Bennett C, Gerin I et al. (2007) Wnt signaling stimulates osteoblastogenesis of mesenchymal precursors by suppressing CCAAT/enhancer-binding protein alpha and peroxisome proliferator-activated receptor gamma. J Biol Chem 282:14515–14524

10. Manolagas S, Almeida M (2007) Gone with the Wnts: beta-catenin, T-cell factor, forkhead box O, and oxidative stress in age-dependent diseases of bone, lipid, and glucose metabolism. Mol Endocrinol 21:2605–2614

11. Nishimura R, Hata K, Yoneda T (2007) Relationship between bone metabolism and adipogenesis. Clin Calcium 17:233–240

12. Nuttall M, Gimble J (2004) Controlling the balance between osteoblastogenesis and adipogenesis and the consequent therapeutic implications. Curr Opin Pharmacol 4:290–294

13. Okazaki R, Inoue D, Shibata M et al. (2002) Estrogen promotes early osteoblast differentiation and inhibits adipocyte differentiation in mouse bone marrow stromal cell lines that express estrogen receptor (ER) alpha or beta. Endocrinology 143:2349–2356

14. Priemel M, Münch C, Beil F et al. (2006) Pathophysiology and pathomorphology of osteoporosis. Radiologe 46:831–838

15. Sambrook P, Cooper C (2006) Osteoporosis. Lancet 367:2010–2018

16. Scheideler M, Elabd C, Zaragosi L et al. (2008) Comparative transcriptomics of human multipotent stem cells during adipogenesis and osteoblastogenesis. BMC Genomics 9:340

17. Schiller P, D'Ippolito G, Brambilla R et al. (2001) Inhibition of gap-junctional communication induces the trans-differentiation of osteoblasts to an adipocytic phenotype in vitro. J Biol Chem 276:14133–14138

18. Sinaki M (1998) Musculoskeletal challenges of osteoporosis. Aging (Milano) 10:249–262

19. Zaidi M, Moonga B, Sun l et al. (2003) Understanding osteoclast formation and function: implications for future therapies for osteoporosis. Curr Opin Orthop 14:341–350

20. Zayzafoon M, Gathings W, McDonald J (2004) Modeled microgravity inhibits osteogenic differentiation of human mesenchymal stem cells and increases adipogenesis. Endocrinology 145:2421–2432

Chapter 4 Subgroups of Osteoporosis

1. Duque G (2008) Bone and fat connection in aging bone. Curr Opin Rheumatol 20:429–434

2. Duque G, Troen B (2008) Understanding the mechanisms of senile osteoporosis: new facts for a major geriatric syndrome. J Am Geriatr Soc 56:935–941

3. Eckstein F, Matsuura M, Kuhn V et al. (2007) Sex differences of human trabecular bone microstructure in aging are site-dependent. J Bone Miner Res 22:817–824

Chapter 5 Risk Factors for Fractures

1. Abolhassani F, Moayyeri A, Naghavi M et al. (2006) Incidence and characteristics of falls leading to hip fracture in Iranian population. Bone 39:408–413

2. Aguirre J, Piotkin L, Stewart S et al. (2006) Osteocyte apoptosis is induced by weightlessness in mice and precedes osteoclast recruitment and bone loss. J Bone Miner Res 21:605–615

3. Aharonoff G, Dennis M, Elshinawy A et al. (2003) Circumstances of falls causing hip fractures in the elderly. J Orthop Trauma 17:S22–S26

4. Andrew T, Macgregor A (2004) Genes and osteoporosis. Curr Osteoporos Rep 2:79–89

5. Barrett-Connor E, Sajjan S, Siris E et al. (2008) Wrist fracture as a predictor of future fractures in younger versus older postmenopausal women: results from the National Osteoporosis Risk Assessment (NORA). Osteoporos Int 19:607–613

6. Berg K, Kunins H, Jackson J et al. (2008) Association between alcohol consumption and both osteoporotic fracture and bone density. Am J Med 121:406–418

7. Burke-Doe A, Hudson A, Werth H et al. (2008) Knowledge of osteoporosis risk factors and prevalence of risk factors for osteoporosis, falls, and fracture in functionally independent older adults. J Geriatr Phys Ther 31:11–17

8. Carbonell Sala S, Brandi M (2007) 2006 update on genetic determinants of osteoporosis. J Endocrinol Invest 30(Suppl 6):2–7

9. Chapurlat R, Bauer D, Nevitt M et al. (2003) Incidence and risk factors for a second hip fracture. The study of osteoporotic fractures. Osteoporos Int 14:130–136

10. Cherniack E, Levis S, Troen B (2008) Hypovitaminosis D: a widespread epidemic. Geriatrics 63:24–30

11. Cummings S (1996) Treatable and untreatable risk factors for hip fracture. Bone 18:165S–167S

12. Douroudis K, Tarassi K, Athanassiades T et al. (2007) HLA alleles as predisposal factors for postmenopausal osteoporosis in a Greek population. Tissue Antigens 69:592–596

13. Fitzpatrick L, Heaney R (2003) Got soda? J Bone Miner Res 18:1570–1571

14. Gerdhem P, Obrant K (2002) Effects of cigarette-smoking on bone mass as assessed by dual-en-

ergy X-ray absorptiometry and ultrasound. Osteoporos Int 13:933–936

15. Gourlay M, Richy F, Reginster J (2003) Strategies for the prevention of hip fractures. Am J Med 115:309–317

16. Guijarro M, Valero C, Paule B et al. (2008) Bone mass in young adults with Down syndrome. J Intellect Disabil Res 52:182–189

17. Hamdi Kara I, Aydin S, Gemalmaz A et al. (2007) Habitual tea drinking and bone mineral density in postmenopausal Turkish women: investigation of prevalence of postmenopausal osteoporosis in Turkey (PPOT Study). Int J Vitam Nutr Res 77:389–397

18. Heanney R (2001) Nutrition and risk for osteoporosis. Osteoporosis 2:669–700

19. Hernández Hernández J, Riancho Moral J, Gonzáles Macias J (2008) Metabolic syndrome: how about bone? Med Clin (Barc) 130:745–750

20. Hodgson J, Devine A, Burke V et al. (2008) Chocolate consumption and bone density in older women. Am J Clin Nutr 87:175–180

21. Javaid M, Lekamwasam S, Clark J et al. (2006) Infant growth influences proximal femoral geometry in adulthood. J Bone Miner Res 21:508–512

22. Kanis J, Borgstrom F, De Laet C et al. (2005) Assessment of fracture risk. Osteoporos Int 16:581–589

23. Kanis J, Johnell O, De Laet C et al. (2004) A meta-analysis of previous fracture and subsequent fracture risk. Bone 35:375–382

24. Kannus P, Parkkari J, Niemi S et al. (2000) Prevention of hip fracture in elderly people with use of a hip protector. N Engl J Med 343:1506–1513

25. Koh J, Park B, Kim D et al. (2007) Identification of novel RANK polymorphisms and their putative association with low BMD among postmenopausal women. Osteoporos Int 18:323–331

26. Krall E, Dawson-Hughes B (1991) Smoking and bone loss among postmenopausal women. J Bone Miner Res 6:331–338

27. Kudlacek S, Freudenthaler O, Weissboeck H et al. (2003) Lactose intolerance: a risk factor for reduced bone mineral density and vertebral fractures? J Gastroenterol 37:1014–1019

28. Langdahl B, Uitterlinden A, Ralston S et al. (2008) Large-scale analysis of association between polymorphisms in the transforming growth factor beta 1 gene (TGFB1) and osteoporosis: the GENOMOS study. Bone 42:969–981

29. Logar D, Komadina R, Prezelj J et al. (2007) Expression of bone resorption genes in osteoarthritis and in osteoporosis. J Bone Miner Metab 25:219–225

30. Majima T, Shimatsu A, Komatsu Y et al. (2008) Increased bone turnover in patients with hypercholesterolemia. Endocr J 55:143–151

31. Makovey J, Nuyen T, Naganathan V et al. (2007) Genetic effects on bone loss in peri- and postmenopausal women: a longitudinal twin study. J Bone Miner Res 22:1773–1780

32. Marshall L, Zmuda J, Chan B et al. (2008) Race and ethnic variation in proximal femur structure and BMD among older men. J Bone Miner Res 23:121–130

33. McGartland C, Robson P, Murray L et al. (2003) Carbonated soft drink consumption and bone mineral density in adolescence: the Northern Ireland Young Hearts Project. J Bone Miner Res 18:1563–1569

34. Mezquita-Raya P, Muñoz-Torres M, Alonso G et al. (2004) Susceptibility for postmenopausal osteoporosis: interaction between genetic, hormonal and lifestyle factors. Calcif Tissue Int 75:373–379

35. Mezuk B, Eaton W, Golden S (2008) Depression and osteoporosis: epidemiology and potential mediating pathways. Osteoporos Int 19:1–12

36. Miazgowski T, Kryźanowska-Świniarska B, Ogonowski J et al. (2008) Does type 2 diabetes predispose to osteoporotic bone fractures? Endokrynol Pol 59:224–229

37. Nguyen TV, Center JR, Sambrook PN et al. (2001) Risk factors for proximal humerus, forearm, and wrist fractures in elderly men and women: The Dubbo Osteoporosis Epidemiology Study. Am J Epidemiol 153:587–595

38. Olmos J, Vázquez L, Amado J et al. (2008) Mineral metabolism in obese patients following vertical banded gastroplasty. Obes Surg 18:197–203

39. Osmancevic A, Landin-Wilhelmsen K, Larkö O et al. (2008) Risk factors for osteoporosis and bone status in postmenopausal women with psoriasis treated with UVB therapy. Acta Derm Venereol 88:240–246

40. Pasco J, Henry M, Sanders K et al. (2004) Beta-adrenergic blockers reduce the risk of fracture partly by increasing bone mineral density: Geelong Osteoporosis Study. J Bone Miner Res 19:19–24

41. Perese E, Perese K (2003) Health problems of women with severe mental illness. J Am Acad Nurse Pract 15:212–219

42. Petronijević M, Petronijević N, Ivković M et al. (2008) Low bone mineral density and high bone metabolism turnover in premenopausal women with unipolar depression. Bone 42:582–590

43. Pignolo R, Suda R, McMillan E et al. (2008) Defects in telomere maintenance molecules impair osteoblast differentiation and promote osteoporosis. Aging Cell 7:23–31

44. Ralston S (2003) Genetic determinants of susceptibility to osteoporosis. Curr Opin Pharmacol 3:286–290

45. Ralston S (2007) Genetics of osteoporosis. Proc Nutr Soc 66:158–165

46. Recker R, Hinders S, Davies K et al. (1996) Correcting calcium nutritional deficiency prevents spine fractures in elderly women. J Bone Miner Res 11:1961–1966

47. Richards J, Rivadeneira F, Inouye M et al. (2008) Bone mineral density, osteoporosis, and osteoporotic fractures: a genome-wide association study. Lancet 371:1505–1512

48. Ridker P, Chasman D, Zee R et al. (2008) Rationale, design, and methodology of the Women's Genome Health Study: a genome-wide association study of more than 25,000 initially healthy American women. Clin Chem 54:249–255

49. Roux X (2001) The genetics of osteoporosis. Joint Bone Spine 68:482–486

50. Savage S, Alter B (2008) The role of telomere biology in bone marrow failure and other disorders. Mech Ageing Dev 129:35–47

51. Sen S, Rives V, Messina O et al. (2005) A risk assessment tool (OsteoRisk) for identifying Latin American women with osteoporosis. J Gen Intern Med 20:245–250

52. Sirola J, Kröger H, Honkanen R et al. (2003) Smoking may impair the bone protective effects of nutritional calcium: a population-based approach. J Bone Miner Res 18:1036–1042

53. Smith S, Heer M (2002) Calcium and bone metabolism during space flight. Nutrition 18:849–852

54. Sneve M, Emaus N, Joakimsen R et al. (2008) The association between serum parathyroid hormone and bone mineral density, and the impact of smoking: the Tromso Study. Eur J Endocrinol 158:401–409

55. Styrkarsdottir U, Halldorsson B, Gretarsdottir S et al. (2008) Multiple genetic loci for bone mineral density and fractures. N Engl J Med 358:2355–2365

56. Tobias J, Hutchinson A, Hunt L et al. (2007) Use of clinical risk factors to indentify postmenopausal women with vertebral fractures. Osteoporos Int 18:35–43

57. van Helden S, van Geel A, Geusens P et al. (2008) Bone and fall-related fracture risk in women and men with a recent clinical fracture. J Bone Joint Surg Am 90:241–248

58. van Meurs J, Trikalinos T, Ralston S et al. (2008) Large-scale analysis of association between LRP5 and LRP6 variants and osteoporosis. JAMA 299:1277–1290

59. Walker M, Novotny R, Bilezikian J et al. (2008) Race and diet interactions in the acquisition, maintenance, and loss of bone. J Nutr 138:1256S–1260S

60. Walsh M, Hunter G, Livingstone M (2006) Sarcopenia in premenopausal and postmenopausal women with osteopenia, osteoporosis and normal bone mineral density. Osteoporos Int 17:61–67

61. Wang X, Deng F, Tan L et al. (2008) Bivariate whole genome linkage analyses for total body lean mass and BMD. J Bone Miner Res 23:447–452

62. Weaver C (2008) The role of nutrition on optimizing peak bone mass. Asia Pac J Clin Nutr 17 (Suppl 1):135–137

63. Williams F, Spector T (2007) The genetics of osteoporosis. Acta Rheumatol Port 32:231–240

64. Wong J, Arango-Viana J, Squires T (2008) Heart, liver and spleen pathology in chronic alcohol and drug users. J Forensic Leg Med 15:141–147

65. Yamada Y, Ando F, Shimokata H (2007) Association of candidate gene polymorphisms with bone mineral density in community-dwelling Japanese women and men. Int J Mol Med 19:791–801

66. Zelzer E, Olsen B (2003) The genetic basis for skeletal diseases. Nature 423:343–348

Chapter 6 Clinical Evaluation of Osteoporosis

1. Demondion X, Boutry N, Khalil C et al. (2008) Plain radiographs of the wrist and hand. J Radiol 89:640–653

2. Kanis J, Burlet N, Cooper C et al. (2008) European guidance for the diagnosis and management of osteoporosis in postmenopausal osteoporosis. Osteoporos Int 19:399–428

3. Orr-Walker B, Evans M, Ames R et al. (1997) Premature hair graying and bone mineral density. J Clin Endocrinol Metab 82:3580–3583

4. Raisz L (2005) Screening for osteoporosis. New Engl J Med 353:164–171

5. Rosen C, Holick M, Millard P (1994) Premature graying of hair is a risk marker for osteopenia. J Clin Endocrinol Metab 79:854–857

Chapter 7 Bone Density in Osteoporosis

1. Banse X (2002) When density fails to predict bone strength. Acta Orthop Scand 73(Suppl):303: S2–S53

2. Damilakis J, Papadokostakis G, Perisinakis K et al. (2003) Can radial bone mineral density and quantitative ultrasound measurements reduce the number of women who need axial density skeletal assessment? Osteoporos Int 14:688–693

3. Faulkner K (2000) Bone matters: are density increases necessary to reduce fracture risk? J Bone Miner Res 15:183–187

4. Feldstein A, Elmer P, Orwoll E et al. (2003) Bone mineral density measurement and treatment for osteoporosis in older individuals with fractures. Arch Intern Med 163:2165–2172

5. Hans D, Shepherd J, Schwartz E et al. (2008) Peripheral dual-energy X-ray absorptiometry in the management of osteoporosis: the 2007 ISCD Official Positions. J Clin Densitom 11:188–206

6. Kanis J, Burlet N, Cooper C et al. (2008) European guidance for the diagnosis and management of osteoporosis in postmenopausal osteoporosis. Osteoporos Int 19:399–428

7. Kaptoge S, da Silva J, Brixen K et al. (2008) Geographical variation in DXA bone mineral density in young European men and women. Results from the network in Europe on male osteoporosis (NEMO) study. Bone 43:332–339

8. Kolta S, Quiligotti S, Ruyssen-Witrand A et al. (2008) In vivo 3D reconstruction of human vertebrae with the three-dimensional X-ray absorptiometry (3D-XA) method. Osteoporos Int 19:185–192

9. Kullenberg R, Falch J (2003) Prevalence of osteoporosis using bone mineral measurements at the calcaneus by dual X-ray and laser (DXL). Osteoporos Int 14:823–827

10. Marshall D, Johnell O, Wedel H et al. (1996) Meta-analysis of how well measures of bone mineral density predict occurrence of osteoporotic fractures. Br Med J 312:1254–1259

11. Miller P, Zapalowski C, Kulak C et al. (1999) Bone densitometry: the best way to detect osteoporosis and to monitor therapy. J Clin Endocrinol Metab 84:1867–1871

12. O'Gradaigh D, Debiram I, Love S et al. (2003) A prospective study of discordance in diagnosis of osteoporosis using spine and proximal femur bone densitometry. Osteoporos Int 14:13–18

13. Roschger P, Paschalis E, Fratzi P et al. (2008) Bone mineralization density distribution in health and disease. Bone 42:456–466

14. Sakar S, Reginster J, Crans G et al. (2004) Relationship between changes in biochemical markers of bone turnover and BMD to predict vertebral fracture risk. J Bone Miner Res 19:391–40

15. Siris E, Chen Y, Abbott T et al. (2004) Bone mineral density thresholds for pharmacological intervention to prevent fractures. Arch Intern Med 164:1108–1112

16. Stone K, Seeley D, Lui L et al. (2003) BMD at multiple sites and risk of fracture of multiple types: long-term results from the study of osteoporotic fractures. J Bone Miner Res 18:1947–1954

17. Szulc P, Delmas P (2001) Biochemical markers of bone turnover in men. Calcif Tissue Int 69:229–230

18. Tao B, Liu J, Li X et al. (2008) An assessment of the use of quantitative ultrasound and the Osteoporosis Self-Assessment Tool for Asians in determining the risk of nonvertebral facture in postmenopausal Chinese women. J Bone Miner Metab 26:60–65

19. Tothill P, Hannan W (2007) Precision and accuracy of measuring changes in bone mineral density by dual-energy X-ray absorptiometry. Osteoporos Int 18:1515–1523

20. Zimering M, Shin J, Shah J et al. (2007) Validation of a novel risk estimation tool for predicting low bone density in Caucasian and African American men veterans. J Clin Densitom 10:289–297

Chapter 8 Laboratory Evaluation of Osteoporosis

1. Akhter M, Lappe J, Davies K et al. (2007) Transmenopausal changes in the trabecular bone structure. Bone 41:111–116
2. Byrd S, Comiskey E (2007) Postnatal maturation and radiology of the growing spine. Neurosurg Clin N Am 18:431–461
3. Carballido-Gamio J, Majumdar S (2006) Clinical utility of microarchitecture measurements of trabecular bone. Curr Osteoporos Rep 4:64–70
4. Eisenberger S, Hoppe G, Pyerin W et al. (2004) High-quality RNA preparation for transcript profiling of osteocytes from native human bone microdissections. Anal Biochem 335:260–266
5. Gomes S, dos Reis L, de Oliveira I et al. (2008) Usefulness of a quick decalcification of bone sections embedded in methyl methacrylate [corrected]: an improved method for immunohistochemistry. J Bone Miner Metab 26:110–113
6. Graiser T, Bernhards J (2007) Tyramide signal amplification: an enhanced method for immunohistochemistry on methyl-methacrylate-embedded bone marrow trephine sections. Acta Haematol 117:122–127
7. Griffith J, Yeung D, Antonio G et al. (2005) Vertebral bone mineral density, marrow perfusion, and fat content in healthy men and men with osteoporosis: dynamic contrast-enhanced MR imaging and MR spectroscopy. Radiology 236:945–951
8. Harper K, Weber T (1998) Secondary osteoporosis. Diagnostic considerations. Endocrinol Metab Clin North Am 27:325–348
9. Jee W (2005) The past, present, and future of bone morphometry: its contribution to an improved understanding of bone biology. J Bone Miner Metab 23(Suppl):1–10
10. Johnell O, Oden A, De Laet C et al. (2002) Biochemical markers and the assessment of fracture probability. Osteoporos Int 13:523–526
11. Kanis J, Burlet N, Cooper C et al. (2008) European guidance for the diagnosis and management of osteoporosis in postmenopausal osteoporosis. Osteoporos Int 19:399–428
12. Knabe C, Kraska B, Koch C et al. (2006) A method for immunohistochemical detection of osteogenic markers in undecalcified bone sections. Biotech Histochem 81:31–39
13. Kunze E, Middel P, Fayyazi A et al. (2008) Immunohistochemical staining of plastic (methylmethacrylate)-embedded bone marrow biopsies applying the biotin-free tyramide signal amplification system. Appl Immunohistochem Mol Morphol 16:76–82
14. Laboux O, Dion N, Arana-Chavez V et al. (2004) Microwave irradiation of ethanol-fixed bone improves preservation, reduces processing time, and allows both light and electron microscopy on the same sample. J Histochem Cytochem 52:1267–1275
15. Ladinsky G, Vasilic B, Popescu A et al. (2008) Trabecular structure quantified with the MRI-based virtual bone biopsy in postmenopausal women contributes to vertebral deformity burden independent of areal vertebral BMD. J Bone Miner Res 23:64–74
16. Ladinsky G, Wehrli F (2006) Noninvasive assessment of bone microarchitecture by MRI. Curr Osteoporos Rep 4:140–147
17. Leslie W (2008) Factors affecting short-term bone density precision assessment and the effect on patient monitoring. J Bone Miner Res 23:199–204
18. Liu J, Zhao H, Ning G et al. (2008) IGF-1 as an early marker for low bone mass or osteoporosis in premenopausal and postmenopausal women. J Bone Miner Metab 26:159–164
19. Miller P, Baran D, Bilezikan J et al. (1999) Practical clinical application of biomarkers of bone turnover. J Clin Densitom 2:323–342
20. Muller M, Mitton D, Talmant M et al. (2008) Nonlinear ultrasound can detect accumulated damage in human bone. J Biomech 41:1062–1068
21. Muller M, Tencate J, Darling T et al. (2006) Bone micro-damage assessment using non-linear resonant ultrasound spectroscopy (NRUS) techniques: a feasibility study. Ultrasonics 44(Suppl 1):e245–e249
22. Qin L, Bumrerraj S, Leung K et al. (2004) Correlation study of scanning acoustic microscope

reflection coefficients and image brightness intensities of micrographed osteons. J Bone Miner Metab 22:86–89

23. Roggero P, Giannì M, Orsi A et al. (2007) Postnatal "speed of sound" decline in preterm infants: an exploratory study. J Pediatr Gastroenterol Nutr 45:615–617

24. Siris E, Chen Y, Abbott T et al. (2004) Bone mineral density thresholds for pharmacological intervention to prevent fractures. Arch Intern Med 164:1108–1112

25. Suvorova E, Petrenko P, Buffat P (2007) Scanning and transmission electron microscopy for evaluation of order/disorder in bone structure. Scanning 29:162–170

26. Tadokoro M, Hattori K, Takakura Y et al. (2006) Rapid preparation of fresh frozen tissue-engineered bone sections for histological, histomorphological and histochemical analyses. Biomed Mater Eng 16:405–413

27. Tang S, Vashishth D (2007) A non-invasive in vitro technique for the three-dimensional quantification of microdamage in trabecular bone. Bone 40:1259–1264

28. Tersigni M (2007) Frozen human bone: a microscopic investigation. J Forensic Sci 52:16–20

29. Wang X, Masse D, Leng H et al. (2007) Detection of trabecular bone microdamage by micro-computed tomography. J Biomech 40:3397–3403

30. Well D, Meier J, Mahne A et al. (2007) Detection of age-related changes in thoracic structure and function by computed tomography, magnetic resonance imaging, and positron emission tomography. Semin Nucl Med 37:103–119

31. Yang R, Davies C, Archer C et al. (2003) Immunohistochemistry of matrix markers in Technovit 9100 New-embedded undecalcified bone sections. Eur Cell Mater 6:57–71

Chapter 9 Prevention of Osteoporosis

1. Berg K, Kunins H, Jackson J et al. (2008) Association between alcohol consumption and both osteoporotic fracture and bone density. Am J Med 121:406–418

2. Bischoff-Ferrari H, Willett W, Wong J et al. (2005) Fracture prevention with vitamin D supplementation. A Meta-analysis of randomized controlled studies. JAMA 293:2257–2264

3. Bügel S (2008) Vitamin K and bone health in adult humans. Vitam Horm 78:393–416

4. Cree M, Juby A, Carriere K (2003) Mortality and morbidity associated with osteoporosis drug treatment following hip fracture. Osteoporos Int 14:722–727

5. Ettinger M (2003) Aging bone and osteoporosis: strategies for preventing fractures in the elderly. Arch Intern Med 163:2237–2246

6. Gourlay M, Richy F, Reginster J (2003) Strategies for the prevention of hip fractures. Am J Med 115:309–317

7. Gourlay M, Richy F, Reginster J (2003) Strategies for the prevention of hip fractures. Am J Med 115:309–317

8. Kubota M, Shimizu H (2008) Calcium in aging, health, and anti-aging. Significance of calcium supplement for anti-aging. Clin Calcium 18:973–979

9. Millward D, Layman D, Tomé D et al. (2008) Protein quality assessment: impact of expanding understanding of protein and amino acid needs for optimal health. Am J Clin Nutr 87:1576S–1581S

10. Van Schoor N, Devillé W, Bouter L et al. (2002) Acceptance and compliance with external hip protectors: a systematic review of the literature. Osteoporos Int 13:917–924

11. Walker M, Novotny R, Bilezikian J et al. (2008) Race and diet interactions in the acquisition, maintenance, and loss of bone. J Nutr 138:1256S–1260S

Chapter 10 Physical Activity and Exercise Programs

1. Alway S, Siu P (2008) Nuclear apoptosis contributes to sarcopenia. Exerc Sport Sci Rev 36:51–57

2. Børsheim E, Bui Q, Tissier S et al. (2008) Effect of amino acid supplementation on muscle mass, strength and physical function in elderly. Clin Nutr 27:189–195

3. Cherkas L, Hunkin J, Kato B et al. (2008) The association between physical activity in leisure time and leukocyte telomere length. Arch Intern Med 168:154–158

4. Crepaldi G, Romanato G, Tonin P et al. (2007) Osteoporosis and body composition. J Endocrinol Invest 30(Suppl 6):42–47

5. Dutta C (1997) Significance of sarcopenia in the elderly. J Nutr 127(Suppl 5):992S–993S

6. Fricke O, Schoenau E (2007) The 'Functional Muscle-Bone Unit': probing the relevance of mechanical signals for bone development in children and adolescents. Growth Horm IGF Res 17:1–9

7. Gerdhem P, Akesson K, Obrant K (2003) Effect of previous and present physical activity on bone mass in elderly women. Osteoporos Int 14:208–212

8. Heaney R, Layman D (2008) Amount and type of protein influences bone health. Am J Clin Nutr 87:1567S–1570S

9. Hourigan S, Nitz J, Brauer S et al. (2008) Positive effects of exercise on falls and fracture risk in osteopenic women. Osteoporos Int 19:1077–1086

10. Huffman K, Slentz C, Johnson J et al. (2008) Impact of hormone replacement therapy on exercise training-induced improvements in insulin action in sedentary overweight adults. Metabolism 57:888–895

11. Huntoon E, Schmidt C, Sinaki M (2008) Significantly fewer refractures after vertebroplasty in patients who engage in back-extensor-strengthening exercises. Mayo Clin Proc 83:54–57

12. Jansen I, Ross R (2005) Linking age-related changes in skeletal muscle mass and composition with metabolism and disease. J Nutr Health Aging 9:408–419

13. Joseph C, Kenny A, Taxel P et al. (2005) Role of endocrine-immune dysregulation in osteoporosis, sarcopenia, frailty and fracture risk. Mol Aspects Med 26:181–201

14. Kadi F, Ponsot E, Piehl-Aulin K et al. (2008) The effects of regular strength training on telomere length in human skeletal muscle. Med Sci Sports Exerc 40:82–87

15. Kemmler W, Engelke K, Weineck J et al. (2003) The Erlangen fitness osteoporosis prevention study: a controlled exercise trial in early postmenopausal women with low bone density-first-year results. Arch Phys Med Rehabil 84:673–682

16. Lee M, Pittler M, Shin B-C, Ernst E (2008) Tai chi for osteoporosis: a systematic review. Osteoporos Int 19:139–146

17. Lips P (2006) Vitamin D physiology. Prog Biophys Mol Biol 92:4–8

18. Marcell T (2003) Sarcopenia: causes, consequences, and preventions. J Gerontol A Biol Sci Med Sci 58:M911–M916

19. Marcus R (1995) Relationship of age-related decreases in muscle mass and strength to skeletal status. J Gerontol A Biol Sci Med Sci 50 Spec No:86–87

20. Marzetti E, Lawler J, Hiona A et al. (2008) Modulation of age-induced apoptotic signaling and cellular remodeling by exercise and calorie restriction in skeletal muscles. Free Radic Biol Med 44:160–168

21. Paddon-Jones D, Short K, Campbell W et al. (2008) Role of dietary protein in the sarcopenia of aging. Am J Clin Nutr 87:1562S–1566S

22. Pedrosa M, Castro M (2005) Role of vitamin D in the neuro-muscular function. Arq Bras Endocrinol Metabol 49:495–502

23. Ponsot E, Lexell J, Kadi F (2008) Skeletal muscle telomere length is not impaired in healthy physically active old women and men. Muscle Nerve 37:467–472

24. Rolland Y, Abellan Van Kan G, Benetos A et al. (2008) Frailty, osteoporosis and hip fracture: causes, consequences and therapeutic perspectives. J Nutr Health Aging 12:335–346

25. Roubenoff R (2007) Physical activity, inflammation, and muscle loss. Nutr Rev 65:S208–S212

26. Schoenau E (2005) From mechanostat theory to development of the "Functional Muscle-Bone-Unit". J Musculoskelet Neuronal Interact 5:232–238

27. Senchina D, Kohut M (2007) Immunological outcomes of exercise in older adults. Clin Interv Aging 2:3–16

28. Uusi-Rasi K, Sievänen H, Pasanen M et al. (2008) Influence of calcium intake and physical activity on proximal femur bone mass and structure among pre- and postmenopausal women. A 10-year prospective study. Calcif Tissue Int 82:171–181

29. Yarasheski K (2003) Exercise, aging, and muscle protein metabolism. J Gerontol A Biol Sci Med Sci 58:M918–M922

30. Zacker R (2006) Health-related implications and management of sarcopenia. JAAPA 19:24–29

Chapter 11 Treatment Strategies in Osteoporosis

1. Bartl R (2007) Practical guidelines for the management of osteoporosis – evidence-based and cost-effective. Dtsch Med Wochenschr 132:995–999
2. Bartl R (2008) Treatment of osteoporosis according to the "European Guidance 2008". Fracture-oriented – economical – cost-effective. Internist 49:1126–1136
3. Cadarette S, Katz J, Brookhart M et al. (2008) Relative effectiveness of osteoporosis drugs for preventing nonvertebral fracture. Ann Intern Med 148:637–646
4. Cooper C, Jakob F, Chinn C et al. (2008) Fracture incidence and changes in quality of life in women with an inadequate clinical outcome from osteoporosis therapy: the Observational Study of Severe Osteoporosis (OSSO). Osteoporos Int 19:493–501
5. Cummings S, Karpf D, Harris F et al. (2002) Improvements in spine bone density and reduction in risk of vertebral fractures during treatment with antiresorptive drugs. Am J Med 114:281–289
6. Freedman K, Kaplan F, Bilker W et al. (2000) Treatment of osteoporosis: are physicians missing an opportunity? J Bone Joint Surg Am 82:1063–1070
7. Häuselmann H, Rizzoli R (2003) A comprehensive review of treatments for postmenopausal osteoporosis. Osteoporos Int 14:2–12
8. Kanis J, Burlet N, Cooper C et al. (2008) European guidance for the diagnosis and management of osteoporosis in postmenopausal osteoporosis. Osteoporos Int 19:399–428
9. Kanis J, Johnell O, Oden A et al. (2005) Intervention threshholds for osteoporosis in men and women: a study based on data from Sweden. Osteoporos Int 16:6–14
10. MacLean C, Newberry S, Maglione M et al. (2008) Systematic review: comparative effectiveness of treatments to prevent fractures in men and women with low bone density or osteoporosis. Ann Intern Med 148:197–213
11. Marcus R, Wong M, Heath H et al. (2002) Antiresorptive treatment of postmenopausal osteoporosis: comparison of study designs and outcomes in large clinical trials with fracture as an endpoint. Endocr Rev 23:16–37
12. Melton L, Heaney R (2003) Osteoporosis: Too much medicine? Or too little? Bone 32:327–331
13. Pasco J, Henry M, Sanders K et al. (2004) Beta-adrenergic blockers reduce the risk of fracture partly by increasing bone mineral density: Geelong Osteoporosis Study. J Bone Miner Res 19:19–24
14. Riggs L, Parfitt M (2005) Drugs used to treat osteoporosis: the critical need for a uniform nomenclature based on their action on bone remodeling. J Bone Miner Res 20:177–184
15. Rodan G, Martin T (2000) Therapeutic approaches to bone diseases. Science 289:1508–1514
16. Rosen C (2005) Postmenopausal osteoporosis. N Engl J Med 353:595–603
17. Sambrook P, Cooper C (2006) Osteoporosis. Lancet 367:2010–2018
18. Seaman E (2003a) Reduced bone formation and increased bone resorption: rational targets for the treatment of osteoporosis. Osteoporos Int 14(Suppl 3):S2–S8
19. Strewler G (2004) Decimal point – osteoporosis therapy at the 10-year mark. N Engl J Med 350:1172–1174
20. Valverde P (2008) Pharmacotherapies to manage bone loss-associated diseases: a quest for the perfect benefit-to-risk ratio. Curr Med Chem 15:284–304
21. Wehren L, Hosking D, Hochberg M (2004) Putting evidence-based medicine into clinical practice: comparing anti-resorptive agents for the treatment of osteoporosis. Curr Med Res Opinion 20:525–531

Chapter 12 Management of Pain in Osteoporosis

1. Buckalew N, Haut M, Morrow L et al. (2008) Chronic pain is associated with brain volume loss in older adults: preliminary evidence. Pain Med 9:240–248
2. Delaney A, Fleetwood-Walker S, Colvin L et al. (2008) Translational medicine: cancer pain mechanisms and management. Br J Anaesth 101:87–94

3. Hippisley-Cox J, Coupland C (2005) Risk of myocardial infarction in patients taking cyclo-oxygenase-2 inhibitors or conventional non-steroidal anti-inflammatory drugs: population based nested case-control analysis. BMJ 330:1366–1375

4. Krocker D, Ullrich H, Buttgereit F et al. (2008) Influence of adjuvant pain medication on quality of life in the treatment of postmenopausal osteoporosis. Orthopaede 37:435–439

5. Rao R, Singrakhia M (2003) Current concepts review: painful osteoporotic vertebral fracture. J Bone Joint Surg 85:2010–2022

6. Schuh T, Lyles K (2003) Osteoporosis considerations in the frail elderly. Curr Opin Rheumatol 15:481–486

Chapter 13 Calcium and Vitamin D

1. Ahn J, Peters U, Albanes D et al. (2008) Serum vitamin D concentration and prostate cancer risk: a nested case-control study. J Natl Cancer Inst 100:796–804

2. Ali M, Vaidya Y (2007) Vitamin D and cancer. J Cancer Res Ther 3:225–230

3. Cantor I (2008) Shedding light on vitamin D and integrative oncology. Integr Cancer Ther 7:81–89

4. Chapuy M, Arlot M, Duboeuf F et al. (1992) Vitamin D3 and calcium to prevent hip fractures in elderly women. N Engl J Med 327:1637–1642

5. Charles P (1992) Calcium absorption and calcium bioavailability. J Intern Med 231:161–168

6. Chevalley T, Rizzoli R, Nydegger V et al. (1994) Effects of calcium supplements on femoral bone mineral density and vertebral fracture rate in vitamin-D-replete elderly patients. Osteoporos Int 4:245–252

7. Dawson Hughes B (2001) The role of calcium in the treatment of osteoporosis. Osteoporosis 2:545–552

8. Dawson-Hughes B, Dallai G, Krall E et al. (1990) A controlled trial of the effects of calcium supplementation on bone density in postmenopausal women. N Engl J Med 323:878–883

9. Dawson-Hughes B, Harris S, Krall E, Dallal G (1997) Effect of calcium and vitamin D supplementation on bone density in men and women 65 years of age or older. N Engl J Med 337:1437–1443

10. Dawson-Hughes B, Heaney R, Holick M et al. (2005) Estimates of optimal vitamin D status. Osteoporos Int 16:713–716

11. Duque G, Macoritto M, Kremer R (2004) 1,25(OH)2D3 inhibits bone marrow adipogenesis in senescence accelerated mice (SAM-P/6) by decreasing the expression of peroxisome proliferator-activated receptor gamma 2 (PPARgamma2). Exp Gerontol 39:333–338

12. Duque G, Macoritto M, Kremer R (2004) Vitamin D treatment of senescence accelerated mice (SAM-P/6) induces several regulators of stromal cell plasticity. Biogerontology 5:421–429

13. Heaney R (2000) Vitamin D: How much do we need, and how much is too much? Osteoporos Int 11:553–555

14. Holden J, Lemar L, Exler J (2008) Vitamin D in foods: development of the US Department of Agriculture database. Am J Clin Nutr 87:1092S–1096S

15. Holick M, Chen T (2008) Vitamin D deficiency: a worldwide problem with health consequences. Am J Clin Nutr 87:1080S–1086S

16. Hubner R, Muir K, Liu J et al. (2008) Dairy products, polymorphisms in the vitamin D receptor gene and colorectal adenoma recurrence. Int J Cancer 123:586–593

17. Huncharek M, Muscat J, Kupelnick B (2008) Dairy products, dietary calcium and vitamin D intake as risk factors for prostate cancer: a meta-analysis of 26,769 cases from 45 observational studies. Nutr Cancer 60:421–441

18. Karami S, Brennan P, Hung R et al. (2008) Vitamin D receptor polymorphisms and renal cancer risk in Central and Eastern Europe. J Toxicol Environ Health A 71:367–372

19. Kochupillai N (2008) The physiology of vitamin D: current concepts. Indian J Med Res 127:256–262

20. Krishnan A, Moreno J, Nonn L et al. (2007) Calcitriol as a chemopreventive and therapeutic agent in prostate cancer: role of anti-inflammatory activity. J Bone Miner Res 22(Suppl 2): V74–V80

21. Lanham-New S (2008) Importance of calcium, vitamin D and vitamin K for osteoporosis prevention and treatment. Proc Nutr Soc 67:163–176

22. Lim S, Kung A, Sompongse S et al. (2008) Vitamin D inadequacy in postmenopausal women in Eastern Asia. Curr Med Res Opin 24:99–106

23. Lips P (2001) Vitamin D deficiency and secondary hyperparathyroidism in the elderly: consequences for bone loss and fractures and therapeutic implications. Endocr Rev 22:477–501

24. Lips P, Graafmans W, Ooms M et al. (1996) Vitamin D supplementation and fracture incidence in elderly persons. A randomized placebo-controlled trial. Ann Intern Med 124:400–406

25. Mayor S (2008) Lack of vitamin D raises risk of heart disease and worsens prognosis for some cancers. BMJ 336:62

26. Menezes R, Cheney R, Husain A et al. (2008) Vitamin D receptor expression in normal, premalignant, and malignant human lung tissue. Cancer Epidemiol Biomarkers Prev 17:1104–1110

27. Montero-Odasso M, Duque G (2005) Vitamin D in the aging musculoskeletal system: an authentic strength preserving hormone. Mol Aspects Med 26:203–219

28. Nabeshima Y, Imura H (2008) alpha-Klotho: a regulator that integrates calcium homeostasis. Am J Nephrol 28:455–464

29. Okuizumi H, Harada A (2006) Effect of vitamin D on bone mineral density: bone strength and fracture prevention. Clin Calcium 16:1115–1121

30. Papadimitropoulos W, Wells G, Shea B et al. (2002) The Osteoporosis Methodology Group, The Osteoporosis Research Advisory Group: VIII: Meta-analysis of the efficacy of vitamin D treatment in preventing osteoporosis in postmenopausal women. Endocr Rev 23:560–569

31. Pérez-López F (2007) Vitamin D: the secosteroid hormone and human reproduction. Gynecol Endocrinol 23:13–24

32. Reid I (2001) Vitamin D and its metabolites in the management of osteoporosis. Osteoporosis 2:553–575

33. Reid I, Ames R, Evans M, Gamble G, Sharpe S (1995) Long-term effect of calcium supplementation on bone loss and fracture in postmenopausal women: a randomized controlled trial. Am J Med 98:331–335

34. Richart T, Li Y, Staessen J (2008) Renal versus extrarenal activation of vitamin D in relation to atherosclerosis, arterial stiffening, and hypertension. Am J Hypertens 20:1007–1015

35. Roux C, Bischoff-Ferrari H et al. (2008) New insights into the role of vitamin D and calcium in osteoporosis management: an expert roundtable discussion. Curr Med Res Opin 24:1363–1370

36. Sambrock P (2005) Vitamin D and fractures: quo vadis? Lancet 365:1599–1600

37. Shea B, Wells G, Cranney A et al. (2002) The Osteoporosis Methodology Group, The Osteoporosis Research Advisory Group: Meta-analysis of calcium supplementation for the prevention of postmenopausal osteoporosis. Endocr Rev 23:552–559

38. Smith S, Heer M (2002) calcium and bone metabolism during space flight. Nutrition 18:849–852

39. Smith S, Wastney M, O'Brien K et al. (2005) Bone markers, calcium metabolism, and calcium kinetics during extended-duration space flight on the Mir Space Station. J Bone Miner Res 20:208–218

40. Strushkevich N, Usanov S, Plotnikov A et al. (2008) Structural analysis of CYP2R1 in complex with vitamin D3. J Mol Biol 380:95–106

41. Torres P, Prié D, Molina-Blétry V et al. (2007) Klotho: an antiaging protein involved in mineral and vitamin D metabolism. Kidney Int 71:730–737

42. Tucker K, Hannan M, Qiao N et al. (2005) Low plasma vitamin B12 is associated with lower BMD: the Framingham Osteoporosis Study. J Bone Miner Res 20:152–158

43. Uusi-Rasi K, Sievänen H, Pasanen M et al. (2008) Influence of calcium intake and physical activity on proximal femur bone mass and structure among pre- and postmenopausal women. A 10-year prospective study. Calcif Tissue Int 82:171–181

44. vanSchoor N, Visser M, Pluijm S et al. (2008) Vitamin D deficiency as a risk factor for osteoporotic fractures. Bone 42:260–266

45. Wigle D, Turner M, Gomes J et al. (2008) Role of hormonal and other factors in human prostate cancer. J Toxicol Environ Health B Crit Rev 11:242–259

46. Witkowski J, Soroczyńska-Cybula M, Bryl E et al. (2007) Klotho – a common link in physiological and rheumatoid arthritis-related aging of human CD4+ lymphocytes. J Immunol 178:771–777

Chapter 14 Hormones for Replacement Therapy

1. Canfell K, Banks E, Moa A et al. (2008) Decrease in breast cancer incidence following a rapid fall in use of hormone replacement therapy in Australia. Med J Aust 188:641–644
2. Chilibeck P, Cornish S (2008) Effect of estrogenic compounds (estrogen or phytoestrogens) combined with exercise on bone and muscle mass in older individuals. Appl Physiol Nutr Metab 33:200–212
3. Coxam V (2008) Phyto-oestrogens and bone health. Proc Nutr Soc 67:184–195
4. Divasta A, Gordon C (2008) Hormone replacement therapy for the adolescent patient. Ann N Y Acad Sci 1135:204–211
5. Grady D (2003) Postmenopausal hormones – therapy for symptoms only. N Engl J Med 348:1835–1837
6. Huot L, Couris C, Tainturier V et al. (2008) Trends in HRT and anti-osteoporosis medication prescribing in a European population after the WHI study. Osteoporos Int 19:1047–1054
7. Krum S, Miranda-Carboni G, Hauschka P et al. (2008) Estrogen protects bone by inducing Fas ligand in osteoblasts to regulate osteoclast survival. EMBO J 27:535–545
8. Lekander I, Borgström F, Ström O et al. (2008) Cost effectiveness of hormone therapy in women at high risks of fracture in Sweden, the US and the UK – results based on the Women's Health Initiative randomised controlled trial. Bone 42:294–306
9. Mei J, Yeung S, Kung A (2001) High dietary phytoestrogen intake is associated with higher bone mineral density in postmenopausal but not premenopausal women. J Clin Endocrinol Metab 86:5217–5221
10. Migliaccio S, Anderson J (2003) Isoflavones and skeletal health: are these molecules ready for clinical application? Osteoporos Int 14:361–368
11. Qiao X, McConnell K, Khalil R (2008) Sex steroids and vascular responses in hypertension and aging. Gend Med 5(Suppl A):S46–S64
12. Setchell K, Lydeking-Olsen E (2003) Dietary phytoestrogens and their effect on bone: evidence from in vitro and in vivo, human observational, and dietary intervention studies. AM J Clin Nutr 78(Suppl):593S–609S
13. Shulman L (2008) Transdermal hormone therapy and bone health. Clin Interv Aging 3:51–54
14. Torgenson D, Bell-Seyer S (2001) Hormone replacement therapy and prevention of nonvertebral fractures: a meta-analysis of randomized trials. JAMA 285:2891–2897
15. Women´s Health Initiative Group (2002) Risks and benefits of estrogen plus progestin in healthy postmenopausal women. JAMA 288:321–333

Chapter 15 Bisphosphonates

1. Abu-Id M, Warnke P, Gottschalk, J et al. (2008) "Bis-phossy jaws" – high and low risk factors for bisphosphonate-induced osteonecrosis of the jaw. J Craniomaxillofac Surg 36:95–103
2. Adami S, Felsenberg D, Christiansen C et al. (2004) Efficacy and safety of ibandronate given by intravenous injection once every 3 months. Bone 34:881–889
3. Allen M, Gineyts E, Leeming D et al. (2008) Bisphosphonates alter trabecular bone collagen cross-linking and isomerization in beagle dog vertebra. Osteoporos Int 19:329–337
4. Bagger Y, Tankó L, Alexandersen P et al. (2003) Alendronate has a residual effect on bone mass in postmenopausal Danish women up to 7 years after treatment withdrawal. Bone 33:301–307
5. Bartl R, Bartl C, Gradinger R (2008) Use of bisphosphonates in orthopaedic surgery. Orthopäde 37:595–614
6. Bartl R, Goette S, Hadji P, Hammerschmidt T (2005) Persistance and compliance with daily- and weekly-administered bisphosphonates for osteoporosis in Germany. Osteoporos Int 16(Suppl 3):P195
7. Bartl R, Mast G (2008) Bisphosphonate-associated osteonecrosis of the jaw: A pathophysiologic approach. Bone 42(Suppl 1):165
8. Bauss F, Russell G (2004) Ibandronate in osteoporosis: preclinical data and rationale for intermittent dosing. Osteoporos Int 15:423–433
9. Bilezikian J (2006) Osteonecrosis of the jaw – do bisphosphonates pose a risk? N Engl J Med 355:2278–2281
10. Black D, Bilezikian J, Ensrud K et al. (2005) One year of alendronate after one year of para-

thyroid hormone (1-84) for osteoporosis. N Engl J Med 353:555–565

11. Black D, Delmas P, Eastell R et al. (2007) Once-yearly zoledronic acid for treatment of postmenopausal osteoporosis. N Engl J Med 356:1809–1822

12. Black D, Schwartz A, Ensrud K (2006) Effects of continuing or stopping alendronate after 5 years of treatment. The fracture intervention trial long-term extension (FLEX): a randomized trial. JAMA 296:2927–2938

13. Bolland M, Grey A, Horne A et al. (2008) Effects of intravenous zoledronate on bone turnover and BMD persist for at least 24 months. J Bone Miner Res 23:1304–1308

14. Bone H, Adami S, Rizzoli R et al. (2000) Weekly administration of alendronate: rationale and plan for clinical assessment. Clin Ther 22:15–28

15. Bone H, Greenspan S, McKeever C et al. (2000) Alendronate and estrogen effects in postmenopausal women with low bone mineral density. J Endocrinol Metab 85:720–726

16. Bone H, Hosking D, Devogelaer J-P et al. (2004) Ten years' experience with alendronate for osteoporosis in postmenopausal women. N Engl J Med 350:1189–1199

17. Borah B, Dufresne T, Chmielewski P et al. (2002) Risedronate preserves trabecular architecture and increases bone strength in vertebra of ovariectomized minipigs as measured by three-dimensional microcomputed tomography. J Bone Miner Res 17:1139–1147

18. Calis K, Pucino F (2007) Zoledronic acid and secondary prevention of fractures. N Engl J Med 357:1861–1862

19. Cartsos V, Zhu S, Zavras A (2008) Bisphosphonate use and the risk of adverse jaw outcomes: a medical claims study of 714,217 people. J Am Dent Assoc 139:23–30

20. Chavassieux P, Arlot M, Reda C et al. (1997) Histomorphometric assessment of the long-term effects of alendronate on bone quality and remodeling in patients with osteoporosis. J Clin Invest 1000:1475–1480

21. Chesnut C, McClung M, Ensrud K et al. (1995) Alendronate treatment of the postmenopausal osteoporotic women: effect of multiple dosages on bone mass and bone remodeling. Am J Med 99:144–152

22. Chesnut C, Skag A, Christiansen C et al. (2004) Effects of oral ibandronate administered daily or intermittently on fracture risk in postmenopausal osteoporosis. J Bone Miner Res 19:1241–1249

23. Colon-Emeric C (2006) Ten vs five years of bisphosphonate treatment for postmenopausal osteoporosis. Enough of a good thing. JAMA 296:2968–2969

24. Coxon F, Thompson K, Roelofs A et al. (2008) Visualizing mineral binding and uptake of bisphosphnate by osteoclast and non-resorbing cells. Bone 42:848–860

25. Cranney A, Guyatt G, Griffith L et al. (2002) IX: Summary of meta-analyses of therapies for postmenopausal osteoporosis. Endocr Rev 23:570–578

26. Cummings S, Black D Thompson D et al. (1998) Effect of alendronate on risk of fracture in women with low bone density but without vertebral fractures. JAMA 280:2077–2082

27. Dagdelen S, Sener D, Bayraktar M (2007) Influence of type 2 diabetes mellitus on bone mineral density response to bisphosphonates in late postmenopausal osteoporosis. Adv Ther 24:1314–1320

28. Dannemann C, Grätz K, Zwahlen R (2008) Bisphosphonate-induced osteonecrosis of the jaws – a guide to diagnosis, therapy and prevention of BON in dental practice. Schweiz Monatsschr Zahnmed 118:113–123

29. Delmas P, McClung M et al. (2008) Efficacy and safety of risedronate 150 mg once a month in the treatment of postmenopausal osteoporosis. Bone 42:36–42

30. Devogelaer J, Brown J, Burckhardt P et al. (2007) Zoledronic acid efficacy and safety over five years in postmenopausal osteoporosis. Osteoporos Int 18:1211–1218

31. Eastell R, Hannon R, Chines A et al. (2003) Relationship of early changes in bone resorption to the reduction in fracture risk with risedronate. J Bone Miner Res 18:1051–1056

32. Ebeling P, Burr D (2008) Positive effects of intravenous zoledronic acid on bone remodeling and structure: Are different effects on osteoblast activity to other oral bisphosphonates responsible? J Bone Mineral Res 23:2–5

33. Eriksen E, Lyles K, Colon-Emeric C et al. (2008) Timing of first infusion of zoledronic acid 5 mg after recent hip fracture affects antifracture efficacy and reduction of mortality. Osteoporos Int 19(Suppl):S14

34. Guney E, Kisakol G, Ozgen A et al. (2008) Effects of bisphosphonates on lipid metabolism. Neuro Endocrinol Lett 29:252–255

35. Harrington J, Ste-Marie L, Brandi M et al. (2004) Risedronate rapidly reduces the risk for nonvertebral fractures in women with postmenopausal osteoporosis. Calcif Tissue Int 74:129–135

36. Hess L, Jeter J et al. (2008) Factors associated with osteonecrosis of the jaw among bisphosphonate users. Am J Med 121:475–483

37. Hoff A, Toth B, Altundag K et al. (2008) Frequency and risk factors associated with osteonecrosis of the jaw in cancer patients treated with intravenous bisphosphonates. J Bone Miner Res 23:826–836

38. Hornby SB, Evans G, Hornby SL et al. (2003) Long-term zoledronic acid treatment increases bone structure and mechanical strength of long bones of ovariectomized adult rats. Calcif Tissue Int 72:519–527

39. Hosking D, Chilvers C, Christiansen C et al. (1998) Prevention of bone loss with alendronate in postmenopausal women under 60 years of age. N Engl J Med 338:485–492

40. Idris A, Rojas J, Greig I et al. (2008) Aminobisphosphonates cause osteoblast apoptosis and inhibit bone nodule formation in vitro. Calcif Tissue Int 82:191–201

41. Jeffcoat M (2006) Safety of oral bisphosphonates: controlled studies on alveolar bone. Int J Oral Maxillofac Implants 21:349–353

42. Kanis J, Adams J, Borgström F et al. (2008) The cost-effectiveness of alendronate in the management of osteoporosis. Bone 42:4–15

43. Kwek E, Goh S, Koh J et al. (2008) An emerging pattern of subtrochanteric stress fractures: a long-term complication of alendronate therapy? Injury 39:224–231

44. Liberman U, Weiss S, Bröll J et al., for the Alendronate Phase III Osteoporois Treatment Study Group (1995) Effect of oral alendronate on bone mineral density and the incidence of fractures in postmenopausal osteoporosis. N Engl J Med 333:1437–1443

45. Lyles K, Conon-Emeric C, Magaziner J et al. (2007) Zoledronic acid and clinical fractures and mortality after hip fracture. N Engl J Med 357:1799–1809

46. Lyles KW, Colon-Emeric CS, Magaziner JS, Adachi JD, Pieper CF, Mautalen C et al., the HORIZON Recurrent Fracture Trial (2007) Zole-

dronic acid and clinical fractures and mortality after hip fracture. N Engl J Med 357:1799–1809

47. Majumdar S (2008) Oral bisphosphonates and atrial fibrillation. BMJ 336:784–785

48. Marcus R, Wong M, Heath H et al. (2002) Antiresorptive treatment of postmenopausal osteoporosis: comparison of study designs and outcomes in large clinical trials with fracture as an endpoint. Endocr Rev 23:16–37

49. McClung M, Wasnich R, Recker R et al. (2004) Oral daily ibandronate prevents bone loss in early postmenopausal women without osteoporosis. J Bone Miner Res 19:11–18

50. Mellström D, Sörensen O, Goemaere S et al. (2004) Seven years of treatment with risedronate in women with postmenopausal osteoporosis. Calcif Tissue Int 75:462–468

51. Nancollas G, Tang R, Gulde S et al. (2002) Mineral binding affinities and zeta potentials of bisphosphonates. J Bone Miner Res 17(S1):5368

52. Neviaser A, Lane J, Lenart B et al. (2008) Low-energy femoral shaft fractures associated with alendronate use. J Orthop Trauma 22:346–350

53. Papapoulos S, Quandt S, Liberman U et al. (2005) Meta-analysis of the efficacy of alendronate for the prevention of hip fractures in postmenopausal women. Osteoporos Int 16:468–474

54. Pazianas M, Blumentals W, Miller P (2008) Lack of association between oral bisphosphonates and osteonecrosis using jaw surgery as a surrogate marker. Osteoporos Int 19:773–778

55. Pazianas M, Miller P, Blumentals W et al. (2007) A review of the literature on osteonecrosis of the jaw in patients with osteoporosis treated with oral bisphosphonates: prevalence, risk factors, and clinical characteristics. Clin Ther 29:1548–1557

56. Recker R, Delmas P, Halse J et al. (2008) Effects of intravenous zoledronic acid once yearly on bone remodeling and bone structure. J Bone Miner Res 23:6–16

57. Recker R, Reginster J, Delmas P (2003) A new dosing concept for bisphosphonate therapy: rationale and design for the Monthly Oral iBandronate In LadiEs (MOBILE) study. J Bone Miner Res 18(Suppl 2):261

58. Recker R, Weinstein R, Chesnut III, C et al. (2004) Histomorphometric evaluation of daily and intermittent oral ibandronate in women with postmenopausal osteoporosis: results from the BONE study. Osteoporos Int 15:231–237

59. Regev E, Lustmann J, Nashef R (2008) Atraumatic teeth extraction in bisphosphonate-treated patients. J Oral Maxillofac Surg 66:1157–1161

60. Reginster J, Minne H, Sorensen O et al. (2000) Randomized trial of the effects of risedronate on vertebral fractures in women with established postmenopausal osteoporosis. Osteoporos Int 11:83–91

61. Reginster J, Wiese C, Wilson K (2005) Oral monthly ibandronate decreases bone turnover in postmenopausal women with low bone mass: results from the Monthly Oral Pilot Study (MOPS). Osteoporos Int 14(Suppl 7):5

62. Reid I, Brown J, Burckhardt P et al. (2002) Intravenous zoledronic acid in postmenopausal women with low bone mineral density. N Engl J Med 346:653–661

63. Reid R (2003) Bisphosphonates: new indications and methods of administration. Curr Opin Rheumatol 15:458–463

64. Riis B, Ise J, von Stein T et al. (2001) Ibandronate: a comparison of oral daily dosing versus intermittent dosing in postmenopausal osteoporosis. J Bone Miner Res 16:1871–1878

65. Ringe J, Dorst A, Faber H et al. (2003) Three-monthly ibandronate bolus injection offers favourable tolerability and sustained efficacy advantage over two years in established corticosteroid-induced osteoporosis. Rheumatology 42:743–749

66. Rizzoli R. Burlet N, Cahall D et al. (2008) Osteonecrosis of the jaw and bisphosphonate treatment for osteoporosis. Bone 42:841–847

67. Roschger P, Rinnerthaler S, Yates J et al. (2001) Alendronate increases degree and uniformity of mineralisation in cancellous bone and decreases the porosity in cortical bone of osteoporotic women. Bone 29:185–191

68. Roschger P, Rinnerthaler S, Yates J et al. (2001) Alendronate increases degree and uniformity of mineralisation in cancellous bone and decreases the porosity in cortical bone of osteoporotic women. Bone 29:185–191

69. Roux C, Seeman E, Eastell R et al. (2004) Efficacy of risedronate on clinical vertebral fractures within six months. Curr Med Res Opin 20:433–439

70. Russell R, Watts N, Ebentino F, Rogers M (2008) Mechanisms of action of bisphosphonates: similarities and differences and their potential influence on clinical efficacy. Osteoporos Int 19:733–759

71. Saito M (2008) Assessment of bone quality. Effects of bisphosphonates, raloxifene, alfacalcidol, and menatetrenone on bone quality: collagen cross-links, mineralization, and microdamage. Clin Calcium 18:364–372

72. Sambrook P, Geusens P, Ribot C et al. (2003) Alendronate produces greater effects than raloxifene on bone density and bone turnover in postmenopausal women with low bone density: results of EFFECT (Efficacy of FOSAMAX® versus EVISTA® Comparison Trial) International. J Intern Med 255:503–511

73. Sebba A (2008) Significance of a decline in bone mineral density while receiving oral bisphosphonate treatment. Clin Ther 30:443–452

74. Shenker N, Jawad A (2007) Bisphosphonates and osteonecrosis of the jaw. Rheumatology 46:1049–1051

75. Silverman S, Watts N, Delmas P et al. (2007) Effectiveness of bisphosphonates on nonvertebral and hip fractures in the first year of therapy: the risedronate and alendronate (REAL) cohort study. Osteoporos Int 18:25–34

76. Sorensen H, Christensen S et al. (2008) use of bisphosphonates among women and risk of atrial fibrillation and flutter: population based case-control study. BMJ 336:813–816

77. Stakkestad J, Benevolenskaya L, Stepan J et al. (2003) Intravenous ibandronate injections given every three months: a new treatment option to prevent bone loss in postmenopausal women. Ann Rheum Dis 62:969–975

78. Tonino R, Meunier P, Emkey R et al. (2000) Skeletal benefits of alendronate: 7-year treatment of postmenopausal osteoporotic women. J Clin Endocrinol Metab 85:3109–3115

79. Watts N, Cooper C, Lindsay R et al. (2004) Relationship between changes in bone mineral density and vertebral fracture risk associated with risedronate: greater increases in bone mineral density do not relate to greater decreases in fracture risk. J Clin Densitom 7:255–261

80. Watts N, Harris S, Genant H et al. (1990) Intermittent cyclical etidronate treatment of postmenopausal osteoporosis. N Engl J Med 323:73–79

81. Wimalawansa S (2008) Insight into bisphosphonate-associated osteomyelitis of the jaw: pathophysiology, mechanisms and clinical management. Expert Opin Drug Saf 7:491–512

82. Woo S, Hellstein J, Kalmar J (2006) Systematic review: bisphosphonates and osteonecrosis of the jaws. Ann Intern Med 144:753–761

Chapter 16 Selective Oestrogen-Receptor Modulators

1. Cauley J, Norton L, Lippman M et al. (2001) Continued breast cancer risk reduction in postmenopausal women treated with raloxifene: 4-year results from the MORE trial. Breast Cancer Res Treat 65:125–134
2. Cummings S, Eckert S, Krueger K et al. (1999) The effect of raloxifene on risk of breast cancer in postmenopausal women. JAMA 281:2189–2197
3. Ettinger B, Black D, Mitlak B et al. (1999) Reduction of vertebral fracture risk in postmenopausal women with osteoporosis treated with raloxifene. Results from a 3-year randomised clinical trial. JAMA 282:637–645
4. Grady D, Cauley J, Geiger M et al. (2008) Reduced incidence of invasive breast cancer with raloxifene among women at increased coronary risk. J Natl Cancer Inst 100:854–861
5. Lazovic G, Radivojevic U, Marinkovic J (2008) Tibolone: the way to beat many a postmenopausal ailments. Expert Opin Pharmacother 9:1039–1047
6. Maricic M, Aachi J, Meunier P et al. (2000) Raloxifene 60mg/day has effects within 12 months in postmenopausal osteoporosis treatment and prevention studies. Arthritis Rheum 43(9 Suppl):197–201
7. Mosca L, Barrett-Connor E, Wenger N et al. (2001) Design and methods of the Raloxifene Use for The Heart (RUTH) study. Am J Cardiol 88:392–395
8. Yang N, Bryant H, Hardicar S et al. (1996) Estrogen and raloxifene stimulate transforming growth factor-β3 gene expression in rat bone: a potential mechanism for estrogen- or raloxifene-mediated bone maintenance. Endocrinology 137:2075–2084
9. Yang N, Hardikar S, Kim J, Sato M (1993) Raloxifene, an "anti-estrogen" stimulates the effects of estrogen on inhibiting bone resorption through regulating TGFβ-3 expression in bone. J Bone Miner Res 8:S118

Chapter 17 Peptides of the Parathyroid Hormone Family

1. Anastasilakis A, Goulis D, Polyzos S et al. (2008) Acute changes in serum osteoprotegerin and receptor activator for nuclear factor-kappaB ligand levels in women with established osteoporosis treated with teriparatide. Eur J Endocrinol 158:411–415
2. Bilezikian J (2008) Combination anabolic and antiresorptive therapy for osteoporosis: opening the anabolic window. Curr Osteoporos Rep 6:24–30
3. Black D, Greenspan S, Ensrud K et al. (2003) The effect of parathyroid hormone and alendronate alone or in combination in postmenopausal osteoporosis. N Engl J Med 349:1207–1215
4. Bodenner D, Redman C, Riggs A (2007) Teriparatide in the management of osteoporosis. Clin Interv Aging 2:499–507
5. Boonen S, Marin F, Mellstrom D et al. (2006) Safety and efficacy of teriparatide in elderly women with established osteoporosis: bone anabolic therapy from a geriatric perspective. J Am Geriatr Soc 54:782–789
6. Canalis E, Giustina A, Bilezikian J (2007) Mechanisms of anabolic therapies for osteoporosis. N Engl J Med 357:905–916
7. Cosman F, Nieves J, Zion M et al. (2005) Daily and cyclic parathyroid hormone in women receiving alendronate. N Engl J Med 353:566–575
8. Dempster D, Cosman F, Kurland E et al. (2001) Effects of daily treatment with parathyroid hormone on bone microarchitecture and turnover in patients with osteoporosis: a paired biopsy study. J Bone Miner Res 16:1846–1853
9. Goltzman D (2008) Studies on the mechanisms of the skeletal anabolic action of endogenous and exogenous parathyroid hormone. Arch Biochem Biophys 473:218–224
10. Greenspan S, Bone H, Ettinger M et al. (2007) Effect of recombinant human parathyroid hormone (1-84) on vertebral fracture and bone mineral density in postmenopausal women with osteoporosis. Ann Intern Med 146:326–339
11. Greenspan S, Bone H, Marriott T et al. (2005) Preventing the first vertebral fracture in post-

menopausal women with low bone mass using PTH(1-84): results from the TOP study. J Bone Miner Res 20(Suppl 1):S56

12. Hodsman A, Bauer D, Dempster D et al. (2005) Parathyroid hormone and teriparatide for the treatment of osteoporosis: a review of the evidence and suggested guidelines for its use. Endocr Rev 26:688–703

13. Jiang Y, Zhao J, Mitlak B et al. (2003) Recombinant human parathyroid hormone (1-34) [teriparatide] improves both cortical and cancellous bone structure. J Bone Miner Res 18:1932–1941

14. Kaufman J-M, Orwoll E, Goemaere S et al. (2005) Teriparatide effects on vertebral fractures and bone mineral density in men with osteoporosis: treatment and discontinuation of therapy. Osteoporos Int 16:510–516

15. Miller P (2008) Safety of parathyroid hormone for the treatment of osteoporosis. Curr Osteoporos Rep 6:12–16

16. Neer R, Arnaud C, Zanchetta J et al. (2001) Effect of parathyroid hormone (1-34) on fractures and bone mineral density in postmenopausal women with osteoporosis. N Engl J Med 344:1434–1441

17. Pettway G, Meganck J, Koh A et al. (2008) Parathyroid hormone mediates bone growth through the regulation of osteoblast proliferation and differentiation. Bone 42:806–818

18. Prince R, Sipos A, Hossain A et al. (2005) Sustained nonvertebral fragility fracture risk reduction after discontinuation of teriparatide treatment. J Bone Miner Res 20:1507–1513

19. Rajzbaum G, Jakob F, Karras D et al. (2008) Characterization of patients in the European Forsteo Observational Study (EFOS): postmenopausal women entering teriparatide treatment in a community setting. Curr Med Res Opin 24:377–384

20. Rosen C, Bilezikian J (2001) Anabolic therapy of osteoporosis. J Clin Endocrinol Metab 86:957–964

21. Rubin M., Cosman F, Lindsay R, Bilezikian J (2002) The anabolic effect of parathyroid hormone. Osteoporos Int 13:267–277

22. Stroup J, Kane M, Abu-Baker A (2008) Teriparatide in the treatment of osteoporosis. Am J Health Syst Pharm 65:532–539

Chapter 18 Strontium Ranelate

1. Ammann P (2005) Strontium ranelate: a novel mode of action leading to renewed bone quality. Osteoporos Int 16:S11–S15

2. Fuleihan G (2004) Strontium Ranelate – a novel therapy for osteoporosis or a permutation of the same? N Engl J Med 350:504–506

3. Marie P (2003) Optimizing bone metabolism in osteoporosis: insight into the pharmacologic profile of strontium ranelate. Osteoporos Int 14(Suppl 3):S9–S12

4. Marie P (2005) Strontium ranelate: a novel mode of action optimizing bone formation and resorption. Osteoporos Int 16:S7–S10

5. Meunier P, Roux C, Seeman E et al. (2004) The effects of strontium ranelate on the risk of vertebral fracture in women with postmenopausal osteoporosis. N Engl J Med 350:459–468

6. Reginster J, Meunier P (2003) Strontium ranelate phase 2 dose-ranging studies: PREVOS and STRATOS studies. Osteoporos Int 14(Suppl 3): S56–S65

7. Seeman E, Devogelaer J, Lorenc R et al. (2008) Strontium ranelate reduces the risk of vertebral fractures in patients with osteopenia. J Bone Miner Res 23:433–438

Chapter 19 Calcitonin and Fluoride

1. Azarpazhooh A, Main P (2008) Fluoride varnish in the prevention of dental caries in children and adolescents: a systematic review. J Can Dent Assoc 74:73–79

2. Boonen S, Marin F, Obermayer-Pietsch B et al. (2008) Effects of previous antiresorptive therapy on the bone mineral density response to two years of teriparatide treatment in postmenopausal women with osteoporosis. J Clin Endocrinol Metab 93:852–860

3. Chesnut C, Azria M, Silverman S et al. (2008) Salmon calcitonin: a review of current and future therapeutic indications. Osteoporos Int 19:479–491

4. Chesnut C, Silverman S, Andriano K et al. (2000) A randomized trial of nasal spray salmon calcitonin in postmenopausal women with established osteoporosis: the Prevent Recurrence

of Osteoporotic Fractures study. Am J Med 109:267–276

5. Cranney A, Guyatt G, Griffith L, Wells G, Tugwell P, Rosen C et al. (2002) Meta-analyses of therapies for postmenopausal osteoporosis. IX. Summary of meta-analyses of therapies for postmenopausal osteoporosis. Endocr Rev 23:570–578

6. Haguenauer D, Welch V, Shea B et al. (2000) Fluoride for the treatment of postmenopausal osteoporotic fractures: a meta-analysis. Osteoporos Int 11:727–738

7. Palmer C, Wolfe S; American Dietetic Association (2005) Position of the American Dietetic Association: the impact of fluoride on health. J Am Diet Assoc 105:1620–1628

8. Pizzo G, Piscopo M, Pizzo I et al. (2007) Community water fluoridation and caries prevention: a critical review. Clin Oral Investig 11:189–193

9. Vestergaard P, Jorgensen N, Schwarz P, Mosekilde L (2008) Effects of treatment with fluoride on bone mineral density and fracture risk – a meta-analysis. Osteoporos Int 19:257–268

10. Yamaguchi M (2007) Fluoride and bone metabolism. Clin Calcium 17:217–223

Chapter 20 Combination and Sequential Therapies

1. Adami S, San Martin J, Muñoz-Torres M et al. (2008) Effect of raloxifene after recombinant teriparatide [hPTH(1-34)] treatment in postmenopausal women with osteoporosis. Osteoporos Int 19:87–94

2. Boonen S, Marin F, Obermayer-Pietsch B et al. (2008) Effects of previous antiresorptive therapy on the bone mineral density response to two years of teriparatide treatment in postmenopausal women with osteoporosis. J Clin Endocrinol Metab 93:852–860

3. Greenspan S, Emkey R, Bone H et al. (2002) Significant differential effects of alendronate, estrogen, or combination therapy on the rate of bone loss after discontinuation of treatment of postmenopausal osteoporosis. Ann Intern Med 137:875–883

4. Heaney R, Recker R (2005) Combination and sequential therapy for osteoporosis. N Engl J Med 353:624–625

5. Johnell O, Scheele W, Reginster J et al. (2002) Additive effects of raloxifen and alendronate on bone density and biochemical markers on bone remodeling in postmenopausal women with osteoporosis. J Clin Endocrinol Metab 87:985–992

6. Khosla S (2003) Parathyroid hormone plus alendronate – a combination that does not add up. N Engl J Med 349:1277–1279

7. Masud T, Mulcahy B, Thompson AV et al. (1998) Effects of cyclical etidronate combined with calcitrol versus cyclical etidronate alone on spine and femoral neck bone mineral density in postmenopausal osteoporotic women. Ann Rheum Dis 57:346–349

8. Miller P (2004) Combination therapy for osteoporosis: parathyroid hormone and bisphosphonates. Curr Opin Orthop 15:389–395

Chapter 21 Future Directions

1. Bekker P, Holloway D, Rasmussen A et al. (2004) A single-dose placebo-controlled study of AMG 162, a fully human monoclonal antibody to RANKL, in postmenopausal women. J Bone Miner Res 19:1059–1066

2. Cohen S, Dore R et al. (2008) Denosumab treatment effects on structural damage, bone mineral density, and bone turnover in rheumatoid arthritis. Arthritis Rheum 58:1299–1309

3. Fouque-Aubert A, Chapurlat R (2008) Influence of RANKL inhibition on immune system in the treatment of bone diseases. Joint Bone Spine 75:5–10

4. Hamdy N (2008) Denosumab: RANKL inhibition in the management of bone loss. Drugs Today (Barc) 44:7–21

5. Mukherjee A, Shalet S (2003) Growth hormone replacement therapy (GHRT) in children and adolescents: skeletal impact. Med Pediatr Oncol 41:235–242

Chapter 22 Adherence and Monitoring of Osteoporosis Therapy

1. Bartl R, Götte S, Hadji P, Hammerschmidt T (2006) Adherence with daily and weekly administration of oral bisphosphonates for osteoporosis therapy. Dtsch med Wochenschr 131:1257–1262

2. Blouin J, Dragomir A, Moride Y et al. (2008) Impact of noncompliance with alendronate and risedronate on the incidence of nonvertebral osteoporotic fractures in elderly women. Br J Clin Pharmacol 66:117–127

3. Briesacher B, Andrade S, Fouayzi H et al. (2008) Comparison of drug adherence rates among patients with seven different medical conditions. Pharmacotherapy 28:437–443

4. Carr AJ, Thompson PW, Cooper C (2006) Factors associated with adherence and persistence to bisphosphonate therapy in osteoporosis: a cross-sectional survey. Osteoporos Int 17:1638–1644

5. Cooper C, Jakob F, Martin-Mola E et al. (2008) Fracture incidence and changes in quality of life in women with an inadequate clinical outcome from osteoporosis therapy: the Observational Study of Severe Osteoporosis (OSSO). Osteoporos Int 19:493–501

1. Cummings S, Karpf D, Harris F et al. (2006) Improvement in spine bone density and reduction in risk of vertebral fractures during treatment with antiresorptive drugs. Am J Med 112:281–289

2. Finkelstein J, Hayes A, Hunzelman J et al. (2003) The effects of parathyroid hormone, alendronate, or both in men with osteoporosis. N Engl J Med 349:1216–1226

3. Hochberg M, Greenspan S, Wasnich R et al. (2002) Changes in bone density and turnover explain the reduction in incidence of nonvertebral fractures that occur during treatment with antiresorptive agents. J Clin Endocrinol Metab 87:1586–1592

4. Hochberg M, Ross P, Cummings S et al. (1999) Larger increases in bone mineral density during alendronate therapy are associated with a lower risk of new vertebral fractures in women with postmenopausal osteoporosis. Fracture Intervention Trial Research Group. Arthritis Rheum 42:1246–1254

5. Kanis J, Burlet N, Cooper C et al. (2008) European guidance for the diagnosis and management of osteoporosis in postmenopausal osteoporosis. Osteoporos Int 19:399–428

6. Lekkerkerker F, Kanis J, Alsyed N et al. (2007) Adherence to treatment of osteoporosis: a need for study. Osteoporos Int 18:1311–1317

7. Massart F, Marcucci G, Brandi M (2008) Pharmacogenetics of bone treatments: the VDR and ERalpha gene story. Pharmacogenomics 9:733–746

8. Penning-van Beest F, Erkens J, Olson M et al. (2008) Loss of treatment benefit due to low compliance with bisphosphonate therapy. Osteoporos Int 19:551–517

9. Rabenda V, Mertens R, Fabri V et al. (2008) Adherence to bisphosphonates therapy and hip fracture risk in osteoporotic women. Osteoporos Int 19:811–818

10. Reginster J, Collette J, Neuprez A et al. (2008) Role of biochemical markers of bone turnover as prognostic indicator of successful osteoporosis therapy. Bone 42:832–836

11. Reginster JY, Rabenda V (2006) Adherence to anti-osteoporotic treatment: does it really matter? Future Rheumatol 1:37–40

12. Wasnich R, Miller P (2000) Antifracture efficacy of antiresorptive agents are related to changes in bone density. J Clin Endocrinol Metab 85:231–236

Chapter 23 Osteoporotic Fractures

1. Aspenberg P, Wermelin K, Tengwall P, Fahlgren A (2008) Additive effects of PTH and bisphosphonates on the bone healing response to metaphyseal implants in rats. Acta Orthopaedica 79:111–115

2. Bachmann D (2003) Osteoporotic patient: what to do after fixing the fracture. Curr Opin Orthop 14:445–449

3. Bartl R, Bartl C, Gradinger R (2008) Use of bisphosphonates in orthopaedic surgery. Orthopäde 37:595–614

4. Cadarette S, Katz J, Brookhart M et al. (2008) Trends in drug prescribing for osteoporosis after hip fracture, 1995-2004. J Rheumatol 35:319–326

5. Cao Y, Mori S, Mashiba T et al. (2002) Raloxifene, estrogen, and alendronate affect the processes of fracture repair differently in ovariectomized rats. J Bone Miner Res 17:2237–2246

6. Cauley J, Thompson D, Ensrud K et al. (2000) Risk of mortality following clinical fractures. Osteoporos Int 11:556–561

7. Chapurlat R, Bauer D, Nevitt M et al. (2003) Incidence and risk factors for a second hip fracture in elderly women. The study of osteoporotic fractures. Osteoporos Int 14:130–136

8. Cree M, Juby A, Carriere K (2003) Mortality and morbidity associated with osteoporosis drug treatment following hip fracture. Osteoporos Int 14:722–727

9. Eriksen E, Lyles K, Colon-Emeric C et al. (2008) Timing of first infusion of zoledronic acid 5 mg after recent hip fracture affects antifracture efficacy and reduction of mortality. Osteoporos Int 19(Suppl):S14

10. Ferrar L, Jiang G, Adams J, Eastell R (2005) Identification of vertebral fractures: an update. Osteoporos Int 16:717–728

11. Fleisch H (2001) Can bisphosphonates be given to patients with fractures? J Bone Miner Res 16:437–440

12. Follin S, Black J, McDermott M (2003) Lack of diagnosis and treatment of osteoporosis in men and women after hip fracture. Pharmacotherapy 23:190–198

13. Franck H, Boszczyk B, Bierschneider M, Jaksche H (2003) Interdisciplinary approach to balloon kyphoplasty in the treatment of osteoporotic vertebral compression fractures. Eur Spine J 12:S163–S167

14. Gardner M, Flik K, Mooar P et al. (2002) Improvement in the undertreatment of osteoporosis following hip fracture. J Bone Joint Surgery 84:1342–1348

15. Gehrig L, Lane J, O'Connor M (2008) Osteoporosis: management and treatment strategies for orthopaedic surgery. J Bone Joint Surg Am 90:1362–1374

16. Gibson M (2008) Evaluation and treatment of bone disease after fragility fracture. Geriatrics 63:21–30

17. Goh S, Yang K, Koh J et al. (2007) Subtrochanteric insufficiency fractures in patients on alendronate therapy. J Bone Joint Surg Br 89-B:349–353

18. Goldhahn J, Suhm N, Goldhahn S et al. (2008) Influence of osteoporosis of fracture fixation – a systematic literature review. Osteoporos Int 19:761–772

19. Grados F, Depriester C, Cayrolle G et al. (2000) Long-term observations of vertebral osteoporotic fractures treated by percutaneous vertebroplasty. Rheumatology 39:1410–1414

20. Haentjens P, Autier P, Collins J et al. (2003) Colles fracture, spine fracture, and subsequent risk of hip fracture in men and women. J Bone Joint Surg 85A:1936–1943

21. Heinemann D (2000) Osteoporosis. An overview of the National Osteoporosis Foundation clinical practice guide. Geriatrics 55:31–36

22. Johnell O, Kannus P, Obrant K et al. (2001) Management of the patient after an osteoporotic fracture: guidelines for orthopedic surgeons. Acta Orthop Scand 72:325–330

23. Juby A, De Geus-Wenceslau C (2002) Evaluation of osteoporosis treatment in seniors after hip fracture. Osteoporos Int 13:205–210

24. Kamel H, Hussain M, Tariq S et al. (2000) Failure to diagnose and treat osteoporosis in elderly patients hospitalized with hip fracture. Am J Med 109:326–328

25. Kanis J, Johnell O, Oden A et al. (2001) Ten year probabilities of osteoporotic fractures according to BMD and diagnostic thresholds. Osteoporosis Int 12:989–995

26. Kanis J, Oden A, Johnell O, De Laet C, Jonsson B, Oglesby AK (2003) The components of excess mortality after hip fracture. Bone 32:468–473

27. Kannus P, Niemi S, Palvanen M et al. (2008) Rising incidence of low-trauma fractures of the calcaneus and foot among Finnish older adults. J Gerontol A Biol Sci Med Sci 63:642–645

28. Kaufman J, Bolander M, Bunta A et al. (2003) Barriers and solutions to osteoporosis care in patients with a hip fracture. J Bone Joint Surg 85A:1837–1843

29. Lenart B, Lorich D, Lane J (2008) Atypical fractures of the femoral diaphysis in postmenopausal women taking alendronate. N Engl J Med 358:1304–1305

30. Little D, Cornell M, Briody J et al. (2001) Intravenous pamidronate reduces osteoporosis and improves formation of the regenerate during distraction osteogenesis. J Bone Joint Surg (B) 83:1069–1074

31. Maher S, Hidaka C, Cunningham M et al. (2008) What's new in orthopaedic research. J Bone Joint Surg Am 90:1800–1808

32. Moroni A, Faldini C, Hoang-Kim A et al. (2007) Alendronate improves screw fixation in osteoporotic bone. J Bone Miner Res 89-A:96–101

33. Namkung-Matthai H, Appleyard R, Jansen J et al. (2001) Osteoporosis influences the early period of fracture healing in a rat osteoporotic model. Bone 28:80–86

34. Peter C, Cook W, Nunamaker D et al. (1996) Effect of alendronate on fracture healing and bone remodeling in dogs. J Orthop Res 14:74–79

35. Rao R, Singrakhia M (2003) Current concepts review: painful osteoporotic vertebral fracture. J Bone Joint Surg 85:2010–2022

36. Shabat S, Gepstein R, Mann G et al. (2003) The second hip fracture – an analysis of 84 elderly patients. J Orthop Trauma 17:613–617

37. Sobelman O, Gibeling J, Stover S et al. (2004) Do microcracks decrease or increase fatigue resistance in cortical bone? J Biomech 37:1295–1303

38. Torgerson D, Dolan P (1998) Prescribing by general practitioners after an osteoporotic fracture. Ann Rheum Dis 57:378–379

39. van Helden S, van Geel A, Geusens P et al. (2008) Bone and fall-related fracture risk in women and men with a recent clinical fracture. J Bone Joint Surg Am 90:241–248

40. Van Staa T, Leufkens H, Cooper C (2002) Does a fracture at one site predict later fractures at other sites? A British cohort study. Osteoporos Int 13:624–629

41. Vuolteenaho K, Moilanen T, Moilanen E (2008) Non-steroidal anti-inflammatory drugs, cyclo-oxygenase-2 and the bone healing process. Basic Clin Pharmacol Toxicol 102:10–14

Chapter 24 Pregnancy and Lactation

1. Di Gregorio S, Danilowicz K, Rubin Z et al. (2000) Osteoporosis with vertebral fractures associated with pregnancy and lactation. Nutrition 16:1052–1055

2. Feigenberg T, Ben-Shushan A, Daka K et al. (2008) Ultrasound-diagnosed puerperal osteopenia in young primiparas. J Reprod Med 53:287–293

3. Hellmeyer L, Kühnert M, Ziller V et al. (2007) The use of i. v. bisphosphonate in pregnancy-associated osteoporosis – case study. Exp Clin Endocrinol Diabetes 115:139–142

4. Lehman D, Chung M, John-Stewart G et al. (2008) HIV-1 persists in breast milk cells despite Bond S (2008) Low levels of vitamin d in women increase the risk of preeclampsia. J Midwifery Womens Health 53:395

5. O'Sullivan S, Grey A, Singh R et al. (2006) Bisphosphonates in pregnancy and lactation-associated osteoporosis. Osteoporos Int 17:1008–1012

6. Pasco J, Wark J, Carlin J et al. (2008) Maternal vitamin D in pregnancy may influence not only offspring bone mass but other aspects of musculoskeletal health and adiposity. Med Hypotheses 71:266–269

7. Smith M, Marcus P, Wurtz L (2008) Orthopaedic issues in pregnancy. Obstet Gynecol Surv 63:103–111

8. Stump U, Kurth A, Windolf J et al. (2007) Pregnancy-associated osteoporosis: an underestimated and underdiagnosed severe disease. A review of two cases in short- and long-term follow-up. Adv Med Sci 52:94–97

Chapter 25 Osteoporosis in Men

1. Bekaert S, Van Pottelbergh I, De Meyer T et al. (2005) Telomere length versus hormonal and bone mineral status in healthy elderly men. Mech Ageing Dev 126:1115–1122

2. Finkelstein J, Hayes A, Hunzelman J et al. (2003) The effects of parathyroid hormone, alendronate, or both in men with osteoporosis. N Engl J Med 349:1216–1226

3. Follin S, Black J, McDermott M (2003) Lack of diagnosis and treatment of osteoporosis in men and women after hip fracture. Pharmacotherapy 23:190–198

4. Haney E, Bliziotes M (2008) Male osteoporosis: new insights in an understudied disease. Curr Opin Rheumatol 20:423–428

5. Kurland E, Cosman F, McMahon D et al. (2000) Parathyroid hormone as a therapy for idiopathic osteoporosis in men: effects on bone mineral density and bone markers. J Clin Endocrinol 85:3069–3076

6. Levy P, Levy E, Audran M et al. (2002) The cost of osteoporosis in men: the French situation. Bone 30:631–636

7. Lim L, Fink H, Kuskowski M et al. (2008) Loop diuretic use and increased rates of hip bone loss in older men: the Osteoporotic Fractures in Men Study. Arch Intern Med 168:735–740

8. Liu H, Paige N, Goldzweig C et al. (2008) Screening for osteoporosis in men: a systematic review for an American College of Physicians guideline. Ann Intern Med 148:685–701

9. Lynn H, Woo J, Leung P et al. (2008) An evaluation of osteoporosis screening tools for the os-

teoporotic fractures in men (MrOS) study. Osteoporos Int 19:1087–1092

10. Marshall L, Zmuda J, Chan B et al. (2008) Race and ethnic variation in proximal femur structure and BMD among older men. J Bone Miner Res 23:121–130

11. Nakai Y, Noth R, Wexler J et al. (2008) Computer-based screening of chest X-rays for vertebral compression fractures as an osteoporosis index in men. Bone 42:1214–1218

12. Orwoll E (2003) Men, bone and estrogen: unresolved issues. Osteoporos Int 14:93–98

13. Orwoll E, Ettinger M, Weiss S et al. (2000) Alendronate for the treatment of osteoporosis in men. N Engl J Med 343:604–610

14. Ringe JD, Dorst A, Faber H, Ibach K (2004) Alendronate treatment of established primary osteoporosis in men: 3-year results of a prospective, comparative, two-arm study. Rheumatol Int 24:110–113

15. Santori C, Ceccanti M, Diacinti D et al. (2008) Skeletal turnover, bone mineral density, and fractures in male chronic abusers of alcohol. J Endocrinol Invest 31:321–326

16. Sharma S, Fraser M, Lovell F et al. (2008) Characteristics of males over 50 years who present with a fracture: epidemiology and underlying risk factors. J Bone Joint Surg Br 90:72–77

17. Smith M, Eastham J, Gleason D et al. (2003) Randomized controlled trial of zoledronic acid to prevent bone loss in men receiving androgen deprivation therapy for nonmetastatic prostate cancer. J Urol 169:2008–2012

18. Stanworth R, Jones T (2008) Testosterone for the aging male: current evidence and recommended practice. Clin Interv Aging 3:25–44

19. Tuck S, Datta H (2007) Osteoporosis in the aging male: treatment options. Clin Interv Aging 2:521–536

20. Weber T, Drezner M (2001) Effect of alendronate on bone mineral density in male idiopathic osteoporosis. Metabolism 50:912–915

Chapter 26 Osteoporosis in Children

1. Ahmed S, Wong J, McGrogan P (2007) Improving growth in children with inflammatory bowel disease. Horm Res 68(Suppl 5):117–121

2. Akcay T, Turan S, Guran T et al. (2008) Alendronate treatment in children with osteogenesis imperfecta. Indian Pediatr 45:105–109

3. Alemzadeh R, Kichler J, Babar G et al. (2008) Hypovitaminosis D in obese children and adolescents: relationship with adiposity, insulin sensitivity, ethnicity, and season. Metabolism 57:183–191

4. Bailey D (1997) The Saskatchewan pediatric bone mineral accrual study: bone mineral acquisition during the growing years. Int J Sports Med 18(Suppl 3):191–194

5. Baim S, Leonard M, Bianchi M et al. (2008) Official positions of the International Society for Clinical Densitometry and executive summary of the 2007 ISCD Pediatric Position Development Conference. J Clin Densitom 11:6–21

6. Bakalov V, Bondy C (2008) Fracture risk and bone mineral density in Turner syndrome. Rev Endocr Metab Disord 9:145–151

7. Binkley T, Berry R, Specker B (2008) Methods for measurement of pediatric bone. Rev Endocr Metab Disord 9:95–106

8. Brumsen C, Hamdyy N, Papapoulos S (1997) Long-term effects of bisphosphonates on the growing skeleton. Studies of young patients with severe osteoporosis. Medicine 76:266–283

9. Brunetti-Pierri N, Doty S, Hicks J et al. (2008) Generalized metabolic bone disease in Neurofibromatosis type I. Mol Genet Metab 94:105–111

10. Chevrel G, Meunier P (2001) Osteogenesis imperfecta: lifelong management is imperative and feasible. Oint Bone Spine 68:125–129

11. Cohran V, Griffiths M, Heubi J (2008) Bone mineral density in children exposed to chronic glucocorticoid therapy. Clin Pediatr (Phila) 47:469–475

12. Davenport M (2008) Moving toward an understanding of hormone replacement therapy in adolescent girls: looking through the lens of Turner syndrome. Ann N Y Acad Sci 1135:126–137

13. Forward K, Cummings E, Blake K (2007) Risk factors for poor bone health in adolescents and adults with CHARGE syndrome. Am J Med Genet A 143A:839–845

14. Frank G (2003) Role of estrogen and androgen in pubertal skeletal physiology. Med Pediatr Oncol 41:217–221

15. Frost H (2003) On the pathogenesis of osteogenesis imperfecta: some insights of the Utah para-

digm of skeletal physiology. J Musculoskelet Neuronal Interact 3:1–7

16. Gandrud L, Cheung J, Daniels M, Bachrach L (2003) Low-dose intravenous pamidronate reduces fractures in childhood osteoporosis. Pediatr Endocrinol Metab 16:887–892

17. Glorieux F (2008) Osteogenesis imperfecta. Best Pract Res Clin Rheumatol 22:85–100

18. Glorieux F, Bishop N et al. (2008) Intravenous zoledronic acid (ZOL) compared to iv pamidronate (PAM) in children with severe osteogenesis imperfecta (OI). Calcif Tissue Int 82(Suppl 1): S85

19. Glorieux F, Bishop N, Plotkin H et al. (1998) Cyclical administration of pamidronate in children with severe osteogenesis imperfecta. N Engl J Med 339:947–952

20. Goulding A (2007) Risk factors for fractures in normally active children and adolescents. Med Sport Sci 51:102–120

21. Hartman C, Hochberg Z, Shamir R (2003) Osteoporosis in pediatrics. IMAJ 5:509–515

22. Helenius I, Remes V, Salminen S et al. (2006) Incidence and predictors of fractures in children after solid organ transplantation: a 5-year prospective, population-based study. J Bone Miner Res 21:380–387

23. Inoue Y, Shimojo N, Suzuki S et al. (2008) Efficacy of intravenous alendronate for the treatment of glucocorticoid-induced osteoporosis in children with autoimmune disease. Clin Rheumatol 27:909–912

24. Iwasaki T, Takei K, Nakamura S et al. (2008) Secondary osteoporosis in long-term bedridden patients with cerebral palsy. Pediatr Int 50:269–275

25. Kamboj M (2007) Metabolic bone disease in adolescents: recognition, evaluation, treatment, and prevention. Adolesc Med State Art Rev 18:24–46

26. Kamoun-Goldrat A, Ginisty D, Le Merrer M (2008) Effects of bisphosphonates on tooth eruption in children with osteogenesis imperfecta. Eur J Oral Sci 116:195–198

27. Kaste S (2008) Skeletal toxicities of treatment in children with cancer. Pediatr Blood Cancer 50(Suppl 2):469–473

28. Key L, Ries W, Madyastha P, Reed F (2003) Juvenile osteoporosis: recognizing the risk. J Pediatr Endocrinol Metab 16(Suppl 3):683–686

29. Krzesiek E, Iwańczak B (2008) Assessment of bone mineral density in children with celiac disease. Pol Merkur Lekarski 24:219–226

30. Lee Y, Low S, Lim L et al. (2001) Cyclic pamidronate infusion improves bone mineralization and reduces fracture incidence in osteogenesis imperfecta. Eur J Pediatr 160:641–644

31. Makitie O, Toiviainen-Salo S, Marttinen E et al. (2008) Metabolic control and growth during exclusive growth hormone treatment in X-linked hypophosphatemic rickets. Horm Res 69:212–220

32. Malmgren B, Aström E, Söderhäll S (2008) No osteonecrosis in jaws of young patients with osteogenesis imperfecta treated with bisphosphonates. J Oral Pathol Med 37:196–200

33. Marini J (2003) Do bisphosphonates make children's bones better or brittle? N Engl J Med 349:423–426

34. Micklesfield L, Norris S, Nelson D et al. (2007) Comparison of body size, composition, and whole body bone mass between North American and South African children. J Bone Miner Res 22:1869–1877

35. Misra M (2008) Bone density in the adolescent athlete. Rev Endocr Metab Disord 9:139–144

36. More J (2008) Children's bone health and meeting calcium needs. J Fam Health Care 18:22–24

37. Morgan T (2007) Turner syndrome: diagnosis and management. Am Fam Physician 76:405–410

38. Mukherjee A, Shalet S (2003) Growth hormone replacement therapy (GHRT) in children and adolescents: skeletal impact. Med Pediatr Oncol 41:235–242

39. Neri A, Lori I, Festini F et al. (2008) Bone mineral density in cystic fibrosis patients under the age of 18 years. Minerva Pediatr 60:147–154

40. Nicklas T, Hayes D (2008) Position of the American Dietetic Association: nutrition guidance for healthy children ages 2 to 11 years. J Am Diet Assoc 108:1038–1044

41. Patel D, Moore M, Greydanus D (2007) Musculoskeletal diagnosis in adolescents. Adolesc Med State Art Rev 18:1–10

42. Ralston S (2008) Juvenile Paget's disease, familial expansile osteolysis and other genetic osteolytic disorders. Best Pract Res Clin Rheumatol 22:101–111

43. Rauch F, Plotkin H, Zeitlin L, Glorieux F (2003) Bone mass, size and density in children and adolescence with osteogenesis imperfecta: effect of intravenous pamidronate therapy. J Bone Miner Res 18:610–614

44. Sanchez C (2008) Mineral metabolism and bone abnormalities in children with chronic renal failure. Rev Endocr Metab Disord 9:131–137

45. Sherman P (2003) Osteoporosis and young women. Curr Opin Orthop 14:440–444

46. Shroff R, Donald A, Hiorns M et al. (2007) Mineral metabolism and vascular damage in children on dialysis. J Am Soc Nephrol 18:2996–3003

47. Sinigaglia R, Gigante C, Bisinella G et al. (2008) Musculoskeletal manifestations in pediatric acute leukemia. J Pediatr Orthop 28:20–28

48. Thornton J, Ashcroft D, O'Neill T et al. (2008) A systematic review of the effectiveness of strategies for reducing fracture risk in children with juvenile idiopathic arthritis with additional data on long-term risk of fracture and cost of disease management. Health Technol Assess 12:1–208

49. Tlacuilo-Parra A, Morales-Zambrano R, Tostado-Rabago N et al. (2008) Inactivity is a risk factor for low bone mineral density among haemophilic children. Br J Haematol 140:562–567

50. van der Sluis I, van den Heuvel-Eibrink M (2008) Osteoporosis in children with cancer. Pediatr Blood Cancer 50(Suppl 2):474–478

51. Wasilewski-Masker K, Kaste S, Hudson M et al. (2008) Bone mineral density deficits in survivors of childhood cancer: long-term follow-up guidelines and review of the literature. Pediatrics 121:e705–e713

52. Wesseling K, Bakkaloglu S, Salusky I (2008) Chronic kidney disease mineral and bone disorder in children. Pediatr Nephrol 23:195–207

Chapter 27 Immobilization Osteoporosis

1. Iwamoto J, Tadeka T, Sato Y (2005) Interventions to prevent bone loss in astronauts during space flight. Keio J Med 54:55–59

2. Iwasaki T, Takei K, Nakamura S et al. (2008) Secondary osteoporosis in long-term bedridden patients with cerebral palsy. Pediatr Int 50:269–275

3. Lloyd S, Travis N, Lu T et al. (2008) Development of a low-dose anti-resorptive drug regimen reveals synergistic suppression of bone formation when coupled with disuse. J Appl Physiol 104:729–738

4. Zérath E, Grynpas M, Holy X et al. (2002) Spaceflight affects bone formation in rhesus monkeys: a histological and cell culture study. J Appl Physiol 93:1047–1056

Chapter 28 Osteoporosis in Medical Disciplines

1. Adewoye A, Chen T, Ma Q et al. (2008) Sickle cell bone disease: response to vitamin D and calcium. Am J Hematol 83:271–274

2. Alsafwah S, Laguardia S, Arroyo M et al. (2007) Congestive heart failure is a systemic illness: a role for minerals and micronutrients. Clin Med Res 5:238–243

3. Bassett J, Williams A, Murphy E et al. (2008) A lack of thyroid hormones rather than excess thyrotropin causes abnormal skeletal development in hypothyroidism. Mol Endocrinol 22:501–512

4. Book C, Karlsson M, Akesson K et al. (2008) Disease activity and disability but probably not glucocorticoid treatment predicts loss in bone mineral density in women with early rheumatoid arthritis. Scand J Rheumatol 337:248–254

5. Childs M, Armstrong D, Edelson G (1998) Is Charcot arthropathy a late sequela of osteoporosis in patients with diabetes mellitus? J Foot Ankle Surg 37:437–439

6. Cohen A, Shane E (2003) Osteoporosis after solid organ and bone marrow transplantation. Osteoporos Int 14:617–630

7. Cushing H (1932) The basophil adenomas of the pituitary body and their clinical manifestations (pituitary basophilism). Bull Johns Hopkins Hosp 50:137–195

8. Da Silva A, Heras-Herzig A, Schiff D (2007) Bone health in patients with brain tumors. Surg Neurol 68:525–533

9. de Vries F, Pouwels S, Bracke M et al. (2007) Use of beta-2 agonists and risk of hip/femur fracture: a population-based case-control study. Pharmacoepidemiol Drug Saf 16:612–619

10. de Vries F, Souverein P, Cooper C et al. (2007) Use of beta-blockers and the risk of hip/femur

fracture in the United Kingdom and The Netherlands. Calcif Tissue Int 80:69–75

11. Ding C, Parameswaran V, Udayan R et al. (2008) Circulating levels of inflammatory markers predict change in bone mineral density and resorption in older adults: a longitudinal study. J Clin Endocrinol Metab 93:1952–1958

12. Djoussé L, Gaziano J (2008) Alcohol consumption and heart failure: a systematic review. Curr Atheroscler Rep 10:117–120

13. Donker M, van Doormaal J, van Dorrmaal F et al. (2008) Biochemical markers predictive for bone marrow involvement in systemic mastocytosis. Haematologica 93:120–123

14. Ebeling P (2007) Transplantation osteoporosis. Curr Osteoporos Rep 5:29–37

15. Epstein S, Inzerillo A, Caminis J, Zaidi M (2003) Review: disorders associated with acute rapid and severe bone loss. J Bone Miner Res 18:2083–2094

16. Fisher A, Lomasky S, Fisher M et al. (2008) Celiac disease and the endocrinologist: a diagnostic opportunity. Endocr Pract 14:381–388

17. Fukai S (2008) Effects of antiosteoporotic agents on glucose and lipid metabolism and cardiovascular system. Clin Calcium 18:677–684

18. Hjerrild B, Mortensen K, Gravholt C (2008) Turner syndrome and clinical treatment. Br Med Bull 86:77–93

19. Hofbauer L, Brueck C, Shanahan C et al. (2007) Vascular calcification and osteoporosis from clinical observation towards molecular understanding. Osteoporos Int 18:251–259

20. Kamanli A, Ardicoglu O, Ozgocmen S et al. (2008) Bone mineral density in patients with Parkinson's disease. Aging Clin Exp Res 20:277–279

21. Kamide N, Fukuda M, Miura H (2008) The relationship between bone density and the physical performance of ambulatory patients with Parkinson's disease. J Physiol Anthropol 27:7–10

22. Katzman D (2003) Osteoporosis in anorexia nervosa: a brittle future? Curr Drug Targets CNS Neurol Disord 2:11–15

23. Kishimoto T, Watanabe K, Shimada N et al. (2008) Antipsychotic-induced hyperprolactinemia inhibits the hypothalamo-pituitary-gonadal axis and reduces bone mineral density in male patients with schizophrenia. J Clin Psychiatry 69:385–391

24. Kovacs C (2008) Hemophilia, low bone mass, and osteopenia/osteoporosis. Transfus Apher Sci 38:33–40

25. Kudlacek S, Freudenthaler O, Weissboeck H et al. (2003) Lactose intolerance: a risk factor for reduced bone mineral density and vertebral fractures? J Gastroenterol 37:1014–1019

26. Langdahl B, Uitterlinden A, Ralston S et al. (2008) Large-scale analysis of association between polymorphisms in the transforming growth factor beta 1 gene (TGFB1) and osteoporisis: the GENOMOS study. Bone 42:969–981

27. Majima T, Shimatsu A, Komatsu Y et al. (2008) Increased bone turnover in patients with hypercholesterolemia. Endocr J 55:143–151

28. Mathioudakis N, Salvatori R (2008) Adult-onset growth hormone deficiency: causes, complications and treatment options. Curr Opin Endocrinol Diabetes Obes 15:352–358

29. McCabe L (2007) Understanding the pathology and mechanisms of type I diabetic bone loss. J Cell Biochem 102:1343–1357

30. Meaney A, O'Keane V (2007) Bone mineral density changes over a year in young females with schizophrenia: relationship to medication and endocrine variables. Schizophr Res 93:136–143

31. Mezuk B, Eaton W, Golden S (2008) Depression and osteoporosis: epidemiology and potential mediating pathways. Osteoporos Int 19:1–12

32. Moosgaard B, Christensen S, Vestergaard P et al. (2008) Vitamin D metabolites and skeletal consequences in primary hyperparathyroidism. Clin Endocrinol (Oxf) 68:707–715

33. Mosekilde L (2008) Primary hyperparathyroidism and the skeleton. Clin Endocrinol (Oxf) 69:1–19

34. Pack A (2008) Bone health in people with epilepsy: is it impaired and what are the risk factors? Seizure 17:181–186

35. Perese E, Perese K (2003) Health problems of women with severe mental illness. J Am Acad Nurse Pract 15:212–219

36. Peterson E, Cho C, von Koch L et al. (2008) Injurious falls among middle aged and older adults with multiple sclerosis. Arch Phys Med Rehabil 89:1031–1037

37. Petrova N, Edmonds M (2008) Charcot neuro-osteoarthropathy-current standards. Diabetes Metab Res Rev 24(Suppl 1):S58–S61

38. Sapone N, Pellicano R, Simondi D et al. (2008) A 2008 panorama on osteoporosis and inflammatory bowel disease. Minerva Med 99:65–71
39. Schwartz A, Sellmeyer D, Ensrud K et al. (2001) Older women with diabetes have an increased risk of fracture: a prospective study. J Clin Endocrinol Metab 86:32–38
40. Sennerby U, Farahmand B, Ahlbom A et al. (2007) Cardiovascular diseases and future risk in hip fracture in women. Osteoporos Int 18:1355–1362
41. Shah A, Wigley F (2008) Often forgotten manifestations of systemic sclerosis. Rheum Dis Clin North Am 34:221–238
42. Shimokata H, Ando F (2008) Genomic approaches to bone and joint diseases. Current state of disease genome research: osteoporosis. Clin Calcium 18:155–161
43. Sørensen H, Christensen S, Mehnert F et al. (2008) Use of bisphosphonates among women and risk of atrial fibrillation and flutter: population based case-control study. BMJ 336:813–816
44. Stazi A, Trecca A, Trinti B (2008) Osteoporosis in celiac disease and in endocrine and reproductive disorders. World J Gastroenterol 14:498–505
45. Styrkarsdottir U, Halldorsson B, Gretarsdottir S et al. (2008) Multiple genetic loci for bone mineral density and fractures. N Engl J Med 358:2355–2365
46. Szulc P, Kiel D, Delmas P (2008) Calcifications in the abdominal aorta predict fractures in men: MINOS study. J Bone Miner Res 23:95–102
47. Tamura Y, Araki A, Chiba Y et al. (2007) Remarkable increase in lumbar spine bone mineral density and amelioration in biochemical markers of bone turnover after parathyroidectomy in elderly patients with primary hyperparathyroidism: a 5-year follow-up study. J Bone Miner Metab 25:226–231
48. Tauchmanovà L, Colao A, Lombardi G et al. (2007) Bone loss and its management in long-term survivors from allogeneic stem cell transplantation. J Clin Endocrinol Metab 92:4536–4545
49. Tig H, Moschen A, Kaser A et al. (2008) Gut, inflammation and osteoporosis: basic and clinical concepts. Gut 57:684–694
50. Trabulus S, Altiparmak M, Apaydin S et al. (2008) Treatment of renal transplant recipients with low bone mineral density: a randomized prospective trial of alendronate, alfacalcidol, and alendronate combined with alfacalcidol. Transplant Proc 40:160–166
51. Varma R, Aronow W, Basis Y et al. (2008) Relation of bone mineral density to frequency of coronary heart disease. Am J Cardiol 101:1103–1104
52. Wada S, Kamiya S, Fukawa T (2008) Bone quality changes in diabetes. Clin Calcium 18:600–605
53. Wiens M, Etminan M, Gill S et al. (2006) Effects of antihypertensive drug treatments on fracture outcomes: a meta-analysis of observational studies. J Intern Med 260:350–362
54. Yamaguchi T, Sugimoto T (2008) Calcium in aging, health, and anti-aging. Calcium homeostasis and osteoporosis in diabetes mellitus and the metabolic syndrome. Clin Calcium 18:904–911
55. Yudoh K, Matsuno H, Osada R et al. (2000) Decreased cellular activity and replicative capacity of osteoblastic cells isolated from the periarticular bone of rheumatoid arthritis patients compared with osteoarthritis patients. Arthritis Rheum 43:2178–2188
56. Yuen S, Rochwerg B, Ouimet J et al. (2008) Patients with scleroderma may have increased risk of osteoporosis. A comparison to rheumatoid arthritis and noninflammatory musculoskeletal conditions. J Rheumatol 35:1073–1078

Chapter 29 Osteoporosis and Drugs

1. Allport J (2008) Incidence and prevalence of medication-induced osteoporosis: evidence-based review. Curr Opin Rheumatol 20:435–441
2. Bartl R (2007) AED-induced osteopathy – subtypes, pathogenesis, prevention, early diagnosis and treatment. Dtsch Med Wochenschr 132:1475–1479
3. Borderi M, Farneti B, Tampellini L et al (2002) HIV-1, HAART and bone metabolism. New Microbiol 25:375–384
4. Canalis E, Mazziotti G, Giustina A, Bilezikian J (2007) Glucocorticoid-induced osteoporosis: pathophysiology and therapy. Osteoporos Int 18:1319–1328

5. Cohen A, Shane E (2003) Osteoporosis after solid organ and bone marrow transplantation. Osteoporos Int 14:617–630

6. Duque G, Rivas D (2007) Alendronate has an anabolic effect on bone through the differentiation of mesenchymal stem cells. J Bone Miner Res 22:1603–1611

7. Emkey R, Delmas P, Goemaere S et al. (2003) Changes in bone mineral density following discontinuation of alendronate therapy of glucocorticoid-treated patients: a retrospective, observational study. Arthritis Rheum 48:1102–1108

8. Grey A (2008) Skeletal consequences of thiazolidinedione therapy. Osteoporos Int 19:129–137

9. Hahn TJ (1976) Bone complications of anticonvulsants. Drugs 12:201–211

10. Heller HJ, Sakhaee (2001) Anticonvulsant-induced bone disease: a plea for monitoring and treatment. Arch Neurol 58:1352–1353

11. Meisinger C, Heier M, Lang O, Döring A (2007) Beta-blocker use and risk of fractures in men and women from the general population: the MONICA/KORA Augsburg cohort study. Osteoporos Int 18:1189–1195

12. Pack AM, Olarte LS, morrell MJ et al. (2003) Bone mineral density in an outpatient population receiving enzyme-inducing antiepileptic drugs. Epilepsy Behav 4:169–174

13. Petty SJ, O'Brian TJ, Wark JD (2007) Antiepileptic medication and bone health. Osteoporos Int 18:129–142

14. Rehman O, Lane N (2003) Effect of glucocorticoids on bone density. Med Pediatr Oncol 41:212–216

15. Richy F, Bousquet J, Eherlich G et al. (2003) Inhaled corticosteroid effects on bone in asthmatic and COPD patients: a quantitative systematic study. Osteoporos Int 14:179–190

16. Ringe J, Dorst A, Faber H et al. (2003) Three-monthly ibandronate bolus injection offers favourable tolerability and sustained efficacy advantage over two years in established corticosteroid-induced osteoporosis. Rheumatology 42:743–749

17. Saag K, Emkey R, Schnitzer T et al. (1998) Alendronate for the treatment of glucocorticoid-induced osteoporosis. N Engl J Med 339:292–299

18. Sambrook P, Kotowicz M, Nash P et al. (2003) Prevention and treatment of glucocorticoid-induced osteoporosis: a comparison of calcitriol, vitamin D plus calcium and alendronate plus calcium. J None Miner Res 18:919–924

19. Siebler T, Shalet S, Robson H (2002) Effects of chemotherapy on bone metabolism and skeletal growth. Horm Res 58(Suppl 1):80–85

20. Sirola J, Honkanen R, Kröger H et al. (2002) Relation of statin use and bone loss: a prospective population-based cohort study in early postmenopausal women. Osteoporos Int 13:537–541

21. Smith I, Dowsett M (2003) Aromatase inhibitors in breast cancer. N Engl J Med 348:2431–2442

22. Takeuchi Y (2008) Do thiazolidinediones harm skeletal integrity? Clin Calcium 18:650–655

23. Van Staa T, Leufkens H, Cooper C (2002) The epidemiology of corticosteroid-induced osteoporosis: a meta-analysis. Osteoporos Int 13:777–787

24. Vermaat H, Kirtschig G (2008) Prevention and treatment of glucocorticoid-induced osteoporosis in daily dermatologic practice. Int J Dermatol 47:737–742

25. Verrotti A, Greco R, Latini G et al. (2002) Increased bone turnover in prepubertal, pubertal and postpubertal patients receiving carbamazepine. Epilepsia 43:1488–1492

26. Vestergaard P (2005) Epilepsy, osteoporosis and fracture risk-a meta-analysis. Acta Neurol Scand 112:277–286

27. Wallach S, Cohen S, Reid D et al. (2000) Effects of risedronate treatment on bone density and vertebral fracture in patients on corticosteroid therapy. Calcif Tissue Int 67:277–285

28. Ziere G, Dieleman J, van der Cammen T et al. (2008) Selective serotonin reuptake inhibiting antidepressants are associated with an increased risk of nonvertebral fractures. J Clin Psychopharmacol 28:411–417

Chapter 30 AIDS Osteopathy

1. Arnsten J, Freeman R, Howard A et al. (2007) Decreased bone mineral density and increased fracture risk in aging men with or at risk for HIV infection. AIDS 21:617–623

2. Borderi M, Farneti B, Tampellini L et al. (2002) HIV-1, HAART and bone metabolism. New Microbiol 25:375–384

3. Cazanave C, Dupon M, Lavignolie-Aurillac V et al. (2008) Reduced bone mineral density in

HIV-infected patients: prevalence and associated factors. AIDS 22:395–402

4. Clay P, Voss L, Williams C et al. (2008) Valid treatment options for osteoporosis and osteopenia in HIV-infected persons. Ann Pharmacother 42:670–679

5. Grunfeld C (2008) Insulin resistance in HIV infection: drugs, host responses, or restoration to health? Top HIV Med 16:89–93

6. Knobel H, Guelar A, Vallecillo G et al. (2001) Osteopenia in HIV-infected patients: is it the disease or is it the treatment? AIDS 15:807–808

7. Mora S, Sala N, Bricalli D et al. (2001) Bone mineral loss through increased bone turnover in HIV-infected children treated with highly active antiresorptive therapy. AIDS 15:1823–1829

8. Mora S, Zamproni I, Cafarelli L et al. (2007) Alterations in circulating osteoimmune factors may be responsible for high bone resorption rate in HIV-infected children and adolescents. AIDS 21:1129–1135

9. Prior J, Burdge D, Maan E et al. (2007) Fragility fractures and bone mineral density in HIV positive women: a case-control population-based study. Osteoporos Int 18:1345–1353

10. Tebas P, Powderly W, Claxton S et al. (2000) Accelerated bone mineral loss in HIV-infected patients receiving potent antiviral therapy. AIDS 14:F63–F67

11. Teichmann J, Lange U, Discher T et al. (2008) Growth hormone and bone mineral density in HIV-1-infected male subjects. Eur J Med Res 13:173–178

12. Thomas J, Doherty S (2003) HIV infection – a risk factor for osteoporosis. J Acquir Immune Defic Syndr 33:281–291

women with CKD. J Am Soc Nephrol 19:1430–1438

4. Komaba H, Tanaka M, Fukagawa M (2008) Treatment of chronic kidney disease-mineral and bone disorder (CKD-MBD). Intern Med 47:989–994

5. Lam A, Shah S, Paparello J (2008) Outpatient management of chronic kidney disease: proteinuria, anemia and bone disease as therapeutic targets. Am J Ther 15:278–286

6. Maertens S, Van Den Noortgate N (2008) Kidney in old age. Acta Clin Belg 63:8–15

7. Mathieu C, Jafari M (2006) Immunomodulation by 1,25-dihydroxyvitamin D3: therapeutic implications in hemodialysis and renal transplantation. Clin Nephrol 66:275–283

8. Nakashima A, Yorioka N, Tanji C et al. (2003) Bone mineral density may be related to atherosclerosis in hemodialysis patients. Osteoporos Int 14:369–373

9. Stavroulopoulos A, Porter C, Roe S et al. (2008) Relationship between vitamin D status, parathyroid hormone levels and bone mineral density in patients with chronic kidney disease stages 3 and 4. Nephrology (Carlton) 13:63–67

10. Ubara Y, Fushimi T, Tagami T et al. (2003) Histomorphometric features of bone in patients with primary and secondary hypoparathyroidism. Kidney Int 63:1809–1816

11. Ubara Y, Tagami T, Nakanishi S et al. (2005) Significance of minimodeling in dialysis patients with adynamic bone disease. Kidney Int 68:833–839

12. Zhang R, Alper B, Simon E et al. (2008) Management of metabolic bone disease in kidney transplant recipients. Am J Med Sci 335:120–125

Chapter 31 Renal Osteopathy

1. Faull R (2007) Managing bone parameters in dialysis patients: international guideline conflicts. Semin Dial 20:191–194

2. Gesek F, Desmond J (2008) Improved patient outcomes in chronic kidney disease: optimizing vitamin D therapy. Nephrol Nurs J 35(Suppl 2):5S–22S

3. Ishani A, Blackwell T, Jamal S et al. (2008) The effect of raloxifene treatment in postmenopausal

Chapter 32 Localized Osteopathies

1. Abelson A (2008) A review of Paget's disease of bone with a focus on the efficacy and safety of zoledronic acid 5 mg. Curr Med Res Opin 24:695–705

2. Allport J (2008) Incidence and prevalence of medication-induced osteoporosis: evidence-based review. Curr Opin Rheumatil 20:435–441

3. Aspenberg P (2006) Pharmacological treatment of osteonecrosis. Acta Orthop 77:175–176

4. Bartl C, Bartl R, Salzmann G, Imhoff A (2008) Treatment of painful bone marrow edema syndrome with intravenous ibandronate. Bone 42(Suppl 1):112

5. Bartl R, Bartl C, Gradinger R (2008) Use of bisphosphonates in orthopaedic surgery. Orthopäde 37:595–614

6. Bolland M (2008) Bilateral transient osteoporosis of the hip in a young man. J Clin Densitom 11:339–341

7. Cardozo J, Andrate D, Santiago M (2008) The use of bisphosphonate in the treatment of avascular necrosis: a systematic review. Clin Rheumatol 27:685–688

8. Dumitrescu C, Collins M (2008) McCune-Albright syndrome. Orphanet J Rare Dis 3:12

9. Gehrig L, Lane J, O'Connor M (2008) Osteoporosis: management and treatment strategies for orthopaedic surgery. J Bone Joint Surg Am 90:1362–1374

10. Helfrich M, Hocking L (2008) Genetics and aetiology of Pagetic disorders of bone. Arch Biochem Biophys 473:172–182

11. Hofman S (1999) Bone marrow oedema in transient osteoporosis, reflex sympathetic dystrophy and osteonecrosis. EFORT 4:138–151

12. Karantanas A, Drakonaki E, Karachalios T et al. (2008) Acute non-traumatic marrow edema syndrome in the knee: MRI findings at presentation, correlation with spinal DEXA and outcome. Eur J Radiol 67:22–33

13. Karantanas A, Nikolakopoulos I, Korompilias A et al. (2008) Regional migratory osteoporosis in the knee: MRI findings in 22 patients and review of the literature. Eur J Radiol 67:34–41

14. Maher S, Hidaka C, Cunningham M et al. (2008) What's new in orthopaedic Research. J Bone Joint Surg Am 90:1800–1808

15. Mont M, Jones L, Hungerford D (2006) Non-traumatic osteonecrosis of the femoral head: ten years later. J Bone Joint Surg 88-A:1117–1132

16. Morris C, Einhorn T (2005) Bisphosphonates in orthopedic surgery. J Bone Joint Surg 87-A:1609–1618

17. Ralston S, Langston A, Reid I (2008) Pathogenesis and management of Paget's disease of bone. Lancet 372:155–163

18. Reid I, Miller P, Lyles K et al. (2005) A single infusion of zoledronic acid improves remission rates in Paget's disease. A randomized controlled comparison with risedronate. N Engl J Med 353:898–908

19. Schott G (1997) Bisphosphonates for pain relief in reflex sympathetic dystrophy? Lancet 350:1117

20. Siminoski K, Fitzgerals A, Flesch G et al. (2000) Intravenous pamidronate for treatment of reflex sympathetic dystrophy during breast feeding. J Bone Miner Res 15:2052–2055

21. Sudeck P (1902) Über die akute (trophoneurotoxische) Knochenatrophie nach Entzündungen und Traumen der Extremitäten. Dtsch Med Wochenschr 28:336–342

22. Vande Berg B, Lecouvet F, Koutaissoff S et al. (2008) Bone marrow edema of the femoral head and transient osteoporosis of the hip. Eur J Radiol 67:68–77

Chapter 33 Periprosthetic Osteoporosis and Aseptic Loosening of Prostheses

1. Bauer TW, Schils J (1999) The pathology of total joint arthroplasty – I. Mechanisms of implant fixation. Skeletal Radiol 28:423–432

2. Bauer TW, Schils J (1999) The pathology of total joint arthroplasty – II. Mechanisms of implant failure. Skeletal Radiol 28:483–497

3. Bhandari M, Bajammal S, Guyatt G et al. (2005) Effect of bisphosphonates on periprosthetic bone mineral density after total joint arthroplasty. J Bone Joint Surg (A) 87:293–301

4. Gehrig L, Lane J, O'Connor M (2008) Osteoporosis: management and treatment strategies for orthopaedic surgery. J Bone Joint Surg Am 90:1362–1374

5. Glowacki J, Hurwitz S, Thornhill T et al. (2003) Osteoporosis and vitamin-D deficiency among postmenopausal women with osteoarthritis undergoing total hip arthropathy. J Bone Joint Surg 85A:2371–2377

6. Goodman S, Trindade M, Ma T et al. (2005) Pharmacologic modulation of periprosthetic osteolysis. Clin Orthopaedics Rel Res 430:39–45

7. Goodship A, Lawes T, Green J et al. (1999) Bisphosphonates can inhibit mechanically related loosening of hip prostheses. J Bone Joint Surg (Br) 81-B(Suppl III):319

8. Gourlay M, Richy F, Reginster J (2003) Strategies for the prevention of hip fractures. Am J Med 115:309–317

9. Gruen T, McNeice G, Amstutz H (1979) "Modes of failure" of cemented stem-type femoral components: a radiographic analysis of loosening. Clin Orthop 141:17–27

10. Haynes D, Crotti T, Zreiqat H (2004) Regulation of osteoclast activity in peri-implant tissue, a review. Biomaterials 25:4877–4885

11. Hennigs T, Arabmotlagh M, Schwarz A, Zichner L (2002) Dose-dependent prevention of early periprosthetic bone loss by alendronate. Z Orthop Grenzgeb 140:42–47

12. Hilding M, Aspenberg P (2007) Local perioperative treatment with a bisphosphonate improves the fixation of total knee prostheses: a randomized, double-blind radiostereometric study of 50 patients. Acta Orthop 78:795–799

13. Kröger H, Venesmaa P, Jurvelin J et al. (1998) Bone density at the proximal femur after total hip arthroplasty. Clin Orthop Rel Res 352:66–74

14. Li M, Nilsson K (2000) Changes in bone mineral density at the proximal tibia after total knee arthroplasty: a 2-year follow-up of 28 knees using dual energy X-ray absorptiometry. J Orthop Res 18:40–47

15. Lyons A (1999) Effects of alendronate in total hip arthroplasty. Proc South African Orthop Ass 81(Suppl 3):313

16. Mandelin J, Li T-F, Liljeström M et al. (2003) Imbalance of RANKL/RANK/OPG system in interface tissue in loosening of total hip replacement. J Bone Joint Surg 85-B:1196–1201

17. Meraw S, Reeve C (1999) Qualitative analysis of peripheral peri-implant bone and influence of alendronate sodium on early bone regeneration. J Periodontol 70:1228–1233

18. Persson P-E, Nilsson O, Berggren A-M (2005) Do non-steroidal anti-inflammatory drugs cause endoprosthetic loosening? Acta Orthopaedica 76:735–740

19. Povoroznjuk V, Mazur I (1998) Alendronate in complex treatment of periodontal diseases. Bone 22(Suppl):18–22

20. Scrammel B (1999) Alendronate prevents periprosthetic bone loss – 2 year results. J Bone Mineral Res 14(Suppl)1:341

21. Soininvaara T, Jurvelin J, Miettinen H et al. (2002) Effect of alendronate on periprosthetic bone loss after total knee arthroplasty: a one-year, randomized, controlled trial of 19 patients. Calcif Tissue Int 71:472–477

22. Sundfeldt M, Carlsson L, Johansson C et al. (2006) Aseptic loosening, not only a question of wear. A review of different theories. Acta Orthop 77:177–197

23. Tanzer M, Kerabasz D, Krygier J et al. (2005) Bone augmentation around and within porous implants by local bisphosphonate elution. Clin Orthop Relat Res 441:30–39

24. Wang C, Wang J, Weng L (2003) The effect of alendronate on bone mineral density in the distal part of the femur and proximal part of the tibia after total knee arthroplasty. J Bone Joint Surg 85:2121–2126

25. Wermelin K, Suska F, Tengvall P et al. (2008) Stainless steel screws coated with bisphosphonates gabe stronger fixation and more surrounding bone. Histomorphometry in rats. Bone 42:365–371

Chapter 34 Oral Bone Loss, Periodontitis and Osteoporosis

1. El-Shinnawi U, El-Tantawy S (2003) The effect of alendronate sodium on alveolar bone loss in periodontitis (clinical trial). J Int Acad Periodontol 5:5–10

2. Jeffcoat M, Reddy M (1996) Alveolar bone loss and osteoporosis: evidence for a common mode of therapy using the bisphosphonate alendronate. In: Davidovitch Z, Norton LA (eds) Biological mechanisms of tooth movement and craniofacial adaptation. Harvard Society for the Advancement of Orthodontics, Boston, pp 365–374

3. Kuo L, Polson A, Kang T (2008) Associations between periodontal diseases and systemic diseases: a review of the inter-relationships and interactions with diabetes, respiratory diseases, cardiovascular diseases and osteoporosis. Public Health 122:417–433

4. Mattson J, Cerutis D, Parrish L (2002) Osteoporosis: a review and its dental implication. Compend Contin Educ Dent 23:1001–1004

5. Meraw S, Reeve C (1999) Qualitative analysis of peripheral peri-implant bone and influence of alendronate sodium on early bone regeneration. J Periodontol 70:1228–1233

6. Reddy M, Jeffcoat M (1995) Inhibition of alveolar bone loss in human periodontitis with alendronate. J Dental Res 109:25
7. Scrammel B (1999) Alendronate prevents periprosthetic bone loss – 2 year results. J Bone Mineral Res 14(Suppl 1):341
8. Shinoda H, Takeyama S, Suzuki K et al. (2008) Pharmacological topics of bone metabolism: a novel bisphosphonate for the treatment of periodontitis. J Pharmacol Sci 106:555–558
9. Wactawski-Wende J (2001) Periodontal disease and osteoporosis: association and mechanisms. Ann Periodontal 6:197–208

Chapter 35 Disorders of Bone due to Tumours

1. Aapro M, Abrahamsson P, Body J et al. (2008) Guidance on the use of bisphosphonates in solid tumours: recommendations of an international expert panel. Ann Oncol 19:420–432
2. Body J, Bartl R, Burckhardt P et al. (1998): Current use of bisphosphonates in oncology: International Bone and Cancer Study Group. J Clin Oncol 16:3890–3899
3. Body J, Bergmann P, Boonen S et al. (2007) Management of cancer treatment-induced bone loss in early breast and prostate cancer – a consensus paper of the Belgian Bone Club. Osteoporos Int 18:1439–1450
4. Coleman R (2008) Risks and benefits of bisphosphonates. Br J Cancer 98:1736–1740
5. Dhillon S, Lyseng-Williamson K (2008) Zoledronic acid: a review of its use in the management of bone metastases of malignancy. Drugs 68:507–534
6. Fromigue O, Lagneaux L, Body J-J (2000) Bisphosphonates induce breast cancer cell death in vitro. J Bone Mineral Res 15:2211–2221
7. Hillner B, Chlebowski R, Gralow J et al. (2003) American Society of Clinical Oncology 2003 update on the role of bisphosphonates and bone health issues in women with breast cancer. J Clin Oncol 21:4042–4057
8. Kominsky S, Doucet M, Brady K et al. (2007) TGF-beta promotes the establishment of renal cell carcinoma bone metastasis. J Bone Miner Res 22:37–44
9. Lipton A, Cook R, Saad F et al. (2008) Normalization of bone markers is associated with improved survival in patients with bone metastases from solid tumors and elevated bone resorption receiving zoledronic acid. Cancer 113:193–201
10. Major P, Lortholary A, Hon J et al. (2001) Zoledronic acid is superior to pamidronate in the treatment of hypercalcemia of malignancy: a pooled analysis of two randomized, controlled clinical trial. J Clin Oncol 19:558–567
11. Melton III J, Rajkumar V, Khosla S et al. (2004) Fracture risk in monoclonal gammopathy of undetermined significance. J Bone Miner Res 19:25–30
12. Santini D, Vespasiani G, Vincenti B (2003) The antineoplastic role of bisphosphonates: from basic research to clinical evidence. Ann Oncol 14:1468–1476
13. Smith I, Dowsett M (2003) Aromatase inhibitors in breast cancer. N Engl J Med 348:2431–2442

Chapter 36 The Metabolic Syndrome – A Major Cause of Osteoporosis in the World Today

1. Assmann G, Schulte H, Seedorf U (2008) Cardiovascular risk assessment in the metabolic syndrome: results from the Prospective Cardiovascular Munster (PROCAM) Study. Int J Obes (Lond) 32(Suppl 2):S11–S16
2. Azfar R, Gelfand J (2008) Psoriasis and metabolic disease: epidemiology and pathophysiology. Curr Opin Rheumatol 20:416–422
3. Benetos A, Thomas F, Pannier B et al. (2008) All-cause and cardiovascular mortality using the different definitions of metabolic syndrome. Am J Cardiol 102:188–191
4. Brown T, Vaidya D, Rogers W et al. (2008) Does prevalence of the metabolic syndrome in women with coronary artery disease differs by the ATP III and IDF criteria? J Womens Health (Larchmt) 17:841–847
5. Chen K, Lindsey J, Khera A et al. (2008) Independent associations between metabolic syndrome, diabetes mellitus and atherosclerosis: observations from the Dallas Heart Study. Diab Vasc Dis Res 5:96–101
6. Chen Y, Kao T, Huang J et al. (2008) Correlation of metabolic syndrome with residual renal function, solute transport rate and peritoneal solute

clearance in chronic peritoneal dialysis patients. Blood Purif 26:138–144

7. Chubb S, Hyde Z, Almeida O et al. (2008) Lower sex hormone-binding globulin is more strongly associated with metabolic syndrome than lower total testosterone in older men: the Health in Men Study. Eur J Endocrinol 158:785–792

8. de Zeeuw D, Bakker S (2008) Does the metabolic syndrome add to the diagnosis and treatment of cardiovascular disease? Nat Clin Pract Cardiovasc Med 5(Suppl 1):S10–S14

9. Després J, Lemieux I, Bergeron J et al. (2008) Abdominal obesity and the metabolic syndrome: contribution to global cardiometabolic risk. Arterioscler Thromb Vasc Biol 28:1039–1049

10. Eisenmann J (2008) On the use of a continuous metabolic syndrome score in pediatric research. Cardiovasc Diabetol 7:17

11. Epstein S, Leroith D (2008) Diabetes and fragility fractures – a burgeoning epidemic? Bone 43:3–6

12. Feinman R, Volek J (2008) Carbohydrate restriction as the default treatment for type 2 diabetes and metabolic syndrome. Scand Cardiovasc J 1:1–8

13. Ferreira I, Boreham C, Twisk J et al. (2007) Clustering of metabolic syndrome risk factors and arterial stiffness in young adults: the Northern Ireland Young Hearts Project. J Hypertens 25:1009–1020

14. Ford E, Li C, Zhao G et al. (2008) Prevalence of the metabolic syndrome among U.S. adolescents using the definition from the International Diabetes Foundation. Diabetes Care 31:587–589

15. Fujita T (2008) The metabolic syndrome in Japan. Nat Clin Pract Cardiovasc Med 5(Suppl 1):S15–S18

16. Gastaldi G, Giacobino J, Ruiz J (2008) Metabolic syndrome, a mitochondrial disease? Rev Med Suisse 4:1387–1388, 1390–1391

17. Gatto N, Henderson V, St John J et al. (2008) Metabolic syndrome and cognitive function in healthy middle-aged and older adults without diabetes. Neuropsychol Dev Cogn B Aging Neuropsychol Cogn 15:627–641

18. Goncharov N, Katsya G, Chagina N et al. (2008) Three definitions of metabolic syndrome applied to a sample of young obese men and their relation with plasma testosterone. Aging Male 17:1–5

19. Hanai K, Babazono T, Iwamoto Y (2008) Renal manifestations of metabolic syndrome in type 2 diabetes. Diabetes Res Clin Pract 79:318–324

20. Hernández-Hernández J, Riancho Moral J, Gonzáles Macias J (2008) Metabolic syndrome: how about bone? Medicina Clínica 130:745–750

21. Iseki K (2008) Metabolic syndrome and chronic kidney disease: a Japanese perspective on a worldwide problem. J Nephrol 21:305–312

22. Janssen I, Powell L, Crawford S et al. (2008) Menopause and the metabolic syndrome: the Study of Women's Health Across the Nation. Arch Intern Med 168:1568–1575

23. Jeffrey A, Murphy M, Metcalf B et al. (2008) Adiponectin in childhood. Int J Pediatr Obes 6:1–11

24. Jiamsripong P, Mookadam M, Honda T et al. (2008) The metabolic syndrome and cardiovascular disease: part I. Prev Cardiol 11:156–161

25. Jullien D (2008) Pathogenesis of the metabolic syndrome. Ann Dematol Venereol 135(Suppl 4):S243–S248

26. Lameira D, Lejeune S, Mourad J (2008) Metabolic syndrome: epidemiology and its risks. Ann Dermatol Venereol 135(Suppl 4):S249–S253

27. Lann D, Gallagher E, Leroith D (2008) Insulin resistance and the metabolic syndrome. Minerva Med 99:253–262

28. Loke K, Lin J, Mabel D (2008) 3rd College of paediatrics and child health lecture – the past, the present and the shape of things to come. Ann Acad Med Singapore 37:429–434

29. McKeown N, Jacques P, Zhang X et al. (2008) Dietary magnesium intake is related to metabolic syndrome in older Americans. Eur J Nutr 47:210–216

30. Morley J (2008) Diabetes and aging: epidemiologic overview. Clin Geriatr Med 24:395–405

31. Morrison J, Ford E, Steinberger J (2008) The pediatric metabolic syndrome. Minerva Med 99:269–287

32. Munukata M, Honma H, Akasi M et al. (2008) Japanese study to organize proper lifestyle modifications for metabolic syndrome (J-STOP-MetS): design and method. Vasc Health Risk Manag 4:415–420

33. Noale M, Maggi S, Marzari C et al. (2006) Components of the metabolic syndrome and incidence of diabetes in elderly Italians: the Italian Longitudinal Study on Aging. Atherosclerosis 187:385–392

34. Pan W, Yeh W, Weng L (2008) Epidemiology of metabolic syndrome in Asia. Asia Pac J Clin Nutr 17(Suppl 1):37–42

35. Räkel A, Sheehy O, Rahme E et al. (2008) Osteoporosis among patients with type 1 and type 2 diabetes. Diabetes Metab 34:193–205

36. Rueda S, Fernández-Fernández C, Romero F et al. (2008) Vitamin D, PTH, and the metabolic syndrome in severely obese subjects. Obes Surg 18:151–154

37. Safaei H, Janghorbani M, Aminorroaya A et al. (2007) Lovastatin effects on bone mineral density in postmenopausal women with type 2 diabetes mellitus. Acta Diabetol 44:76–82

38. Singer G, Setaro J (2008) Secondary hypertension: obesity and the metabolic syndrome. J Clin Hypertens (Greenwich) 10:567–574

39. Sobieszczyk M, Hoover D, Anastos K et al. (2008) Prevalence and predictors of metabolic syndrome among HIV-infected and HIV-uninfected women in the Women's Interagency HIV Study. J Acquir Immune Defic Syndr 48:272–280

40. Wannamethee S (2008) The metabolic syndrome and cardiovascular risk in the British Regional Heart Study. Int J Obes (Lond) 32(Suppl 2):S25–S29

Subject Index

Printing and Binding: Stürtz GmbH, Würzburg